INTRAVASCULAR ULTRASOUND

Edited by **Yasuhiro Honda**

Intravascular Ultrasound
Edited by Yasuhiro Honda

Published by InTech
Janeza Trdine 9, 51000 Rijeka, Croatia

Publishing Process Manager Petra Nenadic

Technical Editor Teodora Smiljanic

Cover Designer InTech Design Team

Additional hard copies can be obtained from orders@intechopen.com

Intravascular Ultrasound, Edited by Yasuhiro Honda
p. cm.
ISBN 978-953-307-900-4

For EU product safety concerns:
IN TECH d.o.o., Prolaz Marije Krucifikse Kozulić 3, 51000 Rijeka, Croatia,
info@intechopen.com or visit our website at intechopen.com.

Meet the editor

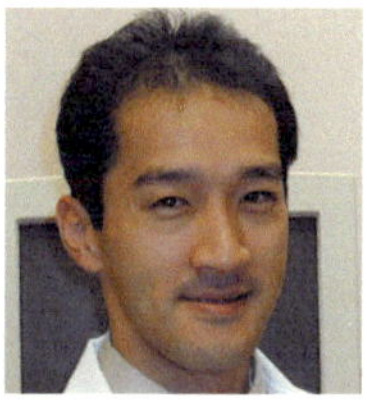

Dr Yasuhiro Honda is a Clinical Associate Professor of Medicine and a faculty member at the Center for Cardiovascular Technology, Stanford University School of Medicine. He received his MD from Kyoto University Faculty of Medicine. After completing cardiology training in Japan, he joined the Division of Cardiovascular Medicine at Stanford University in 1995, and has been serving as Co-Director of the Cardiovascular Core Analysis Laboratory (CCAL) since 2005.

Contents

Preface

In 1971, Bom et al. developed one of the first catheter-based real-time imaging techniques for use in the cardiac system. By placing a set of phased array ultrasound transducers within the cardiac chambers, it was shown that higher frequencies could be used to produce high-resolution images of cardiac structures without interference from bony structures that occurs with transthoracic ultrasound imaging. By the late 1980s, Yock et al. had successfully miniaturized a single-transducer system to enable the transducer placement within coronary arteries. Since then, intravascular ultrasound (IVUS) has become pivotal catheter-based imaging technology, having provided practical guidance for percutaneous interventions as well as scientific insights into vascular biology in clinical settings.

Recent advancements in noninvasive cardiovascular imaging now allow rapid and detailed visualization of cardiovascular structures. However, clinical demand for catheter-based imaging is also growing, largely driven by evolving percutaneous treatment technologies that require precise procedural guidance or real-time assessment of the treatment effects. These technologies include not only a variety of coronary or peripheral vascular interventions, but also percutaneous treatment devices for structural heart disease or heart failure. As illustrated by the late thrombosis issue in drug-eluting stents, the consequences of new treatment may also benefit from in-depth examination of the treated site. Furthermore, the attempt to identify vulnerable plaques significantly stimulates the technical advancements of imaging modalities beyond anatomy.

This book is intended to serve as an up-to-date resource relating to IVUS, not only for practising cardiologists, residents and students, but also for researchers and engineers with aspirations to apply or advance this sophisticated imaging technology. The first section discusses the basic principles and diagnostic applications of the IVUS technology, including the detailed descriptions of advanced tissue characterization and vascular profiling techniques. The second section summarizes the current use of IVUS in interventional applications such as the guidance of complex percutaneous procedures or the assessment of vascular response to new treatments. The third section is dedicated to ongoing technical efforts to further enhance the utility of this imaging technology. It is our hope that this book will prove useful to the medical and engineering community as a comprehensive guide to understanding this rapidly evolving technology and its role in cardiovascular research and patient care.

Being asked to serve as the editor of this book has been a great privilege. However, the successful production has required the support and co-operation of a number of individuals. I would like to express my deep appreciation to all the contributing authors, as well as the staff of the open access publisher InTech, in particular Ms Petra Nenadic, Ms Petra Zobic, and Ms Viktorija Zgela, for their tireless efforts and ongoing encouragement throughout this endeavor. Without their expertise, dedication and time commitment, this book would not have been possible.

Yasuhiro Honda, MD, FACC, FAHA
Clinical Associate Professor of Medicine
Co-Director, Cardiovascular Core Analysis Laboratory
Division of Cardiovascular Medicine
Stanford University School of Medicine
USA

Part 1

Principles and Diagnostic Applications

1

Non-Coronary Vessel Exploration Under Intravascular Ultrasound: Principles and Applicability

Gaël Y. Rochefort
Inserm U658 Ipros Chro, Orleans
France

1. Introduction

Intravascular Ultrasound (IVUS) has become rapidly one of the gold technologies for the endovascular exploration. Next to angiography, which only gives information about the lumen of the investigated vessels, IVUS describes both the luminal and trans-mural anatomy of vascular structures. Actual devices offer several configurations and transducers mounted at the end of an intra-luminal catheter to produce real-time grayscale or color images of blood vessels and cardiac structures. The ultrasound probes miniaturization has permitted closer imaging and magnified details of the vessel wall and plaque. Recent IVUS catheters use phased array imaging where the micro-transducers are enveloped around a catheter tip. Typically, IVUS images show the vessel wall in histological detail: the intima reflects ultrasound brightly and is white, the media is echolucent and dark, and the surrounding adventitia is white.

IVUS has thus become a safe and valuable tool in exploring the disease severity and the treatment completeness during surgical endovascular procedures (Jinzaki et al., 1993; Nishanian et al., 1999), such as assessing the severity of an arterial disease before treatment (Scoccianti et al., 1994), determining the plaque morphology and localization or checking the completeness of stent deployment (Diethrich, 1993; Laskey et al., 1993). Very recently, color flow IVUS and three-dimensional (3D) reconstruction have both introduced significant advances in the understanding of IVUS images (Irshad et al., 2001; Reid et al., 1995; White et al., 1994). The very latest advance, called virtual histology IVUS, provides a color-coded map of the plaque components, thus providing a better understanding of the arterial plaque structure and morphology (Nair et al., 2001; Vince & Davies, 2004).

2. IVUS principle

IVUS gives series of tomographic images of the explored vessel wall. During acquisition, an IVUS catheter is entered into a vessel and then withdrawn through a given vessel segment during simultaneous and continuous imaging, resulting in series of cross section images. Current catheters have frequencies from 30 to 40 MHz, planar resolutions from 50 to 150 µm, and a typical sampling rate of 30 images per second (Di Mario et al., 1995).

2.1 Acquisition using pullback devices

The current methods used to quantify a volumetric IVUS analysis are usually achieved by a simple summation of a targeted subsample of the 2-D images into a volumetric dataset (Chandrasekaran et al., 1994; Rosenfield et al., 1992; Rosenfield et al., 1991). In that case, the accurate volume calculations need the precise localization of each 2-D cross-sectional image used in the longitudinal axis of the vessel segment (Di Mario et al., 1995; Roelandt et al., 1994). To do so, a manual pullback was firstly performed, with recording of the time and length of the acquisition, and the image location was estimated from the pullback start point and the average pullback velocity. Alternatively, displacement sensors were used to record the IVUS catheter translation during the manual pullback procedure (Hagenaars et al., 2000). Since it is obviously difficult to maintain a consistent speed during manual pullback, most current systems have introduced a motorized pullback device with a constant speed (usually around 0.5 mm/s) (Cavaye et al., 1992; Liu et al., 1999; Matar et al., 1994).

2.2 Cardiac synchronization and frame selection

Since images are recorded at 30 frames per second, with a pullback speed of 0.5 mm/s, 60 frames are recorded for each 1-mm vessel segment. Since, a coronary segment of 3 to 10 cm is typically explored, 1800 to 6000 individual frames are usually recorded. Therefore, these large datasets are often sub-sampled using constant intervals (0.5 - 1.0 mm) or using an electrocardiogram gating: the 1-mm interval without respect to the cardiac cycle is often used for manual analysis, whereas computerized algorithms require different sampling intervals (Klingensmith et al., 2000a; von Birgelen et al., 1996a). Therefore, consecutive frames sub-sampled with a 1-mm interval are corresponding to changes in the lumen and vessel areas during the different phases of the cardiac cycle.

A typical "sawtooth" artifact can be seen on longitudinal 2-D pullback displays when the sub-sampling is performed without synchronization to the cardiac cycle. This sawtooth artifact is less marked when the explored vessel exhibit a reduced compliance (such as stented vessels or stenotic vessels). Nevertheless, it is recommended to get the cardiac cycle synchronization since it allows the cyclic cycle artifacts to be eliminated (von Birgelen et al., 1996b; von Birgelen et al., 1997b). In fact, different physiologic, cyclic signals are commonly used to synchronize the IVUS images to the cardiac cycle, including the arterial blood pressure and the electrocardiogram signals (Allan et al., 1998; Sonka et al., 1998).

When operating a retrospective gating, IVUS images and electrocardiogram signals are acquired continuously, since the electrocardiogram signals are required to sort the images and to perform the analysis of the volumetric dataset (Klingensmith et al., 2000a; Kovalski et al., 2000). On the other hand, when operating a prospective gating, the IVUS images are only acquired at a given times of the cardiac cycle and the catheter is then moved to acquire the next gated image (Bruining et al., 1998; von Birgelen et al., 1997a; von Birgelen et al., 1995). This last gating method presents the advantage to not requiring additional steps to perform the analysis of the dataset, and a volumetric dataset is available immediately after the acquisition pullback.

2.3 Transferring the IVUS dataset to an analysis system

The whole raw IVUS data, composed of the reflected acoustic signals, are displayed on IVUS consoles. This dataset could also be stored on S-VHS videotape, on CD-ROM or magneto-optical disks. Recent IVUS consoles have digital output capabilities that allow direct data transfer in digital format, and may provide radiofrequency outputs composed of raw IVUS acoustic signals. This signal processing approach is particularly adapted for a computerized image analysis, since it allows traditional measurements but also radiofrequency-based tissue characterization (Nair et al., 2001; Nair et al., 2002).

3. Devices, recording methods and techniques

3.1 Devices

Typical mechanical IVUS transducers produce cross-sectional images by rotating at the tip of the catheter using a flexible, high-torque cable. These transducers are creating a cone-shaped ultrasound beam that allows the vessel to be imaged slightly forward or in front of the transducer assembly.

An optimized visualization is obtained when using IVUS catheter having appropriate size and frequency. Thus, the clinician has to make a compromise between the highest frequency *vs.* depth of penetration *vs.* catheter size. He also has to consider the wire guide diameter and the guide-wire exchanges utility. IVUS catheters used for most aortic and iliac procedures can be advanced over a 0.035-inch guide wire and range in size and frequency from 6 to 8 Fr and 8 to 20 MHz, respectively. An IVUS probe, ranging between 8 to 15 MHz is commonly used for aortic procedures, allowing an adequate circumferential imaging. The following Table 1 is presenting the current available catheters applicable for peripheral vascular and coronary interventions.

Intravascular Ultrasound Catheters	Size (Fr)	Guide Wire (in)	Frequency (MHz)	Target vessel
Volcano Corporation catheters (phase array)				
Eagle Eye Gold IVUS Imaging (color-flow and virtual histology)	3.5	0.014	20	Carotid renal iliac Femoral
Visions PV 0.018 F/X IVUS Imaging (color-flow)	3.5	0.018	20	Femoral popliteal tibial
Visions PV 8.2F IVUS Imaging	8.2	0.038	8.3	Aorta iliac
Boston Scientific catheters (rotating crystal)				
Atlantis SR Pro	3.2	0.014	40	Femoral popliteal tibial
Atlantis SR Plus	3	0.014	40	Femoral popliteal tibial
Atlantis SR	3.2	0.014	40	Femoral popliteal tibial
Atlantis PV Peripheral Imaging	8	0.035	15	Aorta iliac
Sonicath Ultra Ultrasound	9	0.035	9	Aorta iliac
Sonicath Ultra Ultrasound	3.2	0.018	20	Femoral popliteal tibial
Sonicath Ultra Ultrasound	6	0.035	12.5	Iliac femoral
Sonicath Ultra Ultrasound	6	0.035	20	Femoral popliteal tibial

Table 1. Specifications of commonly used intravascular ultrasound (IVUS) catheters in peripheral occlusive interventions.

3.2 Access to vessels

Depending on the size of the considered vessel (see Table 1), IVUS catheters can be introduced percutaneously through a standard vascular access sheath (5 to 9 Fr). The 8.2 Fr, 10-MHz catheter is one of the most commonly used catheter for aorta-iliac intervention, since it requires a 0.035-inch guide wire and thus can be quickly prepared, introduced, and/or exchanged with other catheters. However, this specific catheter requires a 9 Fr sheath that can be disproportionate for lower extremity interventions.

Most current percutaneous trans-luminal angioplasty balloons and stents targeted for infra-inguinal regions require only 6 Fr sheaths. The 3.4 Fr, 3.2 Fr, or 2.9 Fr catheters, using 0.018-inch and 0.014-inch guide wires, are more suitable for the typical retrograde common femoral artery puncture and access to the contra-lateral femoral-popliteal segments (Hiro et al., 1998; Saketkhoo et al., 2004). In some case, especially with tortuous vessels and when antegrade puncture of the common femoral vessel is required, the 3 Fr catheters are also useful.

Lengths of IVUS catheters are vary from 90 to 150 cm, thus allowing imaging of small tibial vessels from a contra-lateral up-and-over approach. The smaller catheters require 0.018-inch or 0.014-inch guide wires and are commonly used for infra-inguinal interventions, whereas the larger IVUS catheters need 0.035-inch guide wires and used for larger vessel interventions (Hiro et al., 1998).

3.3 Image acquisition and quality

An optimal visualization requires a careful positioning of the catheter tip within the vessel and an appropriate size matching of the device to the artery caliber, meaning that an IVUS intervention necessitates a pre-procedural estimation the target vessel diameters (Figure 1). The best image quality is obtained when the IVUS catheter is parallel to the vessel wall and when the ultrasound beam is perpendicular to the luminal surface. Some artificial differences in the wall thickness measurement may be obtained when the IVUS catheter has an eccentric position, leading to the vessel wall to appear more hyperechoic than the distant wall. Angulations may promote an elliptical image of the vessel lumen, especially when

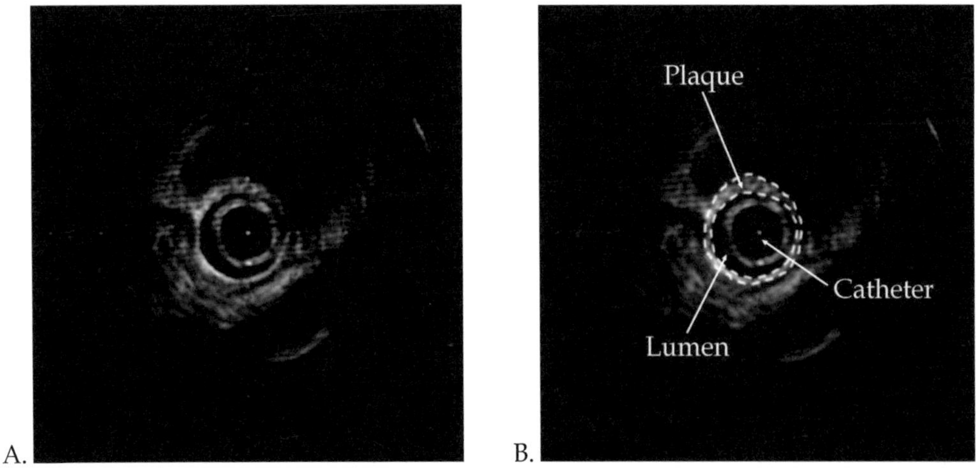

Fig. 1. Illustration of quantitative measurements with IVUS. Examples show an *in vivo* IVUS image digitized from video (A) and the detected borders overlaid (B).

considering tortuous aortas and the thoracic arch. In such cases, the minimal diameter (minor axis) is the best accurate measurement to measure the vessel diameter in angled images and/or tortuous vessels (Roelandt et al., 1994). At last, withdrawing the catheter through the lumen, rather than advancing it, promotes the acquisition of the best-quality images (Danilouchkine et al., 2009).
During the procedure, real-time images of the investigated vessel are displayed on a monitor and are usually recorded digitally. The IVUS devices also allow the on-line and/or off-line measurements of vessel dimensions, luminal diameters, and cross-sectional areas. Recent IVUS units, comprising a motorized and/or automated withdrawing the catheter through the vessel at a controlled rate, may display a longitudinal gray-scale image of the investigated vessel with accurate reconstructed views (Hagenaars et al., 2000). These two-dimensional longitudinal reconstructions allow distances to be measured from one point to another (Liu et al., 1999) and cross-sectional trans-mural wall morphology to be visualized (Di Mario et al., 1995). In fact, the discrimination of plaque, normal tissue, thrombus, dissections, and flaps is often much better appreciated on the two-dimensional longitudinal IVUS reconstructions than on traditional angiographic images (Reid et al., 1995).

4. Data processing and analysis

The dataset for volumetric analysis is represented by image series composed of two-dimensional sections from the investigated vessels. Typically, images are selected at 1-mm inter-slice spacing. Then, to perform a quantitative 3-D reconstruction, the first and most critical step is to precisely identify and trace the anatomical structures of the studied vessel. In fact, identifying the luminal border is essential to discriminate the blood-intima interface, whereas recognizing the external elastic membrane border is important to precisely distinguish the boundary between the media and the adventitia (Kovalski et al., 2000). The space between these 2 borders is the plaque-media complex and is classically used as the measurement for plaque cross-sectional area (Prati et al., 2002).
In stented vessel segments, the lumen/intimal interface and the stent borders are both measured, and the area between these borders is representing the neointimal tissue. In these stented vessel segments, the external elastic membrane border is frequently not distinguished because of signal drop-out behind the stent. In current atherosclerosis research trials, the assessment of stent, luminal and external elastic membrane borders is often performed with manual planimetry using commercially or freely available computer programs. This provides the accurate discrimination of image artifacts and true border locations but this analysis requires the border detection in hundreds of images. Therefore, the use of automated image-processing techniques allows fast online analysis (Sanz-Requena et al., 2007).

4.1 Automated 2-D/3-D border-detection methods

Different approaches have been described to detect the luminal and external elastic membrane borders from 2-D IVUS images, including texture-based methods (Papadogiorgaki et al., 2007), knowledge-based graph searching (Bovenkamp et al., 2009), region growing (Sanz-Requena et al., 2007), radial gradient searching (Luo et al., 2003), and active contours (Sanz-Requena et al., 2007; Takagi et al., 2000). These 2-D border-detection techniques are now used online in newer IVUS imaging consoles, allowing the quantitative evaluation of lumen and plaque measurements. Because the user provides his expertise to augment the algorithm or correct results, the semi-automated techniques typically require

more time but are have a better accuracy. These 2-D border-detection methods are particularly used when the analysis of only a small number of images is required, e.g. during the guidance of interventional procedures (Sarno et al., 2011).
When a fast analysis of many images is required, highly automated techniques for border detection are used and do not require significant user intervention. For example, 3-D border-detection methods using the inter-slice information can provide fast border detection from a large number of images (Cardinal et al., 2010). A graph-searching approach researching the globally optimal contour path through the image data has been developed on the basis of associated cost values (Zhang et al., 1998). Furthermore, this 2-D frame analysis method allows the results to be propagated down the sequence by using the identified 2-D contours in order to limit the search region. Another 2-D border-detection method uses cost values to find longitudinal contours along the volumetric data. Then, these contours guide the cost function minimization in the transverse 2-D images (Koning et al., 2002). Alternatively, several useful approaches use deformable models to perform an active contour detection (Klingensmith et al., 2000a; Kovalski et al., 2000) (Shekhar et al., 1999). One of them uses a balloon force to inflate a model from the catheter outward toward the luminal and medial-adventitial borders (Kovalski et al., 2000). Another deformable model uses a cylindrical model to manually or automatically approximate the structure of the luminal or medial-adventitial surface, and a deformable model algorithm is then used in a 3-D process to attach the defined structure to the surface of interest (Klingensmith et al., 2000a; Shekhar et al., 1999). All these methods allowing the 3-D border-detection have clearly established their overall usefulness for fast border identification in a large sequence of images (Klingensmith et al., 2000a; Kovalski et al., 2000; Shekhar et al., 1999; von Birgelen et al., 1996a; Zhang et al., 1998).
A major limitation of all these 3-D border-detection methods is the lack of a true gold standard for comparison. Histology sections might represent the more powerful gold standard, but they are only available at autopsy, and the required fixation always induces the tissue to shrink (Siegel et al., 1985). Some researchers have tried to evaluate the accuracy of their methods using cylindrical phantoms, but they did not test accuracy in clinical IVUS images (von Birgelen et al., 1996a). Other studies have compared the detected borders with borders traced manually by a single expert, but the obtained inter-observer variability in manual identification of the luminal and medial-adventitial borders might greatly limit the value of these comparisons in IVUS images (Haas et al., 2000; Zhang et al., 1998). At last, some studies have used multiple expert observers for validation, but the number of analyzed images is seriously limited and not sufficient to assess the ability and accuracy of these algorithms (Klingensmith et al., 2000a; Kovalski et al., 2000; Shekhar et al., 1999). Therefore, there is a need of validation of these techniques in large datasets.

4.2 3-D reconstructions of vessel segments

All measurements and evaluations made in 2-D tomographic slices are useful for stent sizing or comparisons of lesions to a reference site, but fail to provide a volumetric perspective. To do such volumetric calculations, the border measurements obtained in consecutive 2-D slices of a vessel segment are integrated, the area enclosed by the luminal border and external elastic membrane border is considered for each slice, and the atheroma area is calculated. The 3-D measurement of lumen, plaque, and vessel volumes are usually calculated with Simpson's rule or trapezoidal integration by the multiplying 2-D area and slice thickness (Finet et al., 2003; von Birgelen et al., 1997a). This last method is suitable for short and straight vessel segments, such as coronary stented lesions, but it does not allow the precise measurement of a longer and curved segment.

The volumetric approach using 3-D border-detection techniques is currently applied in serial IVUS studies examining atherosclerotic disease progression or regression, allowing the assessment of plaque burden in an entire vessel segment through fast analysis of large image sequences. New interventional approaches also use a volumetric IVUS imaging approach to provide new mechanistic insights, such as innovative techniques aimed at the prevention and treatment of in-stent restenosis correlated with histomorphometry measurements (Mehran et al., 1998; Murata et al., 2002); approaches in understanding the effects of radiation therapy and the arterial remodeling on a stented segment (brachytherapy) (Lekston et al., 2008; Weichert et al., 2003; Zimarino et al., 2002; Zimmermann et al., 2005); or using drug-eluting stents on the neointimal hyperplasia development (Jensen et al., 2008; Min et al., 2007; Sano et al., 2006).

4.3 Geometrically correct 3-D IVUS and advanced data processing

Since the curvature of vessels is not taken into account with these straight 3-D IVUS methods, this limitation can be overcome by fusing the curvature information provided by biplane angiography or other techniques with the IVUS border information (Schuurbiers et al., 2009; Sherknies et al., 2005; Tu et al., 2010; Wahle et al., 2006). To do so, one common method is to acquire two separate angiographic images from different angles at the beginning of the ultrasound scanning imaging procedure and to use the catheter outline reconstructed from these images as a template for placement of the IVUS-derived contours (Bourantas et al., 2005; Klingensmith et al., 2000b; Sherknies et al., 2005; von Birgelen et al., 1995; Weichert et al., 2003). Another method consists in following the IVUS transducer in time and space throughout the IVUS pullback using biplane angiography, thus the precise locations of IVUS image acquisitions are recorded in sequence and are used as a reconstruction template (Klingensmith et al., 2000b; Miyazaki et al., 2010; Wallace et al., 2005). However, this method might be difficult because of the cardiac and respiratory motion and the higher radiation exposure during the whole procedure.

Next to the precise location in 3-D space, other geometric considerations of the IVUS probe during image acquisition are important to be taken in account for an accurate 3-D reconstruction (Roelandt et al., 1994; Thrush et al., 1997). For example, the geometry of the reconstructed vessel can be distorted by a rotation of the catheter during pullback. These changes in the angular orientation of the catheter can be corrected by using analytical calculation based on the Frenet-Serret rules and optimizing the fit after projecting the reconstructed lumen from different rotational angles onto the angiogram images (Briguori et al., 2001; Wahle et al., 1999). Axial movements of the catheter due to the cardiac contraction are another cause for 3-D reconstruction inaccuracies. This geometric artifact can be reduced using a cardiac-gating and spatiotemporal location of the IVUS transducer throughout the pullback (Arbab-Zadeh et al., 1999). However, even if some errors in generating 3-D images can potentially surround withy these geometric assumptions, these corrections help improve the interpretability, usefulness and accuracy of the 3-D reconstructions. Repeatability is also a really important consideration in the accuracy and usefulness of 3-D reconstruction techniques. This aspect is however closely related to the reproducibility of the 3-D border-detection process (von Birgelen et al., 1996a).

Offline digitization of IVUS images and retrieval of biplane angiographic images, but also digitization and intense computer processing are both required to obtain a correct geometrically 3-D reconstruction (Prati et al., 1998). Therefore, all these factors, in addition to the artifacts induced by the respiratory and cardiac motions, limit the *in vivo* applicability of the techniques. Other developments of real-time transducer tracking and online radiofrequency IVUS data acquisition can be integrated into the IVUS console to provide accurate 3-D models of investigated vessels within a few minutes after the acquisition (Nair et al., 2002). These add-ons seem really powerful since they could provide an interactive tool for assessing the diagnostic of the pathology, giving an assessment of luminal dimensions, but also vessel and plaque size from any viewing angle and position. Furthermore, these interactive models could allow rotation and manipulation of these virtual 3-D models on the console computer, authorizing the placement of a virtual stent inside the reconstructed artery, thus permitting a stent with the length and size to be appropriately chosen (Atary et al., 2009; Hong et al., 2010).

Other addendum could be integrated into the geometrically correct 3-D models, including analysis of hemodynamic forces, radiofrequency-derived histology, and 3-D stress maps. Therefore, a more precise morphologic plaque classification is possible with the analysis of radiofrequency data. In fact, the back-scattered radiofrequency IVUS data seems to permit the precise characterization of plaque composition, distinguishing the regions of calcified plaque *vs.* calcified necrosis *vs.* collagen (Nair et al., 2001). Another complement might consist on adding the mechanical properties of the investigated tissue. In fact, elastography represents the way a given tissue is responding to an applied force, as a function of its mechanical properties. Thus, the local mechanical properties of the tissue can be determined by comparing the images of a vessel acquired at 2 different levels of static compression (*e.g.* during systole and diastole steps of the cardiac cycle). This strain image (elastogram) may allow a better understanding of the relation between the progression of a disease and the *in vivo* mechanical properties of the vessel (Baldewsing et al., 2007; Cespedes et al., 1997; de Korte & van der Steen, 2002; Liang et al., 2008).

4.4 Comparison of IVUS with other imaging modalities

Even if IVUS might represent the most clinically established technique, other methodologies for vessel investigation are also available, such as angiography or tomographic imaging with magnetic resonance imaging (MRI) and computed tomography (CT). The current IVUS imaging plane resolution achieved in vessel cross sections is of 50 to 150 µm, whereas current frame rates (typically 30 frames/s), pullback speeds (usually 0.5 mm/s), and an ECG-gating or sub-sampling yield images at approximately 0.5- to 1.0-mm intervals (Gatta et al., 2009). On the other hand, the in-plane resolution of magnetic resonance imaging is around 1 mm and the through-plane resolution is between 3 to 5 mm with 2-D techniques (Escolar et al., 2006; Schaar et al., 2007), but the magnetic resonance imaging may allow, under several limitation in spatial resolution and signal-to-noise ratios, the atherosclerotic plaque components to be distinguished (Karmonik et al., 2006). At last, the in-plane resolution of computed tomography is less than 1 mm and the minimum through-plane resolution is approximately 1.25 to 1.50 mm. Some contrast-enhanced protocols are sometimes used to differentiate calcified and non-calcified plaque using contrast agents during computed tomography imaging of vessels (Nasir et al., 2010; Pundziute et al., 2008).

Another important difference between IVUS and the other imaging modalities concerns the orientation of the imaging plane. In fact, since the IVUS probe is inside the vessel during the acquisition, the IVUS imaging plane is oriented perpendicular to the vessel axis, which is optimal for assessing cross-sectional dimensions. On the other hand, magnetic resonance images can be acquired along some body axes (e.g. axial, sagittal, or coronal planes or in a plane oblique to these orthogonal planes) and computed tomography images are typically only acquired in the axial plane, but these images can be reformatted to another orthogonal plane or an oblique plane with image processing techniques (McPherson et al., 2005). Therefore, these plane or oblique images allow only the measurement of relatively short portions of a vessel (only for images that are perpendicular to the vessel axis) and the curvature of the vessel introduces angulation errors in parameter measurement such as the wall thickness (Sherknies et al., 2005).

4.5 Color IVUS and virtual histology IVUS

Color flow IVUS is produced by computer software that detects a difference between the movements of echogenic blood particles from two sequential adjacent frames. Then the blood flow is colored by the software in a red or bleu and is displayed as axial and 3D longitudinal renderings with a very high image resolution (McLeod et al., 2004; Nair et al., 2002). The rendering color of the flow may change from red to orange when there is very fast blood flow (e.g., a tight stenosis). However, the flow velocities cannot be calculated with this technique, image resolution is very high. The color flow IVUS is available on Eagle Eye Gold and the Visions PV 018 catheters (Volcano Corporation, Rancho Cordova, CA) (see Table 1 for specifications). During a color flow IVUS pull-back, the blood flow is displayed in the vessel lumen, pulsing with each cardiac cycle. Unfortunately, the color flow is not gated with the heart rate and cannot be performed when virtual histology images are being acquired. These color flow IVUS are the helpful in distinguishing echolucent disease from luminal blood flow and can also be used to perform peripheral interventions in patients with renal failure or allergy, avoiding the use of contrast media (Goderie et al., 2010; Irshad et al., 2001).
Whereas conventional grayscale ultrasound images are generated from the intensity of the reflected signals that are collected by the probe, virtual histology IVUS images are obtained from the frequency and intensity of the returning signals and frequency varies depending on the tissues (Vince & Davies, 2004). An histological classification has then be realized by comparing the reflected virtual histology data with true histological sections of diseased vessels, and a color-coded map of the different components of the arterial disease has been established (dark green, fibrous; yellow/green, fibro-fatty; white, calcified; red, necrotic lipid core plaque) (McLeod et al., 2004; Nair et al., 2002). This color-coded map is of major importance since it allows the operator to have detailed information about the constituents and the nature of the plaque (Sarno et al., 2011). The virtual histology IVUS is available on Eagle Eye Gold catheter (Volcano Corporation, Rancho Cordova, CA) (see Table 1 for specifications) and is gated with the heartbeat. During the procedure using the "Volcano" setting, the segment length of the vessel to be examined is determined and the luminal border and the external elastic lamina border of the artery are automatically detected by the edge-tracking computer software but might require some manual adjustments. Then, virtual histology images of the delineated plaque can then be processed online with a few minutes, thus allowing clinical decisions to be made promptly, whereas some additional processing can be done offline (Vince & Davies, 2004).

5. Therapeutic interventions

5.1 Percutaneous trans-luminal angioplasty

The accurate measurement of the true luminal diameter, the assessment of the calcific nature of the plaque, the precise delineation of wall morphology, and the ability to carefully visualize the post-balloon result are both required for a successful percutaneous trans-luminal angioplasty of peripheral arterial lesions. In that purpose, IVUS images can delineate the luminal and adventitial surfaces of vessel segments, can discriminate between normal and diseased components, can accurately localization and measurement of the thickness of plaque, and can also differentiate calcified and non-calcified vascular lesions (Pundziute et al., 2008; Rodriguez-Granillo et al., 2006). In fact, since the ultrasound energy is strongly reflected by calcified plaque, it appears as a very bright image with dense acoustic shadowing behind it. Not only luminal dimensions and wall thickness determined by IVUS are accurate to within 0.05 mm (Rodriguez-Granillo et al., 2006), the luminal cross-sectional areas measured from IVUS correlate well with calculated from biplanar angiograms (Cooper et al., 2001; Irshad et al., 2001). Therefore, IVUS allows the sized balloon or stent to be appropriately chosen can whereas conventional angiography is somewhat limited in its ability to provide sensitive data regarding the effects of percutaneous trans-luminal angioplasty. The IVUS advantage is also to provide a precise evaluation of the lesion morphology, such as the luminal dimensions, the trans-mural lesion characteristics and the area of blood flow. Furthermore, the IVUS determination of plaque volume before and after the procedure offers a real quantitative method to estimate the amount of lesion debulking or displacement and a reference point from which to assess the lesion recurrence/restenosis (Kim et al., 2004; Takeda et al., 2003).

The adjunctive use of IVUS during percutaneous trans-luminal angioplasty has been reported on several studies. For example, in patients with lesions of the superficial femoral artery treated with percutaneous trans-luminal angioplasty, IVUS has been reported to accurately detect the presence of dissections, plaque fractures, internal elastic lamina ruptures, and thinning of the media that occurred during the balloon angioplasty (Oshima et al., 1998; Tang et al., 2010). IVUS has also showed that, after a percutaneous trans-luminal angioplasty, the luminal enlargement is mainly produced by stretching of the arterial wall while the volume of the lesion remains relatively constant (Tang et al., 2010).

After a percutaneous trans-luminal angioplasty the restenosis risk has also been correlated to IVUS findings during the initial procedure, providing important information regarding the post-procedural follow-up and surveillance (Montorsi et al., 2004; Xu et al., 1995). The percutaneous trans-luminal angioplasty of a calcific plaque leads to a higher incidence of dissection than a fibrous lesion, whereas fibrous plaques or concentric lesions without signs of fracture or dissection are prone to have late restenosis after a percutaneous trans-luminal angioplasty (Garcia-Garcia et al., 2009; Su et al., 2009). In the same way, IVUS is also able to readily identify that early restenosis following interventions is associated with luminal thrombus, extensive dissection, and oversized balloon dilatation, while late restenosis correlates with residual stenosis, lower residual lumen surface, undersized balloon use, concentric fibrous plaque, absence of dissection, and absence of calcification (Irshad et al., 2001). IVUS is thus able to enhance percutaneous trans-luminal angioplasty procedures by allowing peri-procedural decisions to be made regarding the need for additional interventions.

5.2 Intravascular stents

Dissections, elastic recoil, residual stenosis, a significant residual pressure gradient across the lesion, or plaque ulceration with local thrombus accumulation are common indications for an intravascular stent placement after percutaneous trans-luminal angioplasty. Primary stenting is also commonly used in the treatment of certain lesions, especially common iliac or renal disease (Moise et al., 2009). These intravascular stents are used to increase the

patency of arterial occlusive lesions that have undergone angioplasty by reducing technical failure and restenosis rates. However, placing stents is not without risk since ineffective stent expansion can lead to early thrombosis or a stent migration, whereas overexpansion can result in vessel perforation or excessive intimal hyperplasia (Adlakha et al., 2010).
Establishing the need for stenting as well as the guiding of a stent deployment has been clearly helped by IVUS. Furthermore, defining the appropriate angioplasty diameter endpoint and confirming adequacy of stent deployment have been reported to clearly improve the long-term patency of a vessel undergoing balloon angioplasty and stenting (Waksman et al., 2009).

5.3 Venous interventions

The requirement of IVUS in endovascular interventions of venous disease is not as well described as for arterial lesions, while there are many useful indications for IVUS use in venous obstructive lesions (Raju et al., 2010; Raju & Neglen, 2006). In fact, traditional venography for iliac vein obstruction has numerous limitations, and IVUS imaging yields findings not obvious on venography . In fact, intra-luminal webs or external compression and subsequent deformity represent abnormalities that might disturb the diagnostic. Thus, IVUS can provide an accurate assessment of the degree of vein stenosis whereas the venography can sometimes underestimates this stenosis degree by 30% (Nair et al., 2002). In the same way, IVUS allows more appropriately sized venous stents to be placed after venoplasty. Since more and more venous interventions are being performed for acute deep venous thromboses, effort thromboses, or congenital stenosis, the requirement IVUS might represent a powerful adjunct to delineate the often unclear anatomy related to the venous system (Raju et al., 2010).

6. Conclusion

IVUS requirement has moved rapidly from a purely diagnostic imaging modality to a useful adjunct for vessel endografting to playing an ever-increasing role in peripheral occlusive interventions. This shift has been mainly supported by the miniaturization of the elements, allowing the device and catheter to be as small-profile as the latest stents or balloons, and by the powerful helped that can give IVUS for the most optimal outcomes. While vascular interventions are becoming more and more complex and venture into smaller target vessels, success will be related to the degree of accuracy of the guidance system employed during the procedure. Thus, IVUS is representing an important component of current and future endovascular interventions and should be integrated into the routine practice of the advanced endovascular surgeon and training programs.

7. References

Adlakha, S., Sheikh, M., Wu, J., Burket, M.W., Pandya, U., Colyer, W., Eltahawy, E., & Cooper, C.J. (2010). Stent fracture in the coronary and peripheral arteries. *J Interv Cardiol*, Vol. 23, No. 4, (Publication date: 2010/09/02), pp. 411-419, I.S.S.N.: 1540-8183

Allan, J.J., Smith, R.S., DeJong, S.C., McKay, C.R., & Kerber, R.E. (1998). Intracardiac echocardiographic imaging of the left ventricle from the right ventricle: quantitative experimental evaluation. *J Am Soc Echocardiogr*, Vol. 11, No. 10, (Publication date: 1998/11/06), pp. 921-928, I.S.S.N.: 0894-7317

Arbab-Zadeh, A., DeMaria, A.N., Penny, W.F., Russo, R.J., Kimura, B.J., & Bhargava, V. (1999). Axial movement of the intravascular ultrasound probe during the cardiac cycle: implications for three-dimensional reconstruction and measurements of coronary dimensions. *Am Heart J*, Vol. 138, No. 5 Pt 1, (Publication date: 1999/10/28), pp. 865-872, I.S.S.N.: 0002-8703

Atary, J.Z., Bergheanu, S.C., van der Hoeven, B.L., Atsma, D.E., Bootsma, M., van der Kley, F., Zeppenfeld, K., Jukema, J.W., & Schalij, M.J. (2009). Impact of sirolimus-eluting stent implantation compared to bare-metal stent implantation for acute myocardial infarction on coronary plaque composition at nine months follow-up: a Virtual Histology intravascular ultrasound analysis. Results from the Leiden MISSION! intervention study. *EuroIntervention*, Vol. 5, No. 5, (Publication date: 2010/02/10), pp. 565-572, I.S.S.N.: 1969-6213

Baldewsing, R.A., Schaar, J.A., Mastik, F., & van der Steen, A.F. (2007). Local elasticity imaging of vulnerable atherosclerotic coronary plaques. *Adv Cardiol*, Vol. 44, No. (Publication date: 2006/11/01), pp. 35-61, I.S.S.N.: 0065-2326

Bourantas, C.V., Kourtis, I.C., Plissiti, M.E., Fotiadis, D.I., Katsouras, C.S., Papafaklis, M.I., & Michalis, L.K. (2005). A method for 3D reconstruction of coronary arteries using biplane angiography and intravascular ultrasound images. *Comput Med Imaging Graph*, Vol. 29, No. 8, (Publication date: 2005/11/10), pp. 597-606, I.S.S.N.: 0895-6111

Bovenkamp, E.G., Dijkstra, J., Bosch, J.G., & Reiber, J.H. (2009). User-agent cooperation in multiagent IVUS image segmentation. *IEEE Trans Med Imaging*, Vol. 28, No. 1, (Publication date: 2009/01/01), pp. 94-105, I.S.S.N.: 1558-0062

Briguori, C., Anzuini, A., Airoldi, F., Gimelli, G., Nishida, T., Adamian, M., Corvaja, N., Di Mario, C., & Colombo, A. (2001). Intravascular ultrasound criteria for the assessment of the functional significance of intermediate coronary artery stenoses and comparison with fractional flow reserve. *Am J Cardiol*, Vol. 87, No. 2, (Publication date: 2001/01/12), pp. 136-141, I.S.S.N.: 0002-9149

Bruining, N., von Birgelen, C., de Feyter, P.J., Ligthart, J., Li, W., Serruys, P.W., & Roelandt, J.R. (1998). ECG-gated versus nongated three-dimensional intracoronary ultrasound analysis: implications for volumetric measurements. *Cathet Cardiovasc Diagn*, Vol. 43, No. 3, (Publication date: 1998/04/16), pp. 254-260, I.S.S.N.: 0098-6569

Cardinal, M.H., Soulez, G., Tardif, J.C., Meunier, J., & Cloutier, G. (2010). Fast-marching segmentation of three-dimensional intravascular ultrasound images: a pre- and post-intervention study. *Med Phys*, Vol. 37, No. 7, (Publication date: 2010/09/14), pp. 3633-3647, I.S.S.N.: 0094-2405

Cavaye, D.M., White, R.A., Kopchok, G.E., Mueller, M.P., Maselly, M.J., & Tabbara, M.R. (1992). Three-dimensional intravascular ultrasound imaging of normal and diseased canine and human arteries. *J Vasc Surg*, Vol. 16, No. 4, (Publication date: 1992/10/01), pp. 509-517; discussion 518-509, I.S.S.N.: 0741-5214

Cespedes, E.I., de Korte, C.L., van der Steen, A.F., von Birgelen, C., & Lancee, C.T. (1997). Intravascular elastography: principles and potentials. *Semin Interv Cardiol*, Vol. 2, No. 1, (Publication date: 1997/03/01), pp. 55-62, I.S.S.N.: 1084-2764

Chandrasekaran, K., Sehgal, C.M., Hsu, T.L., Young, N.A., D'Adamo, A.J., Robb, R.A., & Pandian, N.G. (1994). Three-dimensional volumetric ultrasound imaging of arterial pathology from two-dimensional intravascular ultrasound: an in vitro study.

Angiology, Vol. 45, No. 4, (Publication date: 1994/04/01), pp. 253-264, I.S.S.N.: 0003-3197

Cooper, B.Z., Kirwin, J.D., Panetta, T.F., Weinreb, F.M., Ramirez, J.A., Najjar, J.G., Blattman, S.B., Rodino, W., & Song, M. (2001). Accuracy of intravascular ultrasound for diameter measurement of phantom arteries. *J Surg Res*, Vol. 100, No. 1, (Publication date: 2001/08/23), pp. 99-105, I.S.S.N.: 0022-4804

Danilouchkine, M.G., Mastik, F., & van der Steen, A.F. (2009). Reconstructive compounding for IVUS palpography. *IEEE Trans Ultrason Ferroelectr Freq Control*, Vol. 56, No. 12, (Publication date: 2009/12/31), pp. 2630-2642, I.S.S.N.: 1525-8955

de Korte, C.L., & van der Steen, A.F. (2002). Intravascular ultrasound elastography: an overview. *Ultrasonics*, Vol. 40, No. 1-8, (Publication date: 2002/08/06), pp. 859-865, I.S.S.N.: 0041-624X

Di Mario, C., von Birgelen, C., Prati, F., Soni, B., Li, W., Bruining, N., de Jaegere, P.P., de Feyter, P.J., Serruys, P.W., & Roelandt, J.R. (1995). Three dimensional reconstruction of cross sectional intracoronary ultrasound: clinical or research tool? *Br Heart J*, Vol. 73, No. 5 Suppl 2, (Publication date: 1995/05/01), pp. 26-32, I.S.S.N.: 0007-0769

Diethrich, E.B. (1993). Endovascular treatment of abdominal aortic occlusive disease: the impact of stents and intravascular ultrasound imaging. *Eur J Vasc Surg*, Vol. 7, No. 3, (Publication date: 1993/05/01), pp. 228-236, I.S.S.N.: 0950-821X

Escolar, E., Weigold, G., Fuisz, A., & Weissman, N.J. (2006). New imaging techniques for diagnosing coronary artery disease. *CMAJ*, Vol. 174, No. 4, (Publication date: 2006/02/16), pp. 487-495, I.S.S.N.: 1488-2329

Finet, G., Weissman, N.J., Mintz, G.S., Satler, L.F., Kent, K.M., Laird, J.R., Adelmann, G.A., Ajani, A.E., Castagna, M.T., Rioufol, G., & Pichard, A.D. (2003). Mechanism of lumen enlargement with direct stenting versus predilatation stenting: influence of remodelling and plaque characteristics assessed by volumetric intracoronary ultrasound. *Heart*, Vol. 89, No. 1, (Publication date: 2002/12/17), pp. 84-90, I.S.S.N.: 1468-201X

Garcia-Garcia, H.M., Shen, Z., & Piazza, N. (2009). Study of restenosis in drug eluting stents: new insights from greyscale intravascular ultrasound and virtual histology. *EuroIntervention*, Vol. 5 Suppl D, No. (Publication date: 2009/09/17), pp. D84-92, I.S.S.N.: 1774-024X

Gatta, C., Pujol, O., Rodriguez Leor, O., Mauri Ferre, J., & Radeva, P. (2009). Fast rigid registration of vascular structures in IVUS sequences. *IEEE Trans Inf Technol Biomed*, Vol. 13, No. 6, (Publication date: 2009/08/01), pp. 1006-1011, I.S.S.N.: 1558-0032

Goderie, T.P., van Soest, G., Garcia-Garcia, H.M., Gonzalo, N., Koljenovic, S., van Leenders, G.J., Mastik, F., Regar, E., Oosterhuis, J.W., Serruys, P.W., & van der Steen, A.F. (2010). Combined optical coherence tomography and intravascular ultrasound radio frequency data analysis for plaque characterization. Classification accuracy of human coronary plaques in vitro. *Int J Cardiovasc Imaging*, Vol. 26, No. 8, (Publication date: 2010/04/17), pp. 843-850, I.S.S.N.: 1875-8312

Haas, C., Ermert, H., Holt, S., Grewe, P., Machraoui, A., & Barmeyer, J. (2000). Segmentation of 3D intravascular ultrasonic images based on a random field model. *Ultrasound Med Biol*, Vol. 26, No. 2, (Publication date: 2000/03/21), pp. 297-306, I.S.S.N.: 0301-5629

Hagenaars, T., Gussenhoven, E.J., van Essen, J.A., Seelen, J., Honkoop, J., & van der Lugt, A. (2000). Reproducibility of volumetric quantification in intravascular ultrasound images. *Ultrasound Med Biol*, Vol. 26, No. 3, (Publication date: 2000/04/25), pp. 367-374, I.S.S.N.: 0301-5629

Hiro, T., Hall, P., Maiello, L., Itoh, A., Colombo, A., Jang, Y.T., Salmon, S.M., & Tobis, J.M. (1998). Clinical feasibility of 0.018-inch intravascular ultrasound imaging device. *Am Heart J*, Vol. 136, No. 6, (Publication date: 1998/12/08), pp. 1017-1020, I.S.S.N.: 0002-8703

Hong, Y.J., Jeong, M.H., Kim, S.W., Choi, Y.H., Ma, E.H., Ko, J.S., Lee, M.G., Park, K.H., Sim, D.S., Yoon, N.S., Yoon, H.J., Kim, K.H., Park, H.W., Kim, J.H., Ahn, Y., Cho, J.G., Park, J.C., & Kang, J.C. (2010). Relation between plaque components and plaque prolapse after drug-eluting stent implantation--virtual histology-intravascular ultrasound. *Circ J*, Vol. 74, No. 6, (Publication date: 2010/05/11), pp. 1142-1151, I.S.S.N.: 1347-4820

Irshad, K., Reid, D.B., Miller, P.H., Velu, R., Kopchok, G.E., & White, R.A. (2001). Early clinical experience with color three-dimensional intravascular ultrasound in peripheral interventions. *J Endovasc Ther*, Vol. 8, No. 4, (Publication date: 2001/09/13), pp. 329-338, I.S.S.N.: 1526-6028

Jensen, L.O., Maeng, M., Thayssen, P., Christiansen, E.H., Hansen, K.N., Galloe, A., Kelbaek, H., Lassen, J.F., & Thuesen, L. (2008). Neointimal hyperplasia after sirolimus-eluting and paclitaxel-eluting stent implantation in diabetic patients: the Randomized Diabetes and Drug-Eluting Stent (DiabeDES) Intravascular Ultrasound Trial. *Eur Heart J*, Vol. 29, No. 22, (Publication date: 2008/10/04), pp. 2733-2741, I.S.S.N.: 1522-9645

Jinzaki, M., Ido, K., Shinmoto, H., Nakatsuka, S., & Hiramatsu, K. (1993). [Advantages of intravascular ultrasound--preliminary experience in patients with peripheral and renal vascular disease]. *Nippon Igaku Hoshasen Gakkai Zasshi*, Vol. 53, No. 4, (Publication date: 1993/04/25), pp. 478-480, I.S.S.N.: 0048-0428

Karmonik, C., Basto, P., & Morrisett, J.D. (2006). Quantification of carotid atherosclerotic plaque components using feature space analysis and magnetic resonance imaging. *Conf Proc IEEE Eng Med Biol Soc*, Vol. 1, No. (Publication date: 2007/10/20), pp. 3102-3105, I.S.S.N.: 1557-170X

Kim, Y.H., Hong, M.K., Lee, S.W., Lee, C.W., Han, K.H., Kim, J.J., Park, S.W., Mintz, G.S., & Park, S.J. (2004). Randomized comparison of debulking followed by stenting versus stenting alone for ostial left anterior descending artery stenosis: intravascular ultrasound guidance. *Am Heart J*, Vol. 148, No. 4, (Publication date: 2004/10/02), pp. 663-669, I.S.S.N.: 1097-6744

Klingensmith, J.D., Shekhar, R., & Vince, D.G. (2000a). Evaluation of three-dimensional segmentation algorithms for the identification of luminal and medial-adventitial borders in intravascular ultrasound images. *IEEE Trans Med Imaging*, Vol. 19, No. 10, (Publication date: 2000/12/29), pp. 996-1011, I.S.S.N.: 0278-0062

Klingensmith, J.D., Vince, D.G., Kuban, B.D., Shekhar, R., Tuzcu, E.M., Nissen, S.E., & Cornhill, J.F. (2000b). Assessment of coronary compensatory enlargement by three-dimensional intravascular ultrasound. *Int J Card Imaging*, Vol. 16, No. 2, (Publication date: 2000/08/06), pp. 87-98, I.S.S.N.: 0167-9899

Koning, G., Dijkstra, J., von Birgelen, C., Tuinenburg, J.C., Brunette, J., Tardif, J.C., Oemrawsingh, P.W., Sieling, C., Melsa, S., & Reiber, J.H. (2002). Advanced contour detection for three-dimensional intracoronary ultrasound: a validation--in vitro and in vivo. *Int J Cardiovasc Imaging*, Vol. 18, No. 4, (Publication date: 2002/07/19), pp. 235-248, I.S.S.N.: 1569-5794

Kovalski, G., Beyar, R., Shofti, R., & Azhari, H. (2000). Three-dimensional automatic quantitative analysis of intravascular ultrasound images. *Ultrasound Med Biol*, Vol. 26, No. 4, (Publication date: 2000/06/17), pp. 527-537, I.S.S.N.: 0301-5629

Laskey, W.K., Brady, S.T., Kussmaul, W.G., Waxler, A.R., Krol, J., Herrmann, H.C., Hirshfeld, J.W., Jr., & Sehgal, C. (1993). Intravascular ultrasonographic assessment of the results of coronary artery stenting. *Am Heart J*, Vol. 125, No. 6, (Publication date: 1993/06/01), pp. 1576-1583, I.S.S.N.: 0002-8703

Lekston, A., Chudek, J., Gasior, M., Wilczek, K., Wiecek, A., Kokot, F., Gierlotka, M., Niklewski, T., Fijalkowski, M., Szygula-Jurkiewicz, B., Wojnicz, R., Bialas, B., Osuch, M., Maciejewski, B., & Polonski, L. (2008). Angiographic and intravascular ultrasound assessment of immediate and 9-month efficacy of percutaneous transluminal renal artery balloon angioplasty with subsequent brachytherapy in patients with renovascular hypertension. *Kidney Blood Press Res*, Vol. 31, No. 5, (Publication date: 2008/09/06), pp. 291-298, I.S.S.N.: 1423-0143

Liang, Y., Zhu, H., & Friedman, M.H. (2008). Estimation of the transverse strain tensor in the arterial wall using IVUS image registration. *Ultrasound Med Biol*, Vol. 34, No. 11, (Publication date: 2008/07/16), pp. 1832-1845, I.S.S.N.: 1879-291X

Liu, J.B., Bonn, J., Needleman, L., Chiou, H.J., Gardiner, G.A., Jr., & Goldberg, B.B. (1999). Feasibility of three-dimensional intravascular ultrasonography: preliminary clinical studies. *J Ultrasound Med*, Vol. 18, No. 7, (Publication date: 1999/07/10), pp. 489-495, I.S.S.N.: 0278-4297

Luo, Z., Wang, Y., & Wang, W. (2003). Estimating coronary artery lumen area with optimization-based contour detection. *IEEE Trans Med Imaging*, Vol. 22, No. 4, (Publication date: 2003/05/31), pp. 564-566, I.S.S.N.: 0278-0062

Matar, F.A., Mintz, G.S., Douek, P., Farb, A., Virmani, R., Javier, S.P., Popma, J.J., Pichard, A.D., Kent, K.M., Satler, L.F., & et al. (1994). Coronary artery lumen volume measurement using three-dimensional intravascular ultrasound: validation of a new technique. *Cathet Cardiovasc Diagn*, Vol. 33, No. 3, (Publication date: 1994/11/01), pp. 214-220, I.S.S.N.: 0098-6569

McLeod, A.L., Watson, R.J., Anderson, T., Inglis, S., Newby, D.E., Northridge, D.B., Uren, N.G., & McDicken, W.N. (2004). Classification of arterial plaque by spectral analysis in remodelled human atherosclerotic coronary arteries. *Ultrasound Med Biol*, Vol. 30, No. 2, (Publication date: 2004/03/05), pp. 155-159, I.S.S.N.: 0301-5629

McPherson, A., Karrholm, J., Pinskerova, V., Sosna, A., & Martelli, S. (2005). Imaging knee position using MRI, RSA/CT and 3D digitisation. *J Biomech*, Vol. 38, No. 2, (Publication date: 2004/12/16), pp. 263-268, I.S.S.N.: 0021-9290

Mehran, R., Mintz, G.S., Hong, M.K., Tio, F.O., Bramwell, O., Brahimi, A., Kent, K.M., Pichard, A.D., Satler, L.F., Popma, J.J., & Leon, M.B. (1998). Validation of the in vivo intravascular ultrasound measurement of in-stent neointimal hyperplasia volumes. *J Am Coll Cardiol*, Vol. 32, No. 3, (Publication date: 1998/09/19), pp. 794-799, I.S.S.N.: 0735-1097

Min, P.K., Jung, J.H., Ko, Y.G., Choi, D., Jang, Y., & Shim, W.H. (2007). Effect of cilostazol on in-stent neointimal hyperplasia after coronary artery stenting: a quantative coronary angiography and volumetric intravascular ultrasound study. *Circ J*, Vol. 71, No. 11, (Publication date: 2007/10/30), pp. 1685-1690, I.S.S.N.: 1346-9843

Miyazaki, S., Hiasa, Y., & Kishi, K. (2010). Very late thrombosis after subintimal sirolimus-eluting stent implantation during percutaneous coronary intervention for chronic total occlusion. *J Invasive Cardiol*, Vol. 22, No. 8, (Publication date: 2010/08/04), pp. E162-165, I.S.S.N.: 1557-2501

Moise, M.A., Alvarez-Tostado, J.A., Clair, D.G., Greenberg, R.K., Lyden, S.P., Srivastava, S.D., Eagleton, M., Sarac, T.S., & Kashyap, V.S. (2009). Endovascular management of chronic infrarenal aortic occlusion. *J Endovasc Ther*, Vol. 16, No. 1, (Publication date: 2009/03/14), pp. 84-92, I.S.S.N.: 1526-6028

Montorsi, P., Galli, S., Fabbiocchi, F., Trabattoni, D., Ravagnani, P.M., & Bartorelli, A.L. (2004). Randomized trial of conventional balloon angioplasty versus cutting balloon for in-stent restenosis. Acute and 24-hour angiographic and intravascular ultrasound changes and long-term follow-up. *Ital Heart J*, Vol. 5, No. 4, (Publication date: 2004/06/10), pp. 271-279, I.S.S.N.: 1129-471X

Murata, T., Hiro, T., Fujii, T., Yasumoto, K., Murashige, A., Kohno, M., Yamada, J., Miura, T., & Matsuzaki, M. (2002). Impact of the cross-sectional geometry of the post-deployment coronary stent on in-stent neointimal hyperplasia: an intravascular ultrasound study. *Circ J*, Vol. 66, No. 5, (Publication date: 2002/05/28), pp. 489-493, I.S.S.N.: 1346-9843

Nair, A., Kuban, B.D., Obuchowski, N., & Vince, D.G. (2001). Assessing spectral algorithms to predict atherosclerotic plaque composition with normalized and raw intravascular ultrasound data. *Ultrasound Med Biol*, Vol. 27, No. 10, (Publication date: 2001/12/04), pp. 1319-1331, I.S.S.N.: 0301-5629

Nair, A., Kuban, B.D., Tuzcu, E.M., Schoenhagen, P., Nissen, S.E., & Vince, D.G. (2002). Coronary plaque classification with intravascular ultrasound radiofrequency data analysis. *Circulation*, Vol. 106, No. 17, (Publication date: 2002/10/23), pp. 2200-2206, I.S.S.N.: 1524-4539

Nasir, K., Rivera, J.J., Yoon, Y.E., Chang, S.A., Choi, S.I., Chun, E.J., Choi, D.J., Budoff, M.J., Blumenthal, R.S., & Chang, H.J. (2010). Variation in atherosclerotic plaque composition according to increasing coronary artery calcium scores on computed tomography angiography. *Int J Cardiovasc Imaging*, Vol. 26, No. 8, (Publication date: 2010/04/30), pp. 923-932, I.S.S.N.: 1875-8312

Nishanian, G., Kopchok, G.E., Donayre, C.E., & White, R.A. (1999). The impact of intravascular ultrasound (IVUS) on endovascular interventions. *Semin Vasc Surg*, Vol. 12, No. 4, (Publication date: 2000/01/29), pp. 285-299, I.S.S.N.: 0895-7967

Oshima, A., Itchhaporia, D., & Fitzgerald, P. (1998). New developments in intravascular ultrasound. *Vasc Med*, Vol. 3, No. 4, (Publication date: 1999/04/02), pp. 281-290, I.S.S.N.: 1358-863X

Papadogiorgaki, M., Mezaris, V., Chatzizisis, Y.S., Giannoglou, G.D., & Kompatsiaris, I. (2007). Texture Analysis and Radial Basis Function Approximation for IVUS Image Segmentation. *Open Biomed Eng J*, Vol. 1, No. (Publication date: 2007/01/01), pp. 53-59, I.S.S.N.: 1874-1207

Prati, F., Crea, F., Labellarte, A., Sommariva, L., Marino, P., Caradonna, E., Manzoli, A., Pappalardo, A., & Boccanelli, A. (2002). Normal distribution of an intravascular ultrasound index of vessel remodeling. *Ital Heart J*, Vol. 3, No. 12, (Publication date: 2003/03/04), pp. 710-714, I.S.S.N.: 1129-471X

Prati, F., Mallus, M.T., & Lioy, E. (1998). Three-dimensional reconstruction techniques applied to intracoronary images. *G Ital Cardiol*, Vol. 28, No. 4, (Publication date: 1998/06/09), pp. 460-467, I.S.S.N.: 0046-5968

Pundziute, G., Schuijf, J.D., Jukema, J.W., Decramer, I., Sarno, G., Vanhoenacker, P.K., Boersma, E., Reiber, J.H., Schalij, M.J., Wijns, W., & Bax, J.J. (2008). Evaluation of plaque characteristics in acute coronary syndromes: non-invasive assessment with multi-slice computed tomography and invasive evaluation with intravascular ultrasound radiofrequency data analysis. *Eur Heart J*, Vol. 29, No. 19, (Publication date: 2008/08/07), pp. 2373-2381, I.S.S.N.: 1522-9645

Raju, S., Darcey, R., & Neglen, P. (2010). Unexpected major role for venous stenting in deep reflux disease. *J Vasc Surg*, Vol. 51, No. 2, (Publication date: 2009/12/17), pp. 401-408; discussion 408, I.S.S.N.: 1097-6809

Raju, S., & Neglen, P. (2006). High prevalence of nonthrombotic iliac vein lesions in chronic venous disease: a permissive role in pathogenicity. *J Vasc Surg*, Vol. 44, No. 1, (Publication date: 2006/07/11), pp. 136-143; discussion 144, I.S.S.N.: 0741-5214

Reid, D.B., Douglas, M., & Diethrich, E.B. (1995). The clinical value of three-dimensional intravascular ultrasound imaging. *J Endovasc Surg*, Vol. 2, No. 4, (Publication date: 1995/11/01), pp. 356-364, I.S.S.N.: 1074-6218

Rodriguez-Granillo, G.A., McFadden, E.P., Aoki, J., van Mieghem, C.A., Regar, E., Bruining, N., & Serruys, P.W. (2006). In vivo variability in quantitative coronary ultrasound and tissue characterization measurements with mechanical and phased-array catheters. *Int J Cardiovasc Imaging*, Vol. 22, No. 1, (Publication date: 2005/12/20), pp. 47-53, I.S.S.N.: 1569-5794

Roelandt, J.R., di Mario, C., Pandian, N.G., Wenguang, L., Keane, D., Slager, C.J., de Feyter, P.J., & Serruys, P.W. (1994). Three-dimensional reconstruction of intracoronary ultrasound images. Rationale, approaches, problems, and directions. *Circulation*, Vol. 90, No. 2, (Publication date: 1994/08/01), pp. 1044-1055, I.S.S.N.: 0009-7322

Rosenfield, K., Kaufman, J., Pieczek, A.M., Langevin, R.E., Jr., Palefski, P.E., Razvi, S.A., & Isner, J.M. (1992). Human coronary and peripheral arteries: on-line three-dimensional reconstruction from two-dimensional intravascular US scans. Work in progress. *Radiology*, Vol. 184, No. 3, (Publication date: 1992/09/11), pp. 823-832, I.S.S.N.: 0033-8419

Rosenfield, K., Losordo, D.W., Ramaswamy, K., Pastore, J.O., Langevin, R.E., Razvi, S., Kosowsky, B.D., & Isner, J.M. (1991). Three-dimensional reconstruction of human coronary and peripheral arteries from images recorded during two-dimensional intravascular ultrasound examination. *Circulation*, Vol. 84, No. 5, (Publication date: 1991/11/01), pp. 1938-1956, I.S.S.N.: 0009-7322

Saketkhoo, R.R., Razavi, M.K., Padidar, A., Kee, S.T., Sze, D.Y., & Dake, M.D. (2004). Percutaneous bypass: subintimal recanalization of peripheral occlusive disease with IVUS guided luminal re-entry. *Tech Vasc Interv Radiol*, Vol. 7, No. 1, (Publication date: 2004/04/09), pp. 23-27, I.S.S.N.: 1089-2516

Sano, K., Mintz, G.S., Carlier, S.G., Fujii, K., Takebayashi, H., Kimura, M., Costa, J.R., Jr., Tanaka, K., Costa, R.A., Lui, J., Weisz, G., Moussa, I., Dangas, G.D., Mehran, R., Lansky, A.J., Kreps, E.M., Collins, M., Stone, G.W., Moses, J.W., & Leon, M.B. (2006). Volumetric intravascular ultrasound assessment of neointimal hyperplasia and nonuniform stent strut distribution in sirolimus-eluting stent restenosis. *Am J Cardiol*, Vol. 98, No. 12, (Publication date: 2006/12/06), pp. 1559-1562, I.S.S.N.: 0002-9149

Sanz-Requena, R., Moratal, D., Garcia-Sanchez, D.R., Bodi, V., Rieta, J.J., & Sanchis, J.M. (2007). Automatic segmentation and 3D reconstruction of intravascular ultrasound images for a fast preliminar evaluation of vessel pathologies. *Comput Med Imaging Graph*, Vol. 31, No. 2, (Publication date: 2007/01/12), pp. 71-80, I.S.S.N.: 0895-6111

Sarno, G., Garg, S., Gomez-Lara, J., Garcia Garcia, H.M., Ligthart, J., Bruining, N., Onuma, Y., Witberg, K., van Geuns, R.J., de Boer, S., Wykrzykowska, J., Schultz, C., Duckers, H.J., Regar, E., de Jaegere, P., de Feyter, P., van Es, G.A., Boersma, E., van der Giessen, W., & Serruys, P.W. (2011). Intravascular ultrasound radiofrequency analysis after optimal coronary stenting with initial quantitative coronary angiography guidance: an ATHEROREMO sub-study. *EuroIntervention*, Vol. 6, No. 8, (Publication date: 2011/02/19), pp. 977-984, I.S.S.N.: 1969-6213

Schaar, J.A., Mastik, F., Regar, E., den Uil, C.A., Gijsen, F.J., Wentzel, J.J., Serruys, P.W., & van der Stehen, A.F. (2007). Current diagnostic modalities for vulnerable plaque detection. *Curr Pharm Des*, Vol. 13, No. 10, (Publication date: 2007/04/14), pp. 995-1001, I.S.S.N.: 1873-4286

Schuurbiers, J.C., Lopez, N.G., Ligthart, J., Gijsen, F.J., Dijkstra, J., Serruys, P.W., Van der Steen, A.F., & Wentzel, J.J. (2009). In vivo validation of CAAS QCA-3D coronary reconstruction using fusion of angiography and intravascular ultrasound (ANGUS). *Catheter Cardiovasc Interv*, Vol. 73, No. 5, (Publication date: 2009/03/25), pp. 620-626, I.S.S.N.: 1522-726X

Scoccianti, M., Verbin, C.S., Kopchok, G.E., Back, M.R., Donayre, C.E., Sinow, R.M., & White, R.A. (1994). Intravascular ultrasound guidance for peripheral vascular interventions. *J Endovasc Surg*, Vol. 1, No. (Publication date: 1994/09/01), pp. 71-80, I.S.S.N.: 1074-6218

Shekhar, R., Cothren, R.M., Vince, D.G., Chandra, S., Thomas, J.D., & Cornhill, J.F. (1999). Three-dimensional segmentation of luminal and adventitial borders in serial intravascular ultrasound images. *Comput Med Imaging Graph*, Vol. 23, No. 6, (Publication date: 2000/01/14), pp. 299-309, I.S.S.N.: 0895-6111

Sherknies, D., Meunier, J., Mongrain, R., & Tardif, J.C. (2005). Three-dimensional trajectory assessment of an IVUS transducer from single-plane cineangiograms: a phantom study. *IEEE Trans Biomed Eng*, Vol. 52, No. 3, (Publication date: 2005/03/12), pp. 543-549, I.S.S.N.: 0018-9294

Siegel, R.J., Swan, K., Edwalds, G., & Fishbein, M.C. (1985). Limitations of postmortem assessment of human coronary artery size and luminal narrowing: differential effects of tissue fixation and processing on vessels with different degrees of atherosclerosis. *J Am Coll Cardiol*, Vol. 5, No. 2 Pt 1, (Publication date: 1985/02/01), pp. 342-346, I.S.S.N.: 0735-1097

Sonka, M., Liang, W., Kanani, P., Allan, J., DeJong, S., Kerber, R., & McKay, C. (1998). Intracardiac echocardiography: computerized detection of left ventricular borders. *Int J Card Imaging*, Vol. 14, No. 6, (Publication date: 1999/08/24), pp. 397-411, I.S.S.N.: 0167-9899

Su, J.L., Wang, B., & Emelianov, S.Y. (2009). Photoacoustic imaging of coronary artery stents. *Opt Express*, Vol. 17, No. 22, (Publication date: 2009/12/10), pp. 19894-19901, I.S.S.N.: 1094-4087

Takagi, A., Hibi, K., Zhang, X., Teo, T.J., Bonneau, H.N., Yock, P.G., & Fitzgerald, P.J. (2000). Automated contour detection for high-frequency intravascular ultrasound imaging:

a technique with blood noise reduction for edge enhancement. *Ultrasound Med Biol*, Vol. 26, No. 6, (Publication date: 2000/09/21), pp. 1033-1041, I.S.S.N.: 0301-5629

Takeda, Y., Tsuchikane, E., Kobayashi, T., Terai, K., Kobayashi, Y., Nakagawa, T., Sakurai, M., & Awata, N. (2003). Effect of plaque debulking before stent implantation on in-stent neointimal proliferation: a serial 3-dimensional intravascular ultrasound study. *Am Heart J*, Vol. 146, No. 1, (Publication date: 2003/07/10), pp. 175-182, I.S.S.N.: 1097-6744

Tang, G.L., Chin, J., & Kibbe, M.R. (2010). Advances in diagnostic imaging for peripheral arterial disease. *Expert Rev Cardiovasc Ther*, Vol. 8, No. 10, (Publication date: 2010/10/13), pp. 1447-1455, I.S.S.N.: 1744-8344

Thrush, A.J., Bonnett, D.E., Elliott, M.R., Kutob, S.S., & Evans, D.H. (1997). An evaluation of the potential and limitations of three-dimensional reconstructions from intravascular ultrasound images. *Ultrasound Med Biol*, Vol. 23, No. 3, (Publication date: 1997/01/01), pp. 437-445, I.S.S.N.: 0301-5629

Tu, S., Huang, Z., Koning, G., Cui, K., & Reiber, J.H. (2010). A novel three-dimensional quantitative coronary angiography system: In-vivo comparison with intravascular ultrasound for assessing arterial segment length. *Catheter Cardiovasc Interv*, Vol. 76, No. 2, (Publication date: 2010/07/29), pp. 291-298, I.S.S.N.: 1522-726X

Vince, D.G., & Davies, S.C. (2004). Peripheral application of intravascular ultrasound virtual histology. *Semin Vasc Surg*, Vol. 17, No. 2, (Publication date: 2004/06/09), pp. 119-125, I.S.S.N.: 0895-7967

von Birgelen, C., de Feyter, P.J., de Vrey, E.A., Li, W., Bruining, N., Nicosia, A., Roelandt, J.R., & Serruys, P.W. (1997a). Simpson's rule for the volumetric ultrasound assessment of atherosclerotic coronary arteries: a study with ECG-gated three-dimensional intravascular ultrasound. *Coron Artery Dis*, Vol. 8, No. 6, (Publication date: 1997/06/01), pp. 363-369, I.S.S.N.: 0954-6928

von Birgelen, C., Di Mario, C., Li, W., Schuurbiers, J.C., Slager, C.J., de Feyter, P.J., Roelandt, J.R., & Serruys, P.W. (1996a). Morphometric analysis in three-dimensional intracoronary ultrasound: an in vitro and in vivo study performed with a novel system for the contour detection of lumen and plaque. *Am Heart J*, Vol. 132, No. 3, (Publication date: 1996/09/01), pp. 516-527, I.S.S.N.: 0002-8703

von Birgelen, C., Di Mario, C., Reimers, B., Prati, F., Bruining, N., Gil, R., Serruys, P.W., & Roelandt, J.R. (1996b). Three-dimensional intracoronary ultrasound imaging. Methodology and clinical relevance for the assessment of coronary arteries and bypass grafts. *J Cardiovasc Surg (Torino)*, Vol. 37, No. 2, (Publication date: 1996/04/01), pp. 129-139, I.S.S.N.: 0021-9509

von Birgelen, C., Erbel, R., Di Mario, C., Li, W., Prati, F., Ge, J., Bruining, N., Gorge, G., Slager, C.J., Serruys, P.W., & et al. (1995). Three-dimensional reconstruction of coronary arteries with intravascular ultrasound. *Herz*, Vol. 20, No. 4, (Publication date: 1995/08/01), pp. 277-289, I.S.S.N.: 0340-9937

von Birgelen, C., Li, W., Bom, N., & Serruys, P.W. (1997b). Quantitative three-dimensional intravascular ultrasound. *Semin Interv Cardiol*, Vol. 2, No. 1, (Publication date: 1997/03/01), pp. 25-32, I.S.S.N.: 1084-2764

Wahle, A., Lopez, J.J., Olszewski, M.E., Vigmostad, S.C., Chandran, K.B., Rossen, J.D., & Sonka, M. (2006). Plaque development, vessel curvature, and wall shear stress in coronary arteries assessed by X-ray angiography and intravascular ultrasound. *Med*

Image Anal, Vol. 10, No. 4, (Publication date: 2006/04/29), pp. 615-631, I.S.S.N.: 1361-8415

Wahle, A., Prause, P.M., DeJong, S.C., & Sonka, M. (1999). Geometrically correct 3-D reconstruction of intravascular ultrasound images by fusion with biplane angiography--methods and validation. *IEEE Trans Med Imaging*, Vol. 18, No. 8, (Publication date: 1999/10/26), pp. 686-699, I.S.S.N.: 0278-0062

Waksman, R., Erbel, R., Di Mario, C., Bartunek, J., de Bruyne, B., Eberli, F.R., Erne, P., Haude, M., Horrigan, M., Ilsley, C., Bose, D., Bonnier, H., Koolen, J., Luscher, T.F., & Weissman, N.J. (2009). Early- and long-term intravascular ultrasound and angiographic findings after bioabsorbable magnesium stent implantation in human coronary arteries. *JACC Cardiovasc Interv*, Vol. 2, No. 4, (Publication date: 2009/05/26), pp. 312-320, I.S.S.N.: 1876-7605

Wallace, M.J., Ahrar, K., Tinkey, P., & Wright, K.C. (2005). Transvenous extrahepatic portacaval shunt with use of a modified prototype stent-graft: experimental study in animals. *J Vasc Interv Radiol*, Vol. 16, No. 2 Pt 1, (Publication date: 2005/02/17), pp. 261-267, I.S.S.N.: 1051-0443

Weichert, F., Muller, H., Quast, U., Kraushaar, A., Spilles, P., Heintz, M., Wilke, C., von Birgelen, C., Erbel, R., & Wegener, D. (2003). Virtual 3D IVUS vessel model for intravascular brachytherapy planning. I. 3D segmentation, reconstruction, and visualization of coronary artery architecture and orientation. *Med Phys*, Vol. 30, No. 9, (Publication date: 2003/10/08), pp. 2530-2536, I.S.S.N.: 0094-2405

White, R.A., Scoccianti, M., Back, M., Kopchok, G., & Donayre, C. (1994). Innovations in vascular imaging: arteriography, three-dimensional CT scans, and two- and three-dimensional intravascular ultrasound evaluation of an abdominal aortic aneurysm. *Ann Vasc Surg*, Vol. 8, No. 3, (Publication date: 1994/05/01), pp. 285-289, I.S.S.N.: 0890-5096

Xu, S., Nomura, M., Kurokawa, H., Ando, T., Kimura, M., Ishii, J., Hasegawa, H., Kondo, T., Tadiki, S., & Qi, P. (1995). Relationship between coronary angioscopic and intravascular ultrasound imaging and restenosis. *Chin Med J (Engl)*, Vol. 108, No. 10, (Publication date: 1995/10/01), pp. 743-749, I.S.S.N.: 0366-6999

Zhang, X., McKay, C.R., & Sonka, M. (1998). Tissue characterization in intravascular ultrasound images. *IEEE Trans Med Imaging*, Vol. 17, No. 6, (Publication date: 1999/02/27), pp. 889-899, I.S.S.N.: 0278-0062

Zimarino, M., Weissman, N.J., Waksman, R., De Caterina, R., Ahmed, J.M., Pichard, A.D., & Mintz, G.S. (2002). Analysis of stent edge restenosis with different forms of brachytherapy. *Am J Cardiol*, Vol. 89, No. 3, (Publication date: 2002/01/26), pp. 322-325, I.S.S.N.: 0002-9149

Zimmermann, A., Pollinger, B., Rieber, J., Konig, A., Erhard, I., Krotz, F., Sohn, H.Y., Kantlehner, R., Haimerl, W., Duhmke, E., Leibig, M., Theisen, K., Klauss, V., & Schiele, T.M. (2005). Early time course of neointima formation and vascular remodelling following percutaneous coronary intervention and vascular brachytherapy of in-stent restenotic lesions as assessed by intravascular ultrasound analysis. *Z Kardiol*, Vol. 94, No. 4, (Publication date: 2005/04/02), pp. 239-246, I.S.S.N.: 0300-5860

2

Plaque Regression and Stability Evaluated by Intravascular Ultrasound and Coronary Angioscopy: A Review

Satoshi Saito, Takafumi Hiro,
Tadateru Takayama and Atsushi Hirayama
Keiai Hospital & Nihon University
Japan

1. Introduction

Although atherosclerosis seems to be continuously progressive and irreversible, it has been being demonstrated that substantial regression or stabilization of atherosclerotic lesions can occur by some interventions improving its determinants. However, the concepts of plaque regression or stabilization are not so new. It has been reviewed that the first reported observation of plaque regression could be found in the 1920s (Wissler, 1976), in which switching cholesterol-fed rabbits to low-fat chow over 2–3 years resulted in arterial lesions becoming more fibrous with a reduced lipid content. Later on, as the earliest prospective studies, a couple of previous studies in the 1950s have shown distinctive facts of plaque shrinkage or favorable change of its tissue components due to special diet therapy or some specific medications. In 1957 Friedman M et al. documented a result from prospective, interventional study demonstrating substantial shrinkage of atherosclerotic lesions performed in cholesterol-fed rabbits (Friedman, 1957). The dietary regimen raised total plasma cholesterol to around 1,000 mg/dl, and then animals received intravenous injections of phosphatidylcholine. They reported that after less than a week or so the size of the plaques as well as cholesterol stores within the arterial wall were significantly reduced. This striking report with some following supportive studies and reviews (Wissler, 1976; Armstrong, 1976; Malinow, 1983) has been surprisingly ignored for long years because of some beliefs regarding distinctive persistent characteristics of atherosclerosis, the negative history of which was reviewed by Stein Y, et al (Stein , 2001). However, various additional facts of plaque regression by some interventions have been demonstrated in other type of animal studies (Maruffo , 1968; Armstrong , 1970) since then without strong interests among general cardiologists.
The first prospective study demonstrating plaque regression in humans might be the one documented by Ost CR, et al. in 1967(Ost, 1967). In the study, approximately 10% of patients treated with niacin showed improved femoral angiograms. Numerous additional larger trials of lipid lowering have then shown angiographic evidence of regression. However, though statistically significant, the resulted effects were very small (Brown, 1993), in which the improvement of percent stenosis of lumen were at most 2%. Accumulations of clinical evidences demonstrating the benefits of lipid-lowering in clinical outcome therefore yield

this kind of "angiographic paradox". This paradox suggested that the improvement of clinical outcome was not necessarily associated with the improvement of arterial lumen diameter. However, various pathological findings have resolved this enigma. First, the answer came from the recognition of a phenomenon called as vascular remodling (Glagov, 1987). The next answer was regarding the realization that lipid-rich, vulnerable plaques have a central role in acute coronary syndromes (Fuster, 1992; Libby, 1995). Vulnerable plaques are usually small in size and cause less than 50% occlusion. The vulnerable plaques are generally filled with intracellular and extracellular lipid, rich in macrophages and tissue factor, having low concentrations of smooth muscle cells as well as a thin fibrous cap (Shah, 2003; Falk, 1995). Rupture of a vulnerable plaque provokes the formation of a robust thrombosis causing critical lumen occlusion. It has been estimated that lipid lowering, therapy does not induce lumen expansion but rather has most impact on risk reduction by the remodeling and stabilization of small, rupture-prone lesions.

Based on these past histories, a new era of medication strategy had come in late 1980s with an appearance of 3-hydroxy-3-methyl-glutaryl coenzyme A reductase inhibitors (statins) in clinical setting. Many large-scale pivotal clinical trials have then shown that statins remarkably reduced both atherogenic lipoproteins as well as cardiovascular morbidity and mortality (Scandinavian Simvastatin Survival Study Group, 1994; Sacks, 1996; The Long-Term Intervention with Pravastatin in Ischemic Disease (LIPID) Study Group, 1998). However, the angiographic paradox still exists in this era even with a strong statin (Ballantyne, 2008). To overcome the paradox by in-vivo detection of plaque regression and stabilization, new development of commercially available intravascular imaging modalities contributed a lot to understanding the mechanism of statins for reducing cardiovascular events in patients with coronary artery disease. These modalities can visualize plaque size and its serial changes, and can even visualize tissue components within plaque to be able to estimate plaque vulnerability.

In this chapter, readers will be able to describe the imaging mechanisms of intravascular ultrasound and coronary angioscopy especially for observing plaque regression and stabilization. Then, a variety of important evidences of plaque regression and stabilization evaluated by these systems will be introduced in order to understand the clinical feasibility of these modalities as well as to recognize current clinical cutting edge of knowledge regarding plaque regression and stabilization.

2. Assessment of plaque regression and stability

2.1 Assessment with intravascular ultrasound

Intravascular ultrasound (IVUS) can provide gray-scale images with an accurate representation of plaque cross-sectional areas and volumes. Therefore, IVUS can follow in-vivo plaque volumes serially in same patients. IVUS imaging is performed with an automatic catheter-pullback system to acquire consecutive cross-sections of arterial wall. Cross-sectional plaque area for each section can be measured by tracings of lumen-intima border as well as media-adventitia (External elastic membrane area: EEM area). The difference of the two areas corresponds to the plaque area (intima-media complex area). The product of a certain constant distance-related interval and the integration of these plaque areas calculated from each cross-section resulted in total plaque volume of interest. The certain interval varied from 0.1 mm to 10 mm according to the study concept. The IVUS indices used in major clinical trials were as follows: 1) Nominal Change of Percent Plaque

Volume: This is obtained from the absolute nominal change between the baseline and the follow-up period in percent value of plaque volume compared to EEM volume; 2) Percent Change in Plaque Volume: This is calculated from (follow-up plaque volume minus baseline plaque volume) divided by (follow-up plaque volume) times 100. It has been suggested that the former index might be more closely related to clinical outcome (Nicholls, 2010). However, this index would show "regression" even in case of increase in EEM volume (positive remodeling) without any change in plaque volume itself. The latter one may be more reflected to a particular change of a special plaque of interest. Although it has not yet been directly proved that these IVUS parameters are useful surrogate markers for clinical outcome, IVUS have demonstrated a remarkable change in plaque volume by use of statins.

Furthermore, current technologies of IVUS can perform tissue characterization of plaque components with a color-coded image. In Japan, three color-IVUS systems are now commercially available. In addition, various other methods have been proposed with sophisticated mathematical models to detect tissue-specific acoustic properties. An overview of these methods is as follows.

It was originally expected that tissue components within plaque could be identified from the video-intensity pattern of IVUS images. Subsequent studies, however, demonstrated significant limitations of tissue characterization by IVUS intensity patterns alone, especially in discriminating fibrous and fatty tissues or in assessing plaque vulnerability (Hiro, 1996; Hiro, 1997; Kimura, 1995; Jeremias, 1999). To overcome this limitation, special attempts to analyze the echo-signals including the raw radiofrequency (RF) ultrasound signal that comes from plaque segments. The echo signal, which is originally emitted as a pulse wave from the ultrasound catheter tip, is produced at the interface between the two materials having different acoustic impedances. There are several interfaces within plaque, so time-series RF signal is then formed according to the degree of acoustic impedance mismatches and geometrical structure and distribution of each tissue components. Therefore, it can be expected that detection of special acoustic characteristics for each tissue component can allow us to visually identify it. Based upon this hypothesis, several successful studies have been reported, including the three commercially available machines.

2.1.1 Integrated backscatter analysis (IB-IVUS®)

This system visualizes the distribution of quantitative power or energy of echo for each segment of plaque using fast-Fourier transform of time-series RF signal. The total energy range is divided into four local ranges which correspond to four kinds of tissue components. This simple algorithm provides a high accuracy with a reliable sensitivity and specificity (Kawasaki , 2002).

2.1.2 Autoregressive spectral analysis (Virtual histology®)

The echo spectrum is first obtained by autoregressive spectral analysis for each portion of plaque. Autoregressive spectral analysis can obtain a spectrum of time-series signal, which has a different mathematical processing from fast-Fourier transform. Eight kinds of acoustic parameters are then measured for each spectrum. A classification tree which flows according to the values of the eight parameters makes the final diagnosis to discriminate four tissue types. The classification tree is already prepared with previous survey using tissue-known echo-samples (Nair, 2002). (Figure 1)

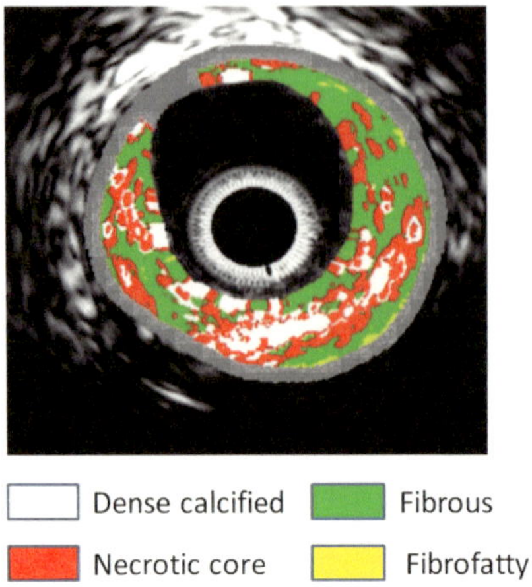

Fig. 1. VH-IVUS
A pre-defined classification tree according to eight acoustic parameters identifies four kind of tissues.

2.1.3 Attenuation-slope analysis

The ultrasound energy is attenuated when running through tissues. The degree of attenuation depends upon the frequency. It is hypothesized that the frequency-dependence of ultrasound attenuation is different according to the tissue type. This system colorized the degree of frequency-dependent of ultrasound attenuation (Wilson , 1994).

2.1.4 Angle-dependence analysis

It has been demonstrated that intravascular ultrasound (IVUS) backscatter from fibrous tissue is strongly dependent on the ultrasound beam angle of incidence (Picano , 1985). It was found that this technique provides an accurate representation of the thickness of the fibrous cap in atherosclerotic plaque, the echo-intensity of which is highly angle-dependent (Hiro , 2001). (Figure 2)

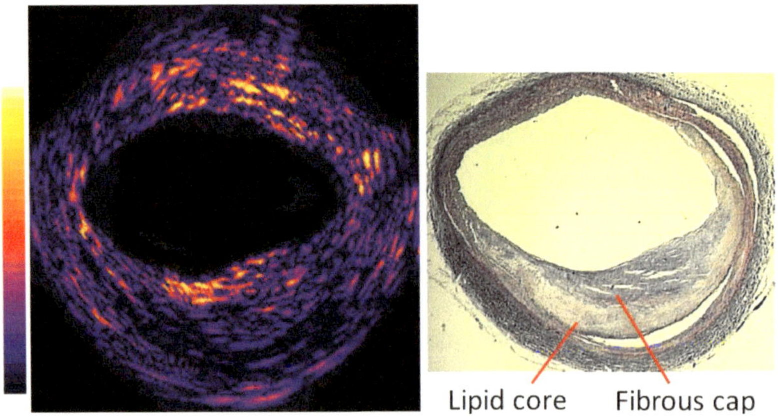

Fig. 2. Angle-dependence analysis
Highly angle-dependent area (yellow) is accurately corresponded to fibrous cap. Incited from (Hiro, 2001)

2.1.5 Fractal analysis

This method obtained the value of fractal dimension, which represents how complex the echo-segment is from each plaque portion. It was found that the echo-signal was more complex from lipidic tissue compared to fibrous tissue (Hiro, 2000).

2.1.6 Wavelet analysis

Wavelet analysis of RF IVUS signals is a novel mathematical model for assessing focal geometrical differences within arterial walls. Color coding of the wavelet correlation coefficient derived from the RF signal allows detection of changes in the geometrical profile of time-series signals to derive an image of plaque components (Figure 3). Murashige et al. showed that lipid-rich plaques could be detected with acceptable sensitivity and specificity using this method (Murashige, 2005). (Figure 3)

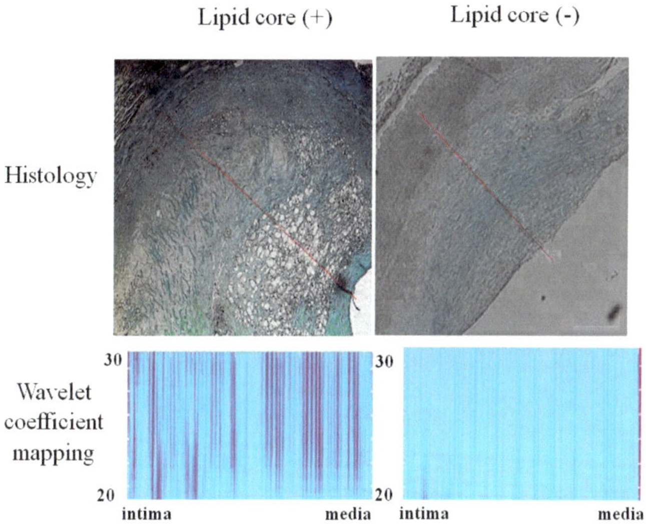

Fig. 3. Wavelet analysis
Wavelet correlation mapping of the RF signal from lipid-rich plaque revealed a unique stripe pattern. Incited from (Murashige, 2005)

2.1.7 Neural network theory

This method analyzes the RF signal with a self-learning system that resembles real neural actions in humans or animals. Kubota used a k-nearest neighbor method to classify tissue types of coronary plaque (Kubota , 2007). The k-nearest neighbor method is like a decision-making system by a majority vote. When a time-series signal is evaluated, there are numerous parameters obtained by a signal-processing system. The parameters (total number = n) from a signal area of interest, therefore, can yield a coordinate as: (x1,x2,x3,.....xn) (Let's call now point P). In such space, previously prepared coordinates obtained from the tissue-known signal exist around the point P. When you look around the point P for a constant distance, you can count the number of tissue-known points. If the majority of tissue-known points is from lipidic tissue, then the point P- corresponded tissue area is considered to be a lipidic tissue. Kubota R et al. modified this k-nearest method to enhance the accuracy of tissue characterization by IVUS. Sathyanarayana S, et al. performed this kind of analysis in analyzing spectral similarity of the RF signal (Sathyanarayana , 2009). It was hypothesized that each tissue component has a special characteristic spectrum shape. This system is now commercially available with a system name, iMap ® (Figure 4). This system can identify four kinds of tissue, which definitions are slightly different from the one used in VH-IVUS. The imaging system is unique, in which the confidence level of identification of tissue types is represented the brightness of each color corresponded to each tissue type. The brightness of confidence level represents the degree of majority in the decision-making space of the k-nearest neighbor method.

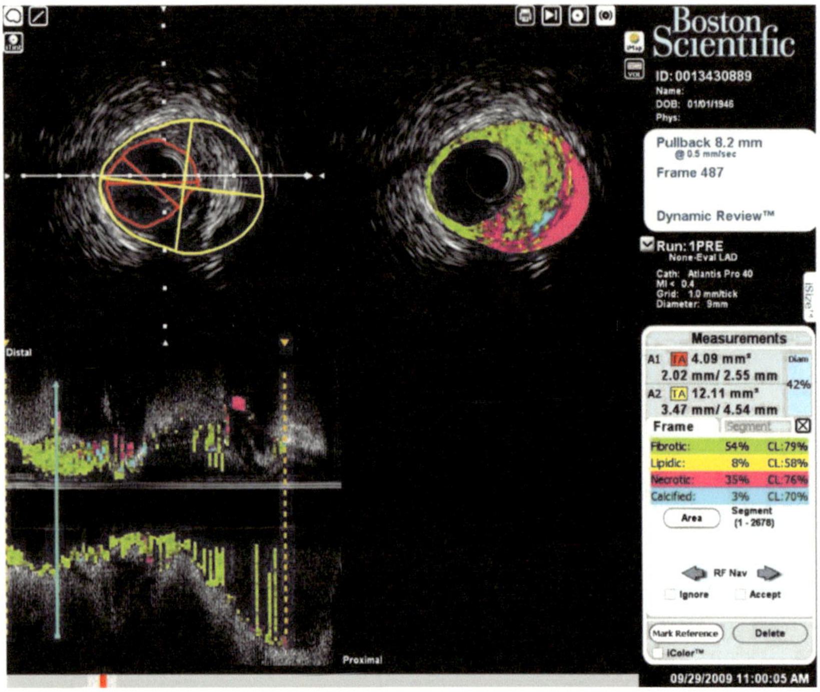

Fig. 4. iMap system.
The system of iMap perform color mapping of four different tissue types. Confidence level of each tissue identification is reflected on the brightness of each color. CL:Confidence level

2.2 Assessment with coronary angioscopy

Coronary angioscopy provides a full-color perspective of the intravascular surface morphology of plaque. This technique also accurately represents the presence of thrombi. In this method, vulnerable plaques are detected as yellow plaques compared to the normal surface which is depicted as white. The degree of yellow grade of the plaque surface is corresponded to how rich lipidic components are under the plaque surface or how thin the thickness of fibrous cap is within the plaque. It has been documented that the degree of yellowness of plaque as well as the number of yellow plaque observed are related to plaque vulnerability and poor patient prognosis in cardiovascular outcome (Kodama , 2000; Ueda , 1997; Ueda , 2004; Naghavi , 2003; Asakura , 2001; Ohtani , 2006; Mizuno, 1992). This modality together with IVUS has provided various aspects of plaque regression and its stability.

2.3 Problems in assessing plaque vulnerability

Naghavi M, and a lot of famous investigators collaborated to try to establish the criteria for defining vulnerable plaques(Naghavi , 2003). As the major criteria, the plaque with the following characteristics can be identified as vulnerable plaque:

- Active inflammation (monocyte/macrophage and sometimes T-cell infiltration)
- Thin cap with large lipid core
- Endothelial denudation with superficial platelet aggregation
- Fissured plaque
- Stenosis more than 90%

As the minor criteria:

- Superficial calcified nodule
- Glistening yellow by coronary angioscopy
- Intraplaque hemorrhage
- Endothelial dysfunction
- Outward (positive) remodelling

So what criteria can we examine generally in all patients?

IVUS and coronary angioscopy can actually represent the thickness of thin fibrous cap and the volume of lipid-rich core. However, Imoto K, et al demonstrated in the study with a biomechanical simulation of in-plaque stress distribution that plaques with the same thickness of fibrous cap does not necessarily indicate the same vulnerability to rupture (Imoto, 2005). Ambrose JA documented a get-to-the-point criticism in search of the vulnerable plaque(Ambrose, 2008). He proposed several prerequisites to establish the way to identify vulnerable plaque for distinctive improving patient vulnerability.

1. "Vulnerable plaque" caused by a thin-capped fibroatheroma can be identified with modern technology.
2. A "vulnerable plaque" caused by plaque erosion should be identifiable.
3. The number of "vulnerable plaques" is known, and the number is limited.
4. The natural history of a "vulnerable plaque" has been identified in patients treated with optimal systemic therapies.
5. An interventional approach applied locally or regionally to an asymptomatic"vulnerable plaque" is proven to reduce future events relative to the best systemic medical therapy.

He criticized that among these prerequisites, only the first is currently possible, but the others are not yet established and require further study. We have to realize that thin-capped fibro-atheroma is not a single cause of acute coronary syndrome. Erosion, inflammatory cell infilitration, intraplaque hemorrhage or local endothelial dysfunction should be also evaluated. Fukumoto Y, et al. has reported that color mapping of shear stress along plaque surface using IVUS images is useful for identifying future rupture point(Fukumoto, 2008), since it was found that local concentration of shear stress is related to a trigger of plaque rupture. Therefore, numerous local risk factor should be considered for identifying the vulnerable plaque. Even when the method is established, still we have additional problems. We have to possess a detailed data on the likelihood of a cardiac event for a proven "vulnerable plaque." For example, if only 5% of a given plaque type as identified will develop an event on follow-up, all 20 of these plaques will need to be treated with a new procedure to prevent 1 event, that is, NNT=20(Ambrose, 2008). Is this allowed in using the expensive stent therapy? Therefore, a well-designed clinical trial should be performed to prove the clinical feasibility of preventive therapy for a particular plaque which is identified as vulnerable.

3. Clinical evidences using intravascular imagings

A number of human studies in a single center demonstrated the beneficial effects of statin or other lipid-lowering drugs in plaque progression/regression and stabilization. For example, Takagi T, et al. documented in 1997 as one of the earliest reports on IVUS observation that administration of pravastatin reduced serum lipid levels and progression of coronary artery atherosclerotic plaque(Takagi, 1997). Kawasaki et al. reported with use three-dimensional color mapping of tissue components with IB-IVUS system that statin therapy reduced the lipid component in patients with stable angina without reducing the degree of stenosis(Kawasaki, 2005). Previous coronary angioscopic studies have demonstrated that statin therapy stabilizes yellow color grade of coronary plaques (Takano, 2003).
Using IVUS and/or coronary angioscopy, various human multicenter trials with statins have offered important information on plaque regression. In the following paragraphs, the trials including REVERSAL(Nissen , 2004), ASTEROID(Nissen , 2006), ESTABLISH(Okazaki, 2004), JAPAN-ACS(Hiro, 2009), COSMOS(Takayama, 2009), TWINS(Hirayama, 2009) and TOGETHAR(Kodama, 2010) are overviewed and discussed. These trials demonstrated not only the degree of regressive effects of statins on plaque, but also key determinants and mechanisms of plaque regression.

3.1 The REVERSAL study (The Reversal of Atherosclerosis with Aggressive Lipid Lowering trial) (Nissen, 2004)

This was to compare the 18-month effect of regimens designed to produce intensive lipid lowering or moderate lipid lowering on coronary artery atheroma burden and progression. Patients with stable coronary artery disease were randomly assigned to receive a moderate lipid lowering regimen consisting of 40 mg of pravastatin or an intensive lipid-lowering regimen consisting of 80 mg of atorvastatin. The primary efficacy parameter was the percentage change in atheroma volume (follow-up minus baseline). Baseline low-density lipoprotein cholesterol level (mean, 150.2 mg/dL in both treatment groups) was reduced to 110 mg/dL in the pravastatin group and to 79 mg/dL in the atorvastatin group ($P<0.001$). It was shown that progression of coronary atherosclerosis occurred in the pravastatin group (median change = 2.7%; 95% CI:0.2% to 4.7%; $P=0.001$) compared with baseline. Progression did not occur in the atorvastatin group (−0.4%; CI−2.4% to 1.5%; $P=0.98$) compared with baseline. It was concluded that for patients with coronary heart disease, intensive lipid-lowering treatment with atorvastatin reduced progression of coronary atherosclerosis compared with pravastatin. In this study, remarkable regression of plaque by statin was not yet clearly indicated.

3.2 The ASTEROID study (A study to Evaluate the Effect of Rosuvastatin on Intravascular Ultrasound-Derived Coronary Atheroma Burden) (Nissen, 2006)

This study was to assess whether very intensive statin therapy could regress coronary atherosclerosis as determined by IVUS imaging. Patients with stable coronary artery disease received intensive statin therapy with rosuvastatin, 40 mg/day. Two primary efficacy parameters were prespecified: the change in percent atheroma volume (PAV) and the change in nominal atheroma volume in the 10-mm subsegment with the greatest disease severity at baseline (observation period: 24 months). Baseline low-density lipoprotein cholesterol level (mean, 130.4 mg/dL) was reduced to 60.8 mg/dL ($P<0.001$). For the primary efficacy parameter of PAV, the mean decrease was −0.98% and the median was −0.79% (P<0.001 compared with baseline). For the second primary efficacy parameter, change in atheroma volume in the 10-mm subsegment with the greatest disease severity, the mean change was −6.1 mm^3, and the median change was −5.6 mm3 (P<0.001 compared with baseline). This change represents a median reduction of 9.1% in atheroma volume in the 10-mm segment with the greatest disease severity. It was concluded that very high-intensity statin therapy using rosuvastatin 40 mg/day achieved significant regression of atherosclerosis .In this study, remarkable regression of plaque by statin was first clearly indicated as a multicenter study result. Regression can be considered to be a completely different process from inhibition of progression, so this result was striking.

3.3 The ESTABLISH study (Early Statin Treatment in Patients with Acute Coronary Syndrome: Demonstration of the Beneficial Effect on Atherosclerotic Lesions by Serial Volumetric Intravascular Ultrasound Analysis during Half a Year after Coronary Event) (Okazaki, 2004)

This was a single-center, but should be discussed, since the results was historical. Most unique part of this study was study population. This study investigated the 6-month effect of early statin treatment by atorvastatin of 20 mg daily on plaque volume of a nonculprit lesion by serial volumetric intravascular ultrasound in patients with ACS. All patients who underwent emergency coronary angiography and percutaneous coronary intervention were randomized to intensive lipid-lowering therapy (n=35; atorvastatin 20 mg/day) or control (n=35) groups after PCI. Volumetric intravascular ultrasound analyses were performed at baseline and 6-month follow-up for a non-PCI site in 48 patients (atorvastatin, n=24; control, n=24). LDL-C level was significantly decreased by 41.7% (124.6 to 70.0 mg/dL) in the atorvastatin group compared with the control group, in which LDL-C was not significantly changed (123.9 to 119.4 mg/dL) (atorvastatin vs. control : P<0.0001). Plaque volume was significantly reduced in the atorvastatin group (mean 13.1% decrease) compared with the control group (8.7 % increase; P<0.0001). These results of the degree of plaque regression by statin were surprisingly remarkable compared to the former reports from foreign countries for patients with stable coronary artery disease. This evidence was then proved by the JAPAN-ACS study which is discussed next.

3.4 The JAPAN-ACS study (Japan Assessment of Pitavastatin and Atorvastatin in Acute Coronary Syndrome) (Hiro, 2009)

This study had almost similar protocol for selecting patients with acute coronary syndrome and measuring protocol to the ESTABLISH study. Major difference was that this was a non-inferiority test with randomization between patients with taking atorvastatin 20 mg/day and patients with pitavastatin of 4 mg/day. Therefore, based on the ESTABLISH study, the objective of this study was to evaluate whether the regressive effects of aggressive lipid-lowering therapy with atorvastatin on coronary plaque volume in patients with acute coronary syndrome are generalized for other statins in multicenter setting (observation period:8-12 months) . The primary end point was the percentage change in nonculprit coronary plaque volume. Baseline low-density lipoprotein cholesterol level (mean, 133.8 and 130.9 mg/dL in atorvastatin, and pitavastatin groups, respectively) was reduced to 84.1 mg/dL (-35.8% decrease: P<0.001, compared to the baseline) in the atorvastatin group and to 81.1 mg/dL (-36.2% decrease: P<0.001)in the pitavastatin group. The mean percentage change in plaque volume was -18.1% and -16.9 % (p=0.5) in the pitavastatin and atorvastatin groups, respectively, which was associated with negative vessel remodeling. The upper limit of 95% confidence interval of the mean difference in percentage change in plaque volume between the two groups did not exceed the pre-defined noninferiority margin of 5%, suggesting noninferiority between the two groups. It was thus proved that the efficacies of both group were equivalent in the percent change of plaque volume. This results supported the data of the ESTABLISH study that early administration of statins after the onset of ACS has the potential to reverse the process of atherosclerosis.This observation also generalized the effect of statins other than atorvastatin on plaque volume in the setting of ACS. The reason why plaques in Japanese patients with ACS shows greater regression by statin compared to the foreign patients with stable coronary artery disease might be shown by the COSMOS study which is summarized later.

Recently interesting results came from a sub-analysis of the JAPAN-ACS study (Hiro , 2010). It demonstrated that the regression of coronary plaque induced by statin therapy after ACS was weaker in diabetic patients than their counterparts, although the reduction of LDL-C level was similar between diabetic group and non-diabetic group. In addition, it was also interesting that significant correlation between % change of PV and low-density lipoprotein cholesterol (LDL-C) level was found in patients with diabetes mellitus ($n=73$, $P<0.05$, $r=0.4$), whereas there was no significant correlation between the 2 parameters in patients without diabetes mellitus ($n=178$). This study was suggesting that there might be LDL-C dependent mechanism and LDL-C non-depedent mechanism in plaque regression by statin. It might be possible that in diabetic patients LDL-C non-dependent mechanism is inhibited by unknown mechanism resulting smaller regression of plaque volume. The mechanism of plaque regression may have various steps and pathways.

3.5 The COSMOS study (The Coronary Atherosclerosis study Measuring Effects of Rosuvastatin Using Intravascular Ultrasound in Japanese Subjects) (Takayama, 2009)

This study was the first multicenter study on IVUS observation of plaque with use of statin for Japanese patients with stable coronary artery disease. This was as a single arm 76-week study to investigate the effect of rosuvastatin on plaque volume in such patients. The patients received first rosuvastatin 2.5mg/day, which could be increased at 4-week intervals to ≤20 mg/day. The primary end point was the percentage change in nonculprit coronary plaque volume. The change in the serum low-density lipoprotein-cholesterol level from baseline to end of follow-up was $-38.6\pm16.9\%$ (mean:140.2 to 82.9 mg/dL, $P<0.0001$). Percent change of plaque volume, the primary endpoint, was $-5.1\pm14.1\%$ ($P<0.0001$). The degree of plaque regression compared to the degree of reduction of LDL-C level was just in-between the results from the foreign patients with stable coronary artery disease and the ones from Japanese patients with acute coronary syndrome (Figure 5). Therefore, Japanese patients as well as patients with acute coronary artery disease can easily show regression of plaque volume compared to the foreign patients and patients with stable coronary artery disease, respectively. This might be due to the difference in plaque tissue characteristics. It has been reported that patients with ACS have many greater-risk nonculprit plaques(Asakura , 2001; Burke , 1997).

3.6 The TWINS study (Hirayama, 2009)

This study as well as the TOGETHAR study were using not only IVUS but also coronary angioscopy to examine the effect of statin on plaque characteristics. The aim of this study

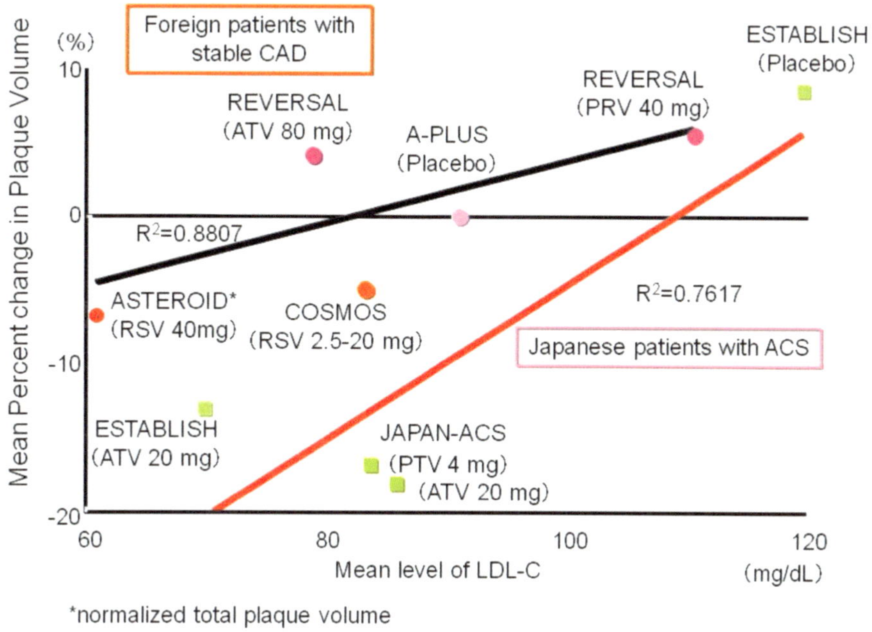

Fig. 5. Meta-regressive analysis of the relationship between LDL-C level and the percent change of plaque volume.
Some data was not the result as the primary endpoint of the study, which was re-estimated by documented data. Black line represents the meta-regression curve for the foreign patients with stable coronary artery disease. Red line represents the one for Japanese patients with ACS. The data of the COSMOS study is just in-between the two lines.
See each protocol and result for each study from the papers by (Takano , 2003; Nissen , 2004; Nissen , 2006; Okazaki , 2004; Hiro , 2009). The data of A-PLUS was obtained from the paper by (Berry , 2007). ATV:atorvastatin, PRV:pravastatin, RSV:rosuvastatin, PTV:pitavastatin.

was to elucidate 80-week time course of atorvastatin-induced changes in vulnerable plaque using angioscopy and intravascular ultrasound (IVUS). Patients with coronary artery disease received atorvastatin of 10-20 mg/day. Mean baseline LDL-C level of 144.4 mg/dL was significantly reduced to 86.4 mg/dL at week 28 and to 89.4 mg/dL at week 80. Angioscopic images were classified into 6 grades (0-5) based on yellow color intensity. The mean angioscopic grade of 58 yellow plaques significantly decreased from 1.5 (95% confidence CI: 1.2 to 1.8) to 1.1 (95%CI 0.9 to 1.3, P=0.012) at week 28 and 1.2 (95%CI :0.9 to 1.4, P=0.024) at week 80, compare to the baseline (no significant difference between week 28 and week 80). Mean volume of 30 lesions, including the 58 yellow plaques, significantly reduced -8.3% (95%CI: -11.5 to -5.2) at week 28 (P<0.001 for baseline vs week 28) and -17.8% (95%CI -23.9 to -11.8) at week 80 (P<0.001) for baseline vs week 80. It should be noted that qualitative changes in plaque occurred relatively early after the beginning of atorvastatin therapy (by week 28), and that quantitative changes in atheroma volume occurred continuously, even after week 28, up to week 80. These non-parallel results suggest that there may be two different, probably independent, mechanisms involved in the reduction of vulnerability, improvement in characteristics, and reduction of the volume of yellow plaques. These different time courses suggested that the improvement in plaque characteristics occurs early, whereas atheroma volume regression occurs over a prolonged period of time.

3.7 The TOGETHAR study (Kodama, 2010)

This multicenter study also revealed that the stabilization and regression of atherosclerotic plaques by statin may differ. This study was performed to assess coronary plaque regression and stabilization following 52 weeks of pitavastatin treatment (2 mg/day). Low-density lipoprotein-cholesterol (LDL-C) was reduced 34.5% (mean: 145.0 to 93.6 mg/dl, $P<0.001$). Yellow grade decreased (2.9 ± 0.8 to 2.6 ± 0.7, $P=0.040$) during 52 weeks. However, percent atheroma volume on IVUS did not change during 52 weeks. It was concluded that fixed dose pitavastatin stabilized vulnerable coronary plaques by the reduction of yellow grade without significant reduction of plaque volume. The fact that plaque volume was not significantly changed was probably due to the characteristics patient populations that did not include patients with ACS. These results suggested that plaque stabilization and plaque regression reflect independent processes mediated by different mechanisms, which has been previously reported(Kawasaki , 2005; Schartl , 2001).

4. Future perspectives

Recently new intravascular imaging modalities have been proposed, including optical coherence tomography. Furthermore, noninvasive imaging system, such as multi-detector CT and MRI, can visualize coronary plaques more vividly than before. Therefore, brilliant future in terms of plaque imaging can be expected. We may have to produce the following future as: Fully understanding of the plaque regression and stabilization in terms of changes in tissue component; Perfect prediction of plaque rupture with an absolute value of its likelihood within a certain period; More detailed elucidation of mechanism of acute coronary syndrome, which is fully imaged by some imaging modalities; Best therapeutic ways which are clarified based on the data of plaque imaging. Therefore, the research world of plaque imaging for plaque regression and stability has still a wide variety of clinical goals.

5. Conclusion

Advanced developments in the field of intravascular ultrasound and angioscopy are offering their capabilities of accurately measuring plaque volume as well as identifying tissue components. These technologies significantly help understand in vivo pathological reactions of plaque by lipid-lowering therapy especially in plaque regression and stabilization. Furthermore, these technologies are providing numerous reliable evidences with multicenter studies.

6. References

Ambrose, J.A. (2008). In search of the "vulnerable plaque": can it be localized and will focal regional therapy ever be an option for cardiac prevention? *J Am Coll Cardiol* Vol.51, No.16, pp.1539-1542

Armstrong, M.L. (1976). Evidence of regression of atherosclerosis in primates and man. *Postgrad Med J* Vol.52, No.609, pp.456-461

Armstrong, M.L., Warner, E.D. & Connor, W.E. (1970). Regression of coronary atheromatosis in rhesus monkeys. *Circ Res* Vol.27, No.1, pp.59-67

Asakura, M., Ueda, Y., Yamaguchi, O., Adachi, T., Hirayama, A., Hori, M. & Kodama, K. (2001). Extensive development of vulnerable plaques as a pan-coronary process in patients with myocardial infarction: an angioscopic study. *J Am Coll Cardiol* Vol.37, No.5, pp.1284-1288

Ballantyne, C.M., Raichlen, J.S., Nicholls, S.J., Erbel, R., Tardif, J.C., Brener, S.J., Cain, V.A. & Nissen, S.E. (2008). Effect of rosuvastatin therapy on coronary artery stenoses assessed by quantitative coronary angiography: a study to evaluate the effect of rosuvastatin on intravascular ultrasound-derived coronary atheroma burden. *Circulation* Vol.117, No.19, pp.2458-2466

Berry, C., L'Allier, P.L., Gregoire, J., Lesperance, J., Levesque, S., Ibrahim, R. & Tardif, J.C. (2007). Comparison of intravascular ultrasound and quantitative coronary angiography for the assessment of coronary artery disease progression. *Circulation* Vol.115, No.14, pp.1851-1857

Brown, B.G., Zhao, X.Q., Sacco, D.E. & Albers, J.J. (1993). Lipid lowering and plaque regression. New insights into prevention of plaque disruption and clinical events in coronary disease. *Circulation* Vol.87, No.6, pp.1781-1791

Burke, A.P., Farb, A., Malcom, G.T., Liang, Y.H., Smialek, J. & Virmani, R. (1997). Coronary risk factors and plaque morphology in men with coronary disease who died suddenly. *N Engl J Med* Vol.336, No.18, pp.1276-1282

Falk, E., Shah, P.K. & Fuster, V. (1995). Coronary plaque disruption. *Circulation* Vol.92, No.3, pp.657-671

Friedman, M., Byers, S.O. & Rosenman, R.H. (1957). Resolution of aortic atherosclerotic infiltration in the rabbit by phosphatide infusion. *Proc Soc Exp Biol Med* Vol.95, No.3, pp.586-588

Fukumoto, Y., Hiro, T., Fujii, T., Hashimoto, G., Fujimura, T., Yamada, J., Okamura, T. & Matsuzaki, M. (2008). Localized elevation of shear stress is related to coronary plaque rupture: a 3-dimensional intravascular ultrasound study with in-vivo color mapping of shear stress distribution. *J Am Coll Cardiol* Vol.51, No.6, pp.645-650

Fuster, V., Badimon, L., Badimon, J.J. & Chesebro, J.H. (1992). The pathogenesis of coronary artery disease and the acute coronary syndromes (1). *N Engl J Med* Vol.326, No.4, pp.242-250

Glagov, S., Weisenberg, E., Zarins, C.K., Stankunavicius, R. & Kolettis, G.J. (1987). Compensatory enlargement of human atherosclerotic coronary arteries. *N Engl J Med* Vol.316, No.22, pp.1371-1375

Hirayama, A., Saito, S., Ueda, Y., Takayama, T., Honye, J., Komatsu, S., Yamaguchi, O., Li, Y., Yajima, J., Nanto, S., Takazawa, K. & Kodama, K. (2009). Qualitative and quantitative changes in coronary plaque associated with atorvastatin therapy. *Circ J* Vol.73, No.4, pp.718-725

Hiro, T., Fujii, T., Matsuzaki, M. & et, al. (2000). Assessment of lipid content of atherosclerotic plaque by intravascular ultrasound using fractal analysis *J Am Coll Cardiol* Vol.35, No.2, pp.38A (abstract)

Hiro, T., Fujii, T., Yasumoto, K., Murata, T., Murashige, A. & Matsuzaki, M. (2001). Detection of fibrous cap in atherosclerotic plaque by intravascular ultrasound by use of color mapping of angle-dependent echo-intensity variation. *Circulation* Vol.103, No.9, pp.1206-1211

Hiro, T., Kimura, T., Morimoto, T., Miyauchi, K., Nakagawa, Y., Yamagishi, M., Ozaki, Y., Kimura, K., Saito, S., Yamaguchi, T., Daida, H. & Matsuzaki, M. (2009). Effect of intensive statin therapy on regression of coronary atherosclerosis in patients with acute coronary syndrome: a multicenter randomized trial evaluated by volumetric intravascular ultrasound using pitavastatin versus atorvastatin (JAPAN-ACS [Japan assessment of pitavastatin and atorvastatin in acute coronary syndrome] study). *J Am Coll Cardiol* Vol.54, No.4, pp.293-302

Hiro, T., Kimura, T., Morimoto, T., Miyauchi, K., Nakagawa, Y., Yamagishi, M., Ozaki, Y., Kimura, K., Saito, S., Yamaguchi, T., Daida, H. & Matsuzaki, M. (2010). Diabetes mellitus is a major negative determinant of coronary plaque regression during statin therapy in patients with acute coronary syndrome--serial intravascular ultrasound observations from the Japan Assessment of Pitavastatin and Atorvastatin in Acute Coronary Syndrome Trial (the JAPAN-ACS Trial). *Circ J* Vol.74, No.6, pp.1165-1174

Hiro, T., Leung, C.Y., De Guzman, S., Caiozzo, V.J., Farvid, A.R., Karimi, H., Helfant, R.H. & Tobis, J.M. (1997). Are soft echoes really soft? Intravascular ultrasound assessment of mechanical properties in human atherosclerotic tissue. *Am Heart J* Vol.133, No.1, pp.1-7

Hiro, T., Leung, C.Y., Russo, R.J., Moussa, I., Karimi, H., Farvid, A.R. & Tobis, J.M. (1996). Variability in tissue characterization of atherosclerotic plaque by intravascular ultrasound: a comparison of four intravascular ultrasound systems. *Am J Card Imaging* Vol.10, No.4, pp.209-218

Imoto, K., Hiro, T., Fujii, T., Murashige, A., Fukumoto, Y., Hashimoto, G., Okamura, T., Yamada, J., Mori, K. & Matsuzaki, M. (2005). Longitudinal structural determinants of atherosclerotic plaque vulnerability: a computational analysis of stress distribution using vessel models and three-dimensional intravascular ultrasound imaging. *J Am Coll Cardiol* Vol.46, No.8, pp.1507-1515

Jeremias, A., Kolz, M.L., Ikonen, T.S., Gummert, J.F., Oshima, A., Hayase, M., Honda, Y., Komiyama, N., Berry, G.J., Morris, R.E., Yock, P.G. & Fitzgerald, P.J. (1999). Feasibility of in vivo intravascular ultrasound tissue characterization in the detection of early vascular transplant rejection. *Circulation* Vol.100, No.21, pp.2127-2130

Kawasaki, M., Sano, K., Okubo, M., Yokoyama, H., Ito, Y., Murata, I., Tsuchiya, K., Minatoguchi, S., Zhou, X., Fujita, H. & Fujiwara, H. (2005). Volumetric quantitative analysis of tissue characteristics of coronary plaques after statin therapy using three-dimensional integrated backscatter intravascular ultrasound. *J Am Coll Cardiol* Vol.45, No.12, pp.1946-1953

Kawasaki, M., Takatsu, H., Noda, T., Sano, K., Ito, Y., Hayakawa, K., Tsuchiya, K., Arai, M., Nishigaki, K., Takemura, G., Minatoguchi, S., Fujiwara, T. & Fujiwara, H. (2002). In vivo quantitative tissue characterization of human coronary arterial plaques by use of integrated backscatter intravascular ultrasound and comparison with angioscopic findings. *Circulation* Vol.105, No.21, pp.2487-2492

Kimura, B.J., Bhargava, V. & DeMaria, A.N. (1995). Value and limitations of intravascular ultrasound imaging in characterizing coronary atherosclerotic plaque. *Am Heart J* Vol.130, No.2, pp.386-396

Kodama, K., Asakura, M., Ueda, Y., Yamaguchi, O. & Hirayama, A. (2000). The role of plaque rupture in the development of acute coronary syndrome evaluated by the coronary angioscope. *Intern Med* Vol.39, No.4, pp.333-335

Kodama, K., Komatsu, S., Ueda, Y., Takayama, T., Yajima, J., Nanto, S., Matsuoka, H., Saito, S. & Hirayama, A. (2010). Stabilization and regression of coronary plaques treated with pitavastatin proven by angioscopy and intravascular ultrasound--the TOGETHAR trial. *Circ J* Vol.74, No.9, pp.1922-1928

Kubota, R., Kunihiro, M., Suetake, N. & et, al (2007). Intravascular ultrasound-based tissue classification of coronary plaque into fibrosis or lipid by k-nearest neighbor method *Proceedings of International Conference on Soft Computing and Human Sciences ?New Horizon beyond the 20th Anniversary of BMFSA-* Vol.SCHS2007, No.1, pp.93-96

Libby, P. (1995). Molecular bases of the acute coronary syndromes. *Circulation* Vol.91, No.11, pp.2844-2850

Malinow, M.R. (1983). Experimental models of atherosclerosis regression. *Atherosclerosis* Vol.48, No.2, pp.105-118

Maruffo, C.A. & Portman, O.W. (1968). Nutritional control of coronary artery atherosclerosis in the squirrel monkey. *J Atheroscler Res* Vol.8, No.2, pp.237-247

Mizuno, K. (1992). Angioscopic examination of the coronary arteries: What we have learned? *Heart Dis Stroke* Vol.1, No.5, pp.320-324

Murashige, A., Hiro, T., Fujii, T., Imoto, K., Murata, T., Fukumoto, Y. & Matsuzaki, M. (2005). Detection of lipid-laden atherosclerotic plaque by wavelet analysis of radiofrequency intravascular ultrasound signals: in vitro validation and preliminary in vivo application. *J Am Coll Cardiol* Vol.45, No.12, pp.1954-1960

Naghavi, M., Libby, P., Falk, E., Casscells, S.W., Litovsky, S., Rumberger, J., Badimon, J.J., Stefanadis, C., Moreno, P., Pasterkamp, G., Fayad, Z., Stone, P.H., Waxman, S., Raggi, P., Madjid, M., Zarrabi, A., Burke, A., Yuan, C., Fitzgerald, P.J., Siscovick, D.S., de Korte, C.L., Aikawa, M., Juhani Airaksinen, K.E., Assmann, G., Becker, C.R., Chesebro, J.H., Farb, A., Galis, Z.S., Jackson, C., Jang, I.K., Koenig, W., Lodder, R.A., March, K., Demirovic, J., Navab, M., Priori, S.G., Rekhter, M.D., Bahr, R.,

Grundy, S.M., Mehran, R., Colombo, A., Boerwinkle, E., Ballantyne, C., Insull, W. Jr, Schwartz, R.S., Vogel, R., Serruys, P.W., Hansson, G.K., Faxon, D.P., Kaul, S., Drexler, H., Greenland, P., Muller, J.E., Virmani, R., Ridker, P.M., Zipes, D.P., Shah, P.K. & Willerson, J.T. (2003). From vulnerable plaque to vulnerable patient: a call for new definitions and risk assessment strategies: Part I. *Circulation* Vol.108, No.14, pp.1664-1672

Nair, A., Kuban, B.D., Tuzcu, E.M., Schoenhagen, P., Nissen, S.E. & Vince, D.G. (2002). Coronary plaque classification with intravascular ultrasound radiofrequency data analysis. *Circulation* Vol.106, No.17, pp.2200-2206

Nicholls, S.J., Hsu, A., Wolski, K., Hu, B., Bayturan, O., Lavoie, A., Uno, K., Tuzcu, E.M. & Nissen, S.E. (2010). Intravascular ultrasound-derived measures of coronary atherosclerotic plaque burden and clinical outcome. *J Am Coll Cardiol* Vol.55, No.21, pp.2399-2407

Nissen, S.E., Nicholls, S.J., Sipahi, I., Libby, P., Raichlen, J.S., Ballantyne, C.M., Davignon, J., Erbel, R., Fruchart, J.C., Tardif, J.C., Schoenhagen, P., Crowe, T., Cain, V., Wolski, K., Goormastic, M. & Tuzcu, E.M. (2006). Effect of very high-intensity statin therapy on regression of coronary atherosclerosis: the ASTEROID trial. *JAMA* Vol.295, No.13, pp.1556-1565

Nissen, S.E., Tuzcu, E.M., Schoenhagen, P., Brown, B.G., Ganz, P., Vogel, R.A., Crowe, T., Howard, G., Cooper, C.J., Brodie, B., Grines, C.L. & DeMaria, A.N. (2004). Effect of intensive compared with moderate lipid-lowering therapy on progression of coronary atherosclerosis: a randomized controlled trial. *JAMA* Vol.291, No.9, pp.1071-1080

Ohtani, T., Ueda, Y., Mizote, I., Oyabu, J., Okada, K., Hirayama, A. & Kodama, K. (2006). Number of yellow plaques detected in a coronary artery is associated with future risk of acute coronary syndrome: detection of vulnerable patients by angioscopy. *J Am Coll Cardiol* Vol.47, No.11, pp.2194-2200

Okazaki, S., Yokoyama, T., Miyauchi, K., Shimada, K., Kurata, T., Sato, H. & Daida, H. (2004). Early statin treatment in patients with acute coronary syndrome: demonstration of the beneficial effect on atherosclerotic lesions by serial volumetric intravascular ultrasound analysis during half a year after coronary event: the ESTABLISH Study. *Circulation* Vol.110, No.9, pp.1061-1068

Ost, C.R. & Stenson, S. (1967). Regression of peripheral atherosclerosis during therapy with high doses of nicotinic acid. *Scand J Clin Lab Invest Suppl* Vol.99, No., pp.241-245

Picano, E., Landini, L., Distante, A., Salvadori, M., Lattanzi, F., Masini, M. & L'Abbate, A. (1985). Angle dependence of ultrasonic backscatter in arterial tissues: a study in vitro. *Circulation* Vol.72, No.3, pp.572-576

Sacks, F.M., Pfeffer, M.A., Moye, L.A. & et, al. (1996). The effect of pravastatin on coronary events after myocardial infarction in patients with average cholesterol levels. Cholesterol and Recurrent Events Trial investigators. *N Engl J Med* Vol.335, No.14, pp.1001-1009

Sathyanarayana, S., Carlier, S., Li, W. & et, al. (2009). Characterisation of atherosclerotic plaque by spectral similarity of radiofrequency intravascular ultrasound signals. *Euro Intervention* Vol.5, No.1, pp.133-139

Scandinavian Simvastatin Survival Study Group (1994). Randomised trial of cholesterol lowering in 4444 patients with coronary heart disease: the Scandinavian Simvastatin Survival Study (4S) *Lancet* Vol.344, No.8934, pp.1383-1389

Schartl, M., Bocksch, W., Koschyk, D.H., Voelker, W., Karsch, K.R., Kreuzer, J., Hausmann, D., Beckmann, S. & Gross, M. (2001). Use of intravascular ultrasound to compare effects of different strategies of lipid-lowering therapy on plaque volume and composition in patients with coronary artery disease. *Circulation* Vol.104, No.4, pp.387-392

Shah, P.K. (2003). Mechanism of plaque vulnerability and rupture *J Am Coll Cardiol 41Suppl* Vol.1, No., pp.15-22

Stein, Y. & Stein, O. (2001). Does therapeutic intervention achieve slowing of progression or bona fide regression of atherosclerotic lesions? *Arterioscler Thromb Vasc Biol* Vol.21, No.2, pp.183-188

Takagi, T., Yoshida, K., Akasaka, T., Hozumi, T., Morioka, S. & Yoshikawa, J. (1997). Intravascular ultrasound analysis of reduction in progression of coronary narrowing by treatment with pravastatin. *Am J Cardiol* Vol.79, No.12, pp.1673-1676

Takano, M., Mizuno, K., Yokoyama, S., Seimiya, K., Ishibashi, F., Okamatsu, K. & Uemura, R. (2003). Changes in coronary plaque color and morphology by lipid-lowering therapy with atorvastatin: serial evaluation by coronary angioscopy. *J Am Coll Cardiol* Vol.42, No.4, pp.680-686

Takayama, T., Hiro, T., Yamagishi, M., Daida, H., Hirayama, A., Saito, S., Yamaguchi, T. & Matsuzaki, M. (2009). Effect of rosuvastatin on coronary atheroma in stable coronary artery disease: multicenter coronary atherosclerosis study measuring effects of rosuvastatin using intravascular ultrasound in Japanese subjects (COSMOS). *Circ J* Vol.73, No.11, pp.2110-2117

The Long-Term Intervention with Pravastatin in Ischemic Disease (LIPID) Study Group (1998). Prevention of cardiovascular events and death with pravastatin in patients with coronary heart disease and a broad range of initial cholesterol levels. The Long-Term Intervention with Pravastatin in Ischaemic Disease (LIPID) Study Group. *N Engl J Med* Vol.339, No.19, pp.1349-1357

Ueda, Y., Asakura, M., Hirayama, A., Adachi, T. & Kodama, K. (1997). Angioscopy of culprit lesions. *Cardiologia* Vol.42, No.8, pp.827-832

Ueda, Y., Ohtani, T., Shimizu, M., Hirayama, A. & Kodama, K. (2004). Assessment of plaque vulnerability by angioscopic classification of plaque color. *Am Heart J* Vol.148, No.2, pp.333-335

Wilson, L.S., Neale, M.L., Talhami, H.E. & Appleberg, M. (1994). Preliminary results from attenuation-slope mapping of plaque using intravascular ultrasound. *Ultrasound Med Biol* Vol.20, No.6, pp.529-542

Wissler, R.W. & Vesselinovitch, D. (1976). Studies of regression of advanced atherosclerosis in experimental animals and man. *Ann N Y Acad Sci* Vol.275, No.1, pp.363-378

3

Integrated Backscatter Intravascular Ultrasound

Masanori Kawasaki
Department of Cardiology,
Gifu University Graduate School of Medicine
Japan

1. Introduction

About 30 years ago, a pathological study by Horie et al. demonstrated that plaque rupture into the lumen of a coronary artery may precede and cause thrombus formation leading to acute myocardial infarction (Horie et al., 1978). In an angioscopic study, Mizuno et al. demonstrated that disruption or erosion of vulnerable plaques and subsequent thromboses are the most frequent cause of acute coronary syndrome (Mizuno et al., 1992). The stability of atherosclerotic plaques is related to the histological composition of plaques and the thickness of fibrous caps. Therefore, recognition of the tissue characteristics of coronary plaques is important to understand and prevent acute coronary syndrome. Accurate identification of the tissue characteristics of coronary plaques *in vivo* may allow the identification of vulnerable plaques before the development of acute coronary syndrome.

In the 1990's, a new technique was developed that could characterize myocardial tissues by integrated backscatter (IB) analysis of ultrasound images. This technique is capable of providing both conventional two-dimensional echocardiographic images and IB images. Ultrasound backscatter power is proportional to the difference of acoustic characteristic impedance that is determined by the density of tissue multiplied by the speed of sound. In studies of the myocardium, calibrated myocardial IB values were significantly correlated with the relative volume of interstitial fibrosis (Picano, 1990 et al.; Naito et al., 1996). In preliminary studies *in vitro*, IB values reflected the structural and biochemical composition of atherosclerotic lesion and could differentiate fibrofatty, fatty and calcification of arterial walls (Barziliai et al., 1987; Urbani et al., 1993; Picano et al., 1988). It was also reported that anisotropy of the direction and backscatter power is related to plaque type (De Kroon et al., 1991). Takiuchi et al. found that quantitative tissue characterization using IB ultrasound could identify lipid pool and fibrosis in human carotid and/or femoral arteries (Takiuchi et al., 2000). However, these studies were done *ex vivo* and different plaque types were measured in only a few local lesions. In the early 2000s, it was reported that IB values measured *in vivo* in human carotid arteries correlated well with postmortem histological classification (Kawasaki et al., 2001). This new non-invasive technique using IB values could characterize the two-dimensional structures of arterial plaques *in vivo*. With this technique, plaque tissues were classified based on histopathology into 6 types, *i.e.* intraplaque hemorrhage, lipid pool, intimal hyperplasia, fibrosis, dense fibrosis, and calcification. This technique was applied in the clinical setting to predict cerebral ischemic lesions after carotid artery stenting. From the analysis of receiver operating characteristic (ROC) curves, a relative intraplaque hemorrhage + lipid pool area of 50% measured by IB ultrasound imaging was the most reliable cutoff value

for predicting cerebral ischemic lesions evaluated by diffusion-weighted magnetic resonance imaging after carotid artery stenting (Yamada et al., 2010).
Since it was difficult to differentiate lipid pool from intimal hyperplasia using IB values, the anatomical features of the lesion were used for this purpose. Because lipid pool is generally located under a fibrous cap, a region of interest (ROI) that was either lipid pool or intimal hyperplasia was classified as lipid pool only when that region was located underneath a ROI with fibrosis. Intimal hyperplasia was identified when a ROI that was either lipid pool or intimal hyperplasia was not covered by a fibrous cap. Most of these two lesion types could be differentiated using this method.

2. IB-IVUS equipment and data acquisition

In the next generation, this ultrasound IB technique was applied to coronary arteries by use of intravascular ultrasound (IVUS) (Kawasaki et al., 2002). A personal computer (Windows XP Professional, CPU: 3.4 GHz) equipped with newly developed custom software was connected to an IVUS imaging system (VISIWAVE, Terumo, Japan) to obtain the radio frequency signal, signal trigger and video image outputs. An analog-to-digital converter digitized the signals at 400 MHz with 8-bit resolution, and the digitized data were stored on the hard drive of the PC for later analysis. In the IVUS analysis, 512 vector lines of ultrasound signal around the circumference were analyzed to calculate the IB values. The IB values for each tissue component were calculated using a fast Fourier transform, and expressed as the average power, measured in decibels (dB), of the frequency component of the backscattered signal from a small volume of tissue. Ultrasound backscattered signals were acquired using a 38 or 43 MHz mechanically-rotating IVUS catheter (ViewIT, Terumo, Tokyo, Japan), digitized and subjected to spectral analysis. The tissue IB values were calibrated by subtracting the IB values from the IB value of a stainless steel needle placed at a distance of 1.5 mm from the catheter. IB-IVUS color-coded maps were constructed based on the IB values by use of custom software written by our group. Conventional IVUS images and IB-IVUS color-coded maps were immediately displayed side-by-side on a monitor. Color-coded maps of the coronary arteries were finally constructed after excluding the vessel lumen and area outside of the external elastic membrane by manually tracing the vessel lumen and external elastic membrane on the conventional IVUS images. With a transducer frequency of 38 or 43 MHz, the wavelength was calculated as 36 or 41 μm, respectively, assuming a tissue sound speed of approximately 1,560 m/sec.

3. Correlation between IB-IVUS and histological images

To compare IB-IVUS images with histological images, coronary cross-sections obtained at autopsy were stained with hematoxylin-eosin, elastic van Gieson and Masson's trichrome. In the training study, three pathologic subsets were identified in each ROI: lipid pool (extracellular lipid, macrophages, microcalcification and/or foam cells), fibrosis and calcification. Necrotic core that consisted of lipid pool, microcalcification and remnants of foam cells and/or dead lymphocytes were classified as lipid pool in the IB-IVUS analysis. In the validation study, coronary arterial cross-sections were classified into three categories: fibrocalcific, fibrous and lipid-rich.
To evaluate overall ultrasound signal attenuation, IB values of the same lesions ($n = 10$) were measured after moving the lesions 2.5 - 4.0 mm from the IVUS catheter. Including the

attenuation by flowing blood, an overall attenuation of 4.0 dB/mm was determined to be the most appropriate, and this value was used to correct for ultrasound signal attenuation. Therefore, when color-coded maps were constructed, each IB value was corrected by adding 4.0 dB/mm when the ROI was located 1.5 mm further away from the catheter and subtracting 4.0 dB/mm when the ROI was located 1.5 mm closer to the catheter. Color-coded maps consisted of four major components: fibrous (green), dense fibrosis (yellow), lipid pool (blue), calcification (red).

The histological analysis of each ROI showed the presence of typical tissue components including calcification (n = 41), fibrosis (n = 102) and lipid pool (n = 99). With the 38 MHz ultrasound mode, the average IB values in each ROI of these tissue components were -7.3 ± 6.5, -27.0 ± 5.3 and -51.2 ± 3.3 dB, respectively; however, with the 43 MHz ultrasound mode, the average IB values were -10.6 ± 6.1, -30.4 ± 4.9 and -54.0 ± 3.9 dB, respectively. The differences among IB values of lipid pool, fibrosis or calcification were significant ($p<0.001$). IB values were highest in calcification and lowest in lipid pool. There was no overlap between the IB values of lipid pool and calcification. According to the analysis of ROC curves, an IB value of ≤ -39 dB (area under curve = 0.98) was the most reliable cutoff point for discriminating lipid pool (90% sensitivity, 92% specificity) and fibrosis (94% sensitivity, 93% specificity), and an IB value of > -17 dB (area under curve = 0.99) was the most reliable cutoff point for discriminating calcification and fibrosis with the 38 MHz mode. An IB value of ≤ -42 dB (area under curve = 0.98) was the most reliable cutoff point for discriminating lipid pool and fibrosis and an IB value of > -20 dB (area under curve = 0.99) was the most reliable cutoff point for discriminating calcification and fibrosis with the 43 MHz mode.

Based on the above cutoff points, two-dimensional color-coded maps of tissue characteristics were constructed. A total of 95 cross-sections were diagnosed as fibrocalcific, fibrous or lipid-rich by the IB-IVUS reader, who was blinded to the histological diagnoses. There was no difference in the diagnosis of the images obtained using either the 38 MHz or 43 MHz ultrasound signal. The overall agreement between the classifications made by IB-IVUS and histology (lipid-rich: n = 35, fibrous: n = 33 and fibrocalcific: n = 27) was excellent (Cohen's κ = 0.83, 95% CI: 0.73 - 0.92).

4. Comparison between IB-IVUS and virtual hostology IVUS

Virtual histology IVUS (Virtual Histology Version 1.4, Volcano Corp., CA, USA) images were acquired by a VH-IVUS console with a 20 MHz phased-array catheter and stored on CD-ROM for offline analysis. To clarify the rotational and cross-sectional position of the included segment, multiple surgical needles were carefully inserted into the coronary arteries before IB-IVUS and VH-IVUS imaging to serve as reference points to compare the two imaging modalities.

In qualitative comparison, small (0.3mm x 0.3mm) region-of-interest (ROI)s were set on the same sites of histological and IVUS images. In quantitative comparison, histological images from cross-sections that were stained with Masson's trichrome were digitized, and the areas that were stained blue were automatically selected by a multipurpose image processor (LUZEX F, Nireco Co., Tokyo, Japan). Then the relative fibrous area (fibrous area / plaque area) was automatically calculated by the LUZEX F system.

In the direct qualitative comparison, the overall agreement between the histological and IB-IVUS diagnoses was higher (Cohen's κ = 0.81, 95% CI: 0.74-0.90) than between the histological and VH-IVUS diagnoses (Cohen's κ = 0.30, 95% CI: 0.14-0.41) (Okubo et al., 2008 (a); Okubo et al., 2008 (b)).

In the direct quantitative comparison, the % fibrosis area determined by IB-IVUS was significantly correlated with the relative area of fibrosis based on histology (r=0.67, p<0.001), whereas the % fibrous area and % fibrous area + % fibro-fatty area determined by VH-IVUS were not correlated with the relative area of fibrosis based on histology (Figure 1) (Okubo et al., 2008).

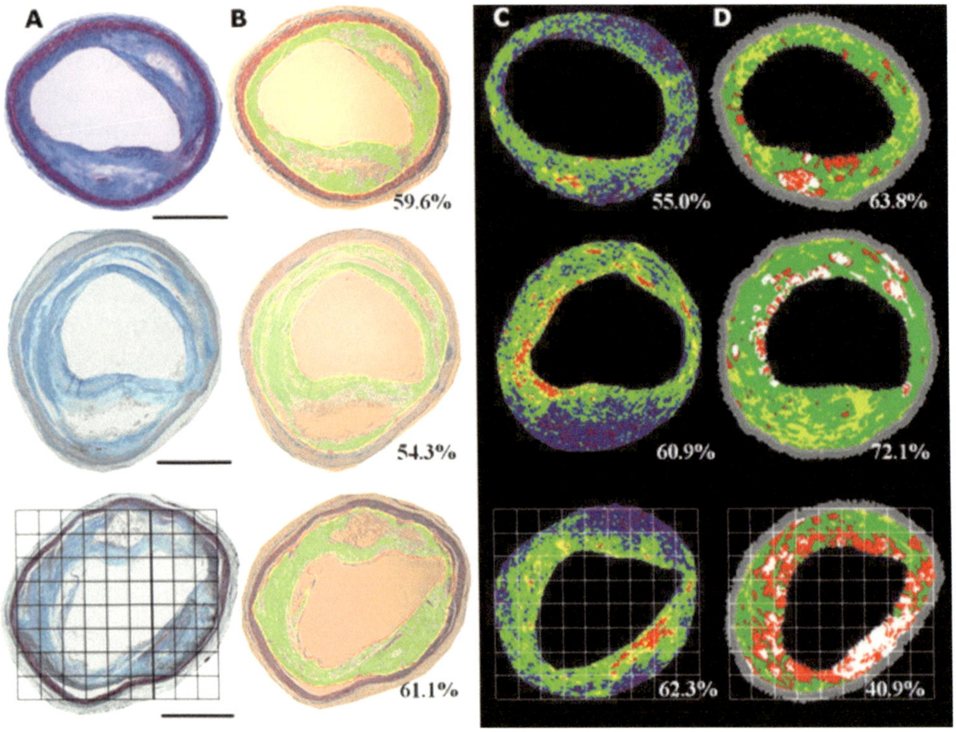

Fig. 1. Representative lesion used in the direct comparison study. A: histological images stained with Masson's trichrome. Bar = 1 mm. B: Images after quantification by the image processor. Areas that were stained blue by Masson's trichrome were automatically selected (green area) by the multipurpose image processor (LUZEX F) and the relative fibrous area (fibrous area / plaque area) was automatically calculated by the system. C: IB-IVUS images corresponding to sections analyzed by histology. D: IVUS-VH images corresponding to sections analyzed by histology. Percentages indicate the relative fibrous areas determined by each method.

5. Comparison of the thickness of the fibrous cap measured by IB-IVUS and optical coherence tomography in vivo

During routine selective percutaneous coronary intervention in 42 consecutive patients, a total of 28 cross-sections that consisted of lipid overlaid by a fibrous cap were imaged by both IVUS and optical coherence tomography in 24 patients with stable angina pectoris. A 0.016-inch optical coherence tomography catheter (Imagewire, LightLab Imaging, Inc.,

Westford, MA) was advanced into the coronary arteries. IB-IVUS and optical coherence tomography (M2 OCT Imaging system, LightLab Imaging, Inc., Westford, MA) were performed in each patient at the same site without significant stenosis as described below. IB-IVUS images were obtained every one second using an automatic pullback device at a rate of 0.5 mm/sec. optical coherence tomography images were obtained using an automatic pullback system at a rate of 0.5 mm/sec. IB-IVUS images were obtained at 0.5 mm intervals, whereas optical coherence tomography images were obtained at 0.03 mm intervals. Therefore, the segments of coronary artery to compare between the two methods were selected based on the IB-IVUS images. Then, these same coronary segments were identified in optical coherence tomography using the distance from easily-definable side branches and calcification as reference markers to ensure that IB-IVUS and optical coherence tomography were compared at the same site. The cross-sections that did not have sufficient imaging quality to analyze tissue characteristics were excluded from the comparison. In the IB-IVUS analysis, images were processed by a smoothing method that averaged nine IB values in nine pixels located in a square field of the color-coded maps to reduce uneven surfaces of tissue components produced by signal noise.

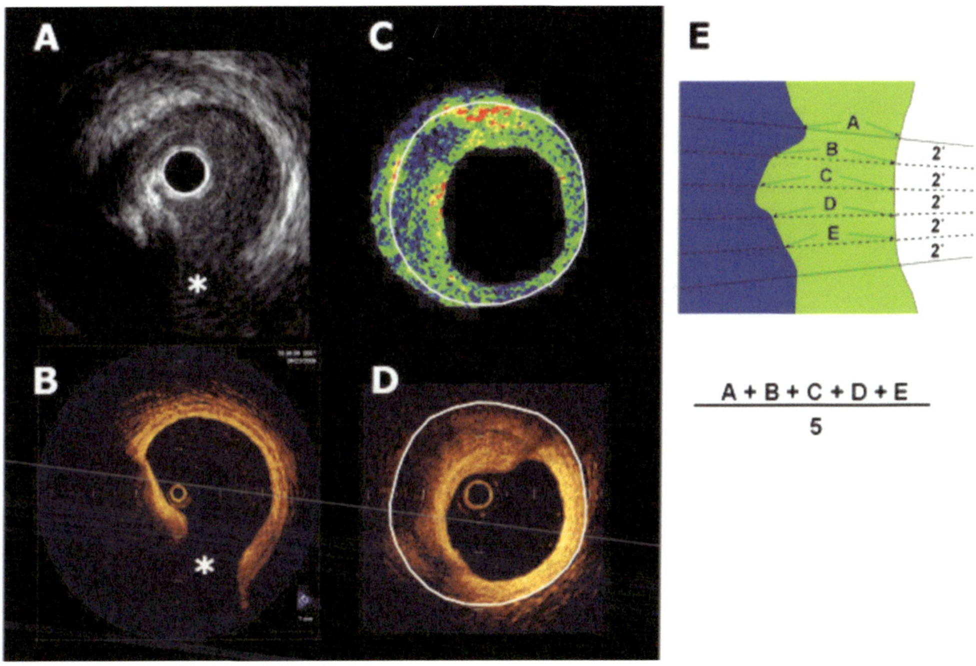

Fig. 2. The same coronary segments were selected for imaging using the distance from easily-identifiable side branches and calcification as reference markers to ensure that integrated backscatter intravascular ultrasound (IB-IVUS) and optical coherence tomography (OCT) were compared at the same site. (A) Conventional IVUS image. (B) Corresponding OCT image. (C) IB-IVUS image. (D) Corresponding OCT image. (E) Fibrous caps that overlaid lipid pool were divided into regions-of-interest (ROIs) (every 10° from the center of the vessel) and the thickness of fibrous caps was measured as an average. The average thickness of fibrous cap was measured by averaging the thickness of fibrous cap every 2° within ROIs. *: septal branch.

Fibrous caps that overlaid lipid pool were divided into ROI (every 10° rotation from the center of the vessel lumen) and the average thickness was determined. The average thickness of fibrous cap was determined by averaging the thickness of fibrous cap every 2° within the ROIs (Figure 2). The areas where the radial axis from the center of the vessel lumen crossed the tangential line of the vessel surface with an angle less than a 80° were excluded from the comparison.

The thickness of fibrous cap measured by IB-IVUS was significantly correlated with that measured by optical coherence tomography ($y = 0.99x - 0.19$, $r = 0.74$, $p<0.001$) (Figure 3) (Kawasaki et al., 2010).

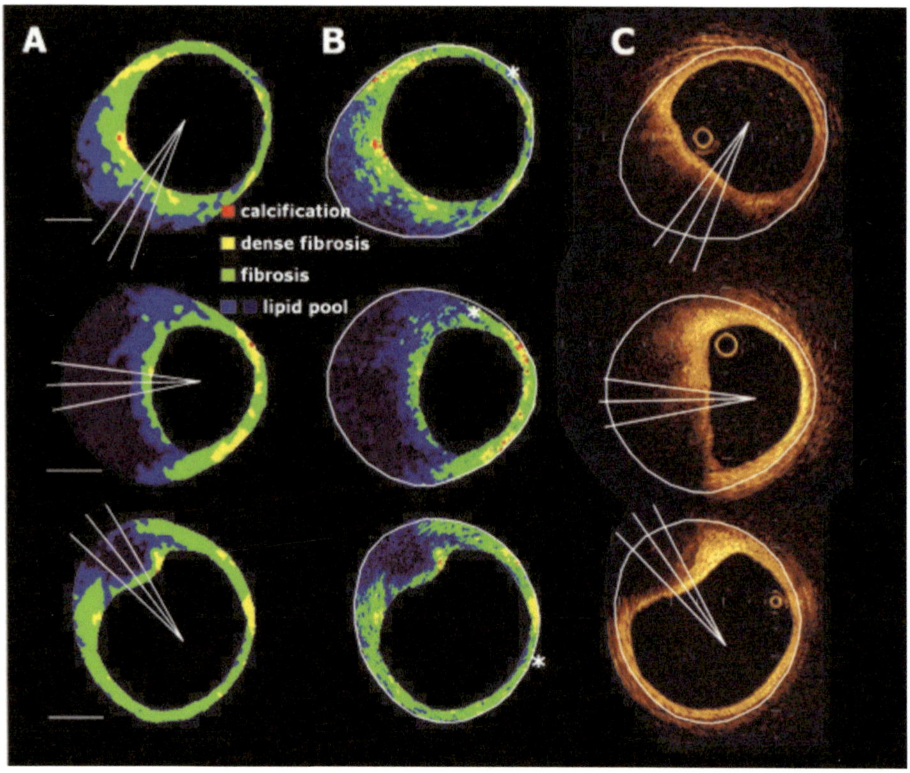

Fig. 3. (A) Representative integrated backscatter intravascular ultrasound (IB-IVUS) images processed by a smoothing method. (B) Original IB-IVUS images (C) Corresponding optical coherence tomography. *: attenuation by guide wire. Bar = 1mm.

A Bland-Altman plot showed that the mean difference between the thickness of fibrous cap measured by IB-IVUS and optical coherence tomography (IB-IVUS - optical coherence tomography) was -2 ± 147 μm (Figure 4). The difference between the two methods appeared to increase as the thickness of the fibrous cap increased. Optical coherence tomography has a better potential for characterizing tissue components located on the near side of the vessel lumen, whereas IB-IVUS has a better potential for characterizing tissue components of entire plaques (Kawasaki et al., 2006).

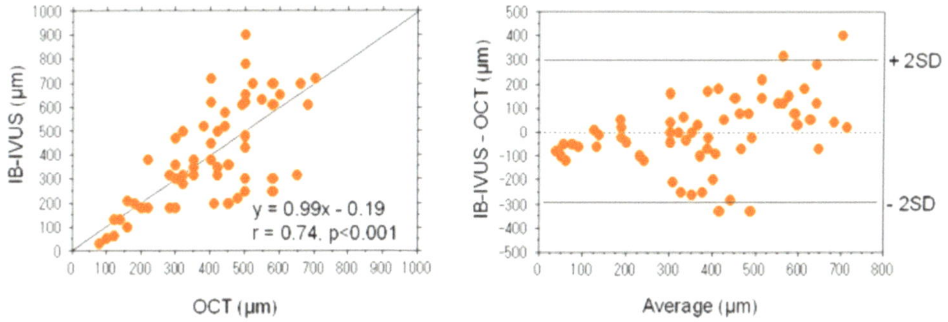

Fig. 4. Left: Correlation between the thickness of fibrous cap measured by integrated backscatter intravascular ultrasound and optical coherence tomography. Right: Bland-Altman plot.

6. Clinical studies conducted by use of IB-IVUS

There have been many clinical studies performed using IB-IVUS. In a prospective study, IB-IVUS was performed in 140 patients with stable angina pectoris in one or two arterial segments without significant stenosis (Sano et al., 2006). The % lipid area was greater in plaques that caused acute coronary syndrome than in plaques that did not cause acute coronary syndrome (72 ± 10 versus 50 ± 16%, $p<0.001$). The % fibrous area was smaller in plaques that caused acute coronary syndrome than in plaques that did not cause acute coronary syndrome (23 ± 6 versus 47 ± 14%, $p<0.001$) (Figure 5).

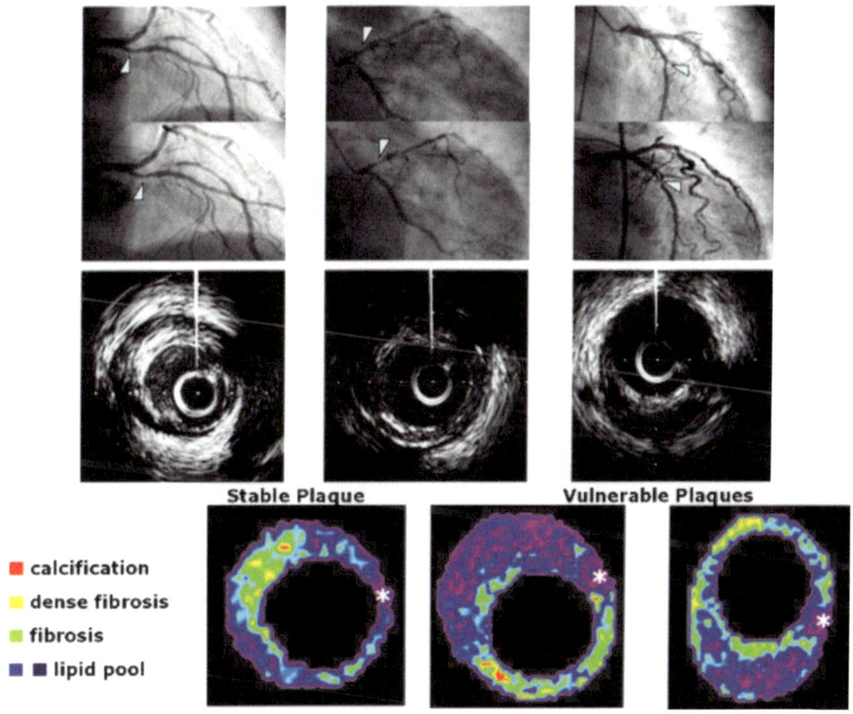

Fig. 5. Images of lesion in patients with (right) and without (left) acute coronary syndrome. (*) indicates the guidewire artifact.

The optimum cutoffs for the calculation of diagnostic accuracy to classify plaques that caused acute coronary syndrome were obtained from the ROC curve. The optimal cutoffs of % fibrous area and % lipid area were 25% and 65% respectively. Regarding remodeling index, Takeuchi et al. reported that % lipid volume in the positive remodeling plaques was greater than the non-positive remodeling plaques (40.5 ± 14.8 versus 26.4 ± 15.9%, $p<0.001$) and they concluded that positive remodeling lesions contain more lipid-rich components compared with non-positive remodeling lesions, which may account for the higher incidence of acute coronary syndrome and plaque vulnerability (Takeuchi et al., 2009).

During percutaneous coronary intervention, 107 non-culprit intermediate plaques in left anterior descending coronary arteries were analyzed by IB-IVUS (Komura et al., 2010). Plaques in the proximal segment had a higher % lipid content than did plaques in the distal segment (36.1 ± 12.3 versus 18.6 ± 13.1%, $p<0.01$). A total of 155 consecutive patients who underwent percutaneous coronary intervention were investigated by IB-IVUS. Lipid-rich plaques measured by IB-IVUS proved to be an independent morphologic predictor of non-target ischemic events after percutaneous coronary intervention, and the risk was particularly increased in patients with elevated serum C-reactive protein levels (Amano et at., 2011). Amano et al. reported that patients with metabolic syndrome showed a significant increase in % lipid area (38 ± 19% versus 30 ± 19%, $p=0.02$) and metabolic syndrome was associated with lipid-rich plaques, contributing to an increase of plaque vulnerability (Amano et al., 2007). Kimura et al. demonstrated that the ratio of LDL to HDL cholesterol was an independent predictor of lipid area / non- lipid area (Kimura et al., 2010).

A substantial reduction of acute cardiac events has been shown in most lipid-lowering trials, despite only a minimal geometric regression of plaque (Brown BG et al., 1993; Fernández-Ortiz A et al., 1994). These findings suggest that plaque stability was increased by the removal of lipids from lipid-rich plaques. Three-dimensional IB-IVUS demonstrated that statin therapy for 6 months reduced the lipid volume in patients with stable angina (pravastatin: 25.5 ± 5.7 to 21.9 ± 5.3%, $p<0.05$; atorvastatin: 26.5 ± 5.2 to 19.9 ± 5.5%, $p<0.01$) without reducing the degree of stenosis. To improve the accuracy of the volumetric analysis, polar coordinates in the two-dimensional color-coded maps were transformed into Cartesian coordinates (64 x 64 pixels) using computer software, because the size of each ROI was different in the polar coordinates. Three-dimensional IB-IVUS offers the potential for quantitative volumetric tissue characterization of coronary atherosclerosis (Kawasaki et al., 2005) (Figure 6).

Otagiri et al. investigated the effectiveness of rosuvastatin in patients with acute coronary syndrome using IB-IVUS. They demonstrated that reduction rate of % lipid volume after 6 months of rosuvastatin therapy was significantly correlated with the baseline values ($r = -0.498$, $p=0.024$) (Otagiri et al., 2011). Early intervention with rosuvastatin in acute coronary syndrome patients caused significant reduction of the non-culprit plaque during 6 months. This regression was mainly due to the decrease in the lipid component measured by IB-IVUS.

7. Technical consideration

The fixation and processing of arterial samples for histopathology decreases the total vessel and luminal cross-sectional area, but the absolute wall area (total vessel cross-sectional area minus luminal cross-sectional area) does not change in vessels with minimal atherosclerotic narrowing (Lockwood et al., 1991; Siegel et al., 1985). Several studies have documented that formalin fixation does not significantly affect the morphology and quantitative echo characteristic of plaque tissue from human aortic walls (Kawasaki et al., 2001; Picano et al., 1983).

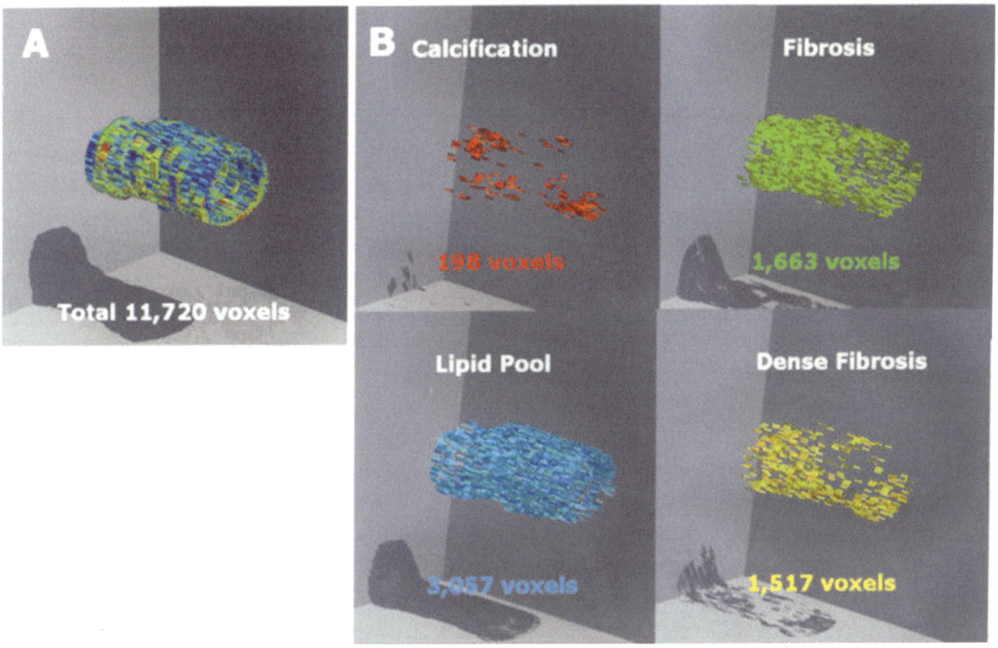

Fig. 6. A: Three-dimensional color-coded maps of coronary arterial plaques constructed by three-dimensional IB-IVUS. B: Three-dimensional color-coded maps of each characteristic. The number of voxels of each tissue characteristic was automatically calculated.

IB-IVUS occasionally underestimates calcified lesions and overestimates lipid pool behind calcification due to the acoustic shadow derived from calcification. Acoustic shadow caused by calcification hinders the precise determination of the tissue characteristics of coronary plaques. However, there were many cases in which lesions that were classified as lipid pool by IB-IVUS due to the acoustic shadow behind calcification actually included lipid core in the same lesion analyzed by histology (n = 16/21, 76%). Our results are consistent with previous results that showed that necrotic core and fibrofatty components were located behind calcification (83 - 89%) (Kume et al., 2007). Since calcification usually originates in lesions with lipid accumulation, the diagnosis of lipid pool by IB-IVUS in lesions behind calcification was usually accurate.

8. Limitations

There were a few limitations of the ultrasound method. First, the angle-dependence of the ultrasound signal makes tissue characterization unstable when lesions are not perpendicular to the ultrasound axis. Picano et al. reported that angular scattering behavior is large in calcified and fibrous tissues, whereas it is slight to nonexistent in normal and fatty plaques (Picano et al., 1985). According to that report, although there was no crossover of IB values between fibrous and fibrofatty within an angle span of 10°, or between fibrous and fatty within an angle span of 14°, this angle-dependence of the ultrasound signal might be partially responsible for the variation of IB values obtained from each tissue component. There was also a report that demonstrated the degree of angle-dependence of 30 MHz ultrasound in detail (Courtney et al., 2002). In that report, the angle-dependence of 30 MHz ultrasound in the

arterial intima and media was 1.11dB/10°. When the 40 MHz catheter was used, the angle dependence increased in arterial tissue. This angle-dependence of the ultrasound signal may decrease the diagnostic accuracy for differentiating tissue components.
Second, the guidewire was not used in the process of imaging because the present studies were performed *ex vivo*. Imaging artifacts *in vivo* due to the guidewire may decrease the diagnostic accuracy. However, removal of the guidewire during imaging after completing the intervention procedure and/or excluding the area behind calcification from the analysis may be necessary in the clinical setting to eliminate this problem. Finally, detecting thrombus from a single IVUS cross-section was not possible because we usually look at multiple IVUS images over time for speckling, scintillation, motion and blood flow in the "microchannel" (Mintz et al., 2001). The analysis of IB values in multiple cross-sections over time is required for the detection of thrombus.

9. References

Amano T, Matsubara T, Uetani T, Nanki M, Marui N, Kato M, Arai K, Yokoi K, Ando H, Ishii H, Izawa H, Murohara T. (2007). Impact of metabolic syndrome on tissue characteristics of angiographically mild to moderate coronary lesions integrated backscatter intravascular ultrasound study. *J Am Coll Cardiol* Vol 49:1149-56.

Amano T, Matsubara T, Uetani T, Kato M, Kato B, Yoshida T, Harada K, Kumagai S, Kunimura A, Shinbo Y, Ishii H, Murohara T. (2011). Lipid-rich plaques predict non-target-lesion ischemic events in patients undergoing percutaneous coronary intervention. *Circ J* Vol 75;157-66.

Barziliai B, Shffitz JE, Miller JG, Sobel BE. (1987). Quantitative ultrasonic characterization of the nature of atherosclerotic plaques in human aorta. *Circ Res.*Vol 60: 459-63.

Brown BG, Zhao XQ, Sacco DE, Albers JJ. (1993). Lipid lowering and plaque regression. New insights into prevention of plaque disruption and clinical events in coronary disease. *Circulation*. Vol 87:1781-91.

Courtney BK, Robertson AL, Maehara A, Luna J, Kitamura K, Morino Y, et al. (2002). Effect of transducer position on backscattered intensity in coronary arteries. *Ultrasound in Med & Biol*. Vol 28:81-91.

De Kroon MGM, van der Wal LF, Gussenhoven WJ, Rijsterborgh H, Bom N. (1991). Backscatter directivity and integrated backscatter power of arterial tissue. *Int J Card Imaging*.Vol 6:265-75.

Fernández-Ortiz A, Badimon JJ, Falk E, Fuster V, Meyer B, Mailhac A, Weng D, Shah PK, Badimon L. (1994). Characterization of the relative thrombogenecity of atherosclerotic plaque components: implications for consequences of plaque rapture. *J Am Coll Cardiol* Vol 23:1562-9.

Horie, T., Sekiguchi, M., Hirosawa, K. (1978). Coronary thrombosis in pathogenesis of acute myocardial infarction. Histopathological study of coronary arteries in 108 necropsied cases using serial section. *Br Heart J* Vol. 40:153-61.

Kawasaki M, Takatsu H, Noda T, Ito Y, Kunishima A, Arai M, Nishigaki K, Takemura G, Morita N, Minatoguchi S, Fujiwara H. (2001). Non-invasive tissue characterization of human atherosclerotic lesions in carotid and femoral arteries by ultrasound integrated backscatter. -Comparison between histology and integrated backscatter images before and after death- *J Am Coll Cardiol.* Vol 38:486-92

Kawasaki M, Takatsu H, Noda T, et al. (2002) In vivo quantitative tissue characterization of human coronary arterial plaques using integrated backscatter intravascular ultrasound and comparison with angioscopic findings. Circulation Vol 105:2487-92.

Kawasaki M, Sano K, Okubo M, Yokoyama H, Ito Y, Murata I, Tsuchiya K, Minatoguchi S, Zhou X, Fujita H, Fujiwara H. (2005). Volumetric quantitative analysis of tissue characteristics of coronary plaques after statin therapy using three dimensional integrated backscatter intravascular ultrasound. *J Am Coll Cardiol* Vol 45:1946-1953.

Kawasaki M, Bouma BE, Bressner J, Houser SL, Nadkarni SK, MacNeill BD, Jang IK, Fujiwara H, Tearney GJ. (2006). Diagnostic accuracy of optical coherence tomography and integrated backscatter intravascular ultrasound images for tissue characterization of human coronary plaques. *J Am Coll Cardiol* Vol 48:81-8.

Kawasaki M, Hattori A, Ishihara Y, Okubo M, Nishigaki K, Takemura G, Saio M, Takami T, Minatoguchi S. (2010). Tissue characterization of coronary plaques and assessment of thickness of fibrous cap using integrated backscatter intravascular ultrasound. Comparison with histology and optical coherence tomography. *Circ J* Vol 74:2641-48.

Kimura T, Itoh T, Fusazaki T, Matsui H, Sugawara S, Ogino Y, Endo H, Kobayashi K, Nakamura M. (2010). Low-density lipoprotein-cholesterol/high-density lipoprotein-cholesterol ratio predicts lipid-rich coronary plaque in patients with coronary artery disease--integrated-backscatter intravascular ultrasound study. *Circ J* Vol 74:1392-8.

Komura N, Hibi K, Kusama I, Otsuka F, Mitsuhashi T, Endo M, Iwahashi N, Okuda J, Tsukahara K, Kosuge M, Ebina T, Umemura S, Kimura K. (2010). Plaque location in the left anterior descending coronary artery and tissue characteristics in angina pectoris: an integrated backscatter intravascular ultrasound study. *Circ J* Vol 74: 142-7.

Kume T, Okura H, Kawamoto T, Akasaka T, Toyota E, Neishi Y, et al. (2007). Assessment of the histological characteristics of coronary arterial plaque with severe calcification. *Circ J*. Vol 71:643-7.

Lockwood GR, Ryan LK, Hunt JW, Foster FS. (1991). Measurement of the ultrasound properties of vascular tissue and blood from 35-65Mhz. *Ultrasound Med Biol*. Vol 17:653-66.

Mintz GS, Nissen SE, Anderson WD, Bailey SR, Erbel R, Fitzgerald PJ, et al. (2001). American College of Cardiology clinical expert consensus document on standards for acquisition, measurement and reporting of intravascular ultrasound studies (IVUS). A report of the American College of Cardiology task force on clinical expert consensus documents developed in collaboration with the European society of cardiology endorsed by the society of cardiac angiography and interventions. *J Am Coll Cardiol*. Vol 37:1478-92.

Mizuno K, Satomura K, Miyamoto A, Arakawa K, Shibuya T, Arai T, Kurita A, Nakamura H, Ambrose JA. (1992). Angioscopic evaluation of coronary artery thrombi in acute coronary syndromes. *N Engl J Med* Vol 326:287-91.

Naito J, Masuyama T, Mano T, Kondo H, Yamamoto K, Nagano R, Doi Y, Hori M, Kamada T. (1996). Ultrasound myocardial tissue characterization in the patients with dilated cardiomyopathy: Value in noninvasive assessment of myocardial fibrosis. *Am Heart J*. Vol 131:115-21.

Okubo M, Kawasaki M, Ishihara Y, Takeyama U, Kubota T, Yamaki T, Ojio S, Nishigaki K, Takemura G, Saio M, Takami T, Minatoguchi S, Fujiwara H. (2008). Development of integrated backscatter intravascular ultrasound for tissue characterization of coronary plaques. *Ultrasound Med Biol.* Vol 34:655-63. (a)

Okubo M, Kawasaki M, Ishihara Y, Takeyama U, Yasuda S, Kubota T, Tanaka S, Yamaki T, Ojio S, Nishigaki K, Takemura G, Saio M, Takami T, Fujiwara H, Minatoguchi S. (2008). Tissue characterization of coronary plaques: comparison of integrated backscatter intravascular ultrasound with virtual histology intravascular ultrasound. *Circ J* Vol 72:1631-9. (b)

Otagiri K, Tsutsui H, Kumazaki S, Miyashita Y, Aizawa K, Koshikawa M, Kasai H, Izawa A, Tomita T, Koyama J, Ikeda U. (2011). Early intervention with rosuvastatin decreases the lipid components of the plaque in acute coronary syndrome: analysis using integrated backscatter IVUS (ELAN study). *Circ J* Vol 75:633-41.

Picano E, Landini L, Distante A, Sarnelli R, Benassi A, L'Abbate A. (1983). Different degreed of atherosclerosis detected by backscattered ultrasound: An in vitro study on fixed human aortic walls. *J Clin ultrasound.* Vol 11:375-379.

Picano E, Landini L, Distante A, Salvadori M, Lattanzi F, Masini M, et al. (1985). Angle dependence of ultrasonic backscatter in arterial tissues: a study in vitro. *Circulation.*Vol 72:572-6.

Picano E, Landini L, Lattanzi F, Salvadori M, Benassi A, L'Abbate A. (1988). Time domain echo pattern evaluation from normal and atherosclerotic arterial walls: a study in vitro. *Circulation.* Vol 77:654-9.

Picano E, Pelosi G, Marzilli M, Lattanzi F, Benassi A, Landini L, L'Abbate A. (1990). In vivo quantitative ultrasonic evaluation of myocardial fibrosis in humans. *Circulation.* Vol 81:58-64.

Sano K, Kawasaki M, Ishihara Y, Okubo M, Tsuchiya K, Nishigaki K, Zhou X, Minatoguchi S, Fujita H, Fujiwara H. (2006). Assessment of vulnerable plaques causing acute coronary syndrome using integrated backscatter intravascular ultrasound. *J Am Coll Cardiol* Vol 47:734-41.

Siegel RJ, Swan K, Edwalds G, Fishbein MC. (1985). Limitations of postmorterm assessment of human coronary artery size and luminal narrowing: differential effects of tissue fixation and processing on vessel with different degrees of atherosclerosis. *J Am Coll Cardiol.* Vol 5:342-346

Takeuchi H, Morino Y, Matsukage T, Masuda N, Kawamura Y, Kasai S, Hashida T, Fujibayashi D, Tanabe T, Ikari Y. (2009). Impact of vascular remodeling on the coronary plaque compositions: an investigation with in vivo tissue characterization using integrated backscatter-intravascular ultrasound *Atherosclerosis.* Vol 202:476-8

Takiuchi S, Rakugi H, Honda K, Masuyama T, Hirata N, Ito H, Sugimoto K, Yanagitani Y, Moriguchi K, Okamura A, Higaki J, Ogihara T. (2000). Quantitative ultrasonic tissue characterization can identify high-risk atherosclerotic alteration in human carotid arteries. *Circulation* Vol 102:766-70.

Urbani MP, Picano E, Parenti G, Mazzarisi A, Fiori L, Paterni M, Pelosi G, Landini L. (1993). In vivo radiofrequency-based ultrasonic tissue characterization of the atherosclerotic plaque. *Stroke.* Vol 24:1507-12.

Yamada K, Kawasaki M, Yoshimura S, Enomoto Y, Asano T, Minatoguchi S, Iwama T. (2010). Prediction of silent ischemic lesions after carotid artery stenting using integrated backscatter ultrasound and magnetic resonance imaging. *Atherosclerosis* Vol 208:161-6

4

IVUS Role in Studies Assessing Atherosclerosis Development

T. Kovarnik[1], A. Wahle[2], R.W. Downe[2] and M. Sonka[2]
[1]2nd Department of Medicine - Department of Cardiovascular Medicine, First Faculty of Medicine, Charles University in Prague and General University Hospital in Prague,
[2]Dept. of Electrical and Computer Engineering, The University of Iowa, Iowa City IA,
[1]Czech Republic
[2]USA

1. Introduction

Atherosclerosis is known as a chronic progressive disease with accumulation of atherosclerotic plaque inside the vessel wall. Angiography studies revealed small (1-2%) increase of lumen during high dose lipid-lowering therapy, but angiography is not the appropriate tool for plaque analysis and has many limitations for precise lumen measurement due to its projective nature. In contrast, intravascular ultrasound or IVUS can accurately measure lumen and vessel diameters, and consequently determine local plaque burden. Careful mechanical pullback allows volume measurements of the lumen, vessel and plaque over a vessel segment. Serial measurements (baseline and follow-up after several months, typically 12±3 months) allow to evaluate changes of these volumes, thus to search for plaque progression or plaque regression and assess their mechanisms (for example decrease of plaque volume or increase of vessel volume), type of vessel reaction (positive and negative remodeling), development of risky plaque features like plaque ulceration and plaque ruptures.

Studies with intravascular ultrasound have shown that disease progression can be stopped (GAIN[1], REVERSAL[2]) or reversed (ASTEROID[3], ESTABLISH[4], COSMOS[5]), especially in response to aggressive lipid-lowering treatment. The mean changes of plaque volume in the treated groups were quite small; on the other hand, large scale lipid-lowering trials have shown significant reduction of ischemic events. This discrepancy between the clinical benefits and the small changes in plaque mass can be explained by plaque stabilization (changes of plaque composition from a high risk profile to a low risk profile). However, conventional grayscale IVUS has significant limitations in the assessment of plaque composition. Virtual histology (VH) based on spectral analysis of IVUS radiofrequency data was developed to quantify coronary plaque components[6].

Risk factors for atherosclerosis are same for all coronary arteries, but some regions are more affected then others like the proximal third of the arteries, ostial regions, and bifurcations. There must be some local factor playing an important role. Local wall shear stress has been identified as such a factor, which is caused by friction between virtual layers of blood inside arteries (the velocity of blood flow is maximal in the middle part of arteries and minimal just next to the endothelium). Shear stress induces deformation of endothelial cells and activates many pro-atherosclerotic genes (VCAM, ICAM, endothelin etc).

This chapter summarizes results of several aforementioned studies and their impact on routine daily practice. Further, it explains how to perform serial IVUS study with precise measurement of plaque volume changes and plaque risk feature changes. Second part of this chapter is focused on 3D vessel reconstruction based of angiography, IVUS, virtual histology and shear stress analysis fusion, which is the technique used for better detailed analyses of the atherosclerotic development.

2. Atherosclerosis

2.1 Atherosclerosis development

Atherosclerosis and its complications are the most frequent causes of mortality and morbidity in the developed countries. The atherosclerotic research made a great progress in investigation of atherosclerosis development, but the regression of atherosclerosis is still a process, which is not well understood.

The best description of atherosclerosis development was proposed by H. Stary et al.[7], who recognized eight stages of atherosclerotic plaque maturation:

- type I - *initial lesion* (adaptive intimal thickening)
- type II - fatty streaks (intimal xantomas, intima is infiltrated by macrophages, which change their phenotype into foam cells)
- type III - preatheroma (pathologic intimal thickening, lysis of foam cells and extracellular accumulation of lipid droplets and lipid pools)
- type IV - *atheroma* (formatting of lipid core)
- type V - *fibroatheroma* (lipid core is covered by a fibrous cap)
- type VI - *complicated lesion* (development of plaque fissures and plaque rupture, bleeding to plaque from vasa vasorum)
- type VII - calcified lesion
- type VIII - fibrous lesion

Types I-II are also called initial lesions, types IV and V developed lesion, type VI is called a complicated lesion and types VII and VIII chronic lesions[8]. This description of atherosclerosis development was done by examinations of post mortem specimens from adults and children. One of the most important findings is that the atherosclerotic mass is located in the vessel wall, and that the lumen area is preserved by positive remodeling up to a specific threshold when luminal narrowing starts to occur. This finding was also confirmed *in vivo* by IVUS[9]. The process of remodeling cannot be observed during coronary angiography, given that only the lumen is visualized and its patency is originally retained. While positive remodeling preserves the lumen, at the same time it constitutes a risk factor for development of an acute coronary syndrome. A likely common pathway is the effect of metalloproteases (enzymes which can breakdown collagen). They allow vessel enlargement, but also increase risk of plaque rupture due to the decrease of collagen amount inside the plaque[10].

Further morphologic features indicating vulnerable plaque are plaque rupture and higher content of necrotic tissue. A very specific type of the rupture-prone plaque is called thin cap fibroatheroma (TCFA). Pathologic description of this type of plaque consist of a large necrotic core with an overlying thin and disrupted fibrous cap infiltrated by macrophages. The smooth muscle cell components within the cap are absent or sparse. The thickness of such a thin fibrous cap is less than 65 μm[11,12], so thin that it may not be identifiable even with IVUS.

2.2 Shear stress

While the entire coronary arteries are exposed to the systemic risk factors, atherosclerotic lesions frequently form at specific regions such as at the vicinity of side branches, along the outer wall of bifurcations, and on the inner wall of curved vessels. An important local factor contributing to lesion formation in these locations is the effective endothelial shear stress (ESS)[13], also called wall shear stress (WSS). Many studies confirmed the mechanistic role of low ESS in the development of atherosclerosis[14-17]. ESS is the tangential force derived from the friction of the flowing blood on the endothelial surface of the arterial wall and is proportional to the product of the blood viscosity (μ) and the spatial gradient of blood velocity at the wall.

Viscosity can be measured or calculated from the measured hematocrit. Intracoronary blood flow can be calculated directly from the time required for the volume of blood contained within the vascular section to leave this section and be displaced by radio-opaque material during a contrast injection[18].

Normal ESS is pulsatile and unidirectional with magnitude that vary within a range of 15-70 dyne/cm^2 over the cardiac cycle[17]. Stone et al.[19] published that plaque progression in minimally diseased coronary artery subsegments occurs almost exclusively in the areas of low ESS. At the same time, the vessels react on plaque progression by positive remodeling in the regions with a low ESS. However, the positive remodeling was also found in regions with high ESS with no plaque progression. It is important to keep in mind that imaging may be performed at a time when the ESS distribution, which leads to a specific plaque development, may have already been altered by plaque development at this or an adjacent location[20]. There are likely multiple stimuli and mechanistic pathway responsible for such positive remodeling. Low ESS contributes not only to plaque progression, but also increases the plaque vulnerability[21]. On the contrary, Helderman et al.[22] found higher numbers of macrophages and higher metalloproteases activity in the region with high ESS. The question how the low ESS contributes to the plaque vulnerability has not been reliably answered yet. The mechanisms how low ESS influences local atherosclerosis likely includes activation of mechanoreceptors in the membrane of the endothelial cells and this signal activates or inhibits mechanosensitive genes. The atheroprotective genes are suppressed, whereas the pro-atherogenic genes are upregulated in the regions with a low ESS[23].

2.3 Atherosclerosis regression

The atherosclerosis was thought to be a one-way process for many years. However, atherosclerosis regression was seen in autopsy findings from children, in angiographic studies and in studies conducted with IVUS.

Fatty streaks in the aorta and the coronary arteries can been seen even in one year old children. These changes disappear at the age of four years and have an unquestionable relationship with breast feeding. Until now, it is not clear whether these findings reflect normal physiologic changes or whether they exhibit signs of premature atherosclerosis[24].

2.4 Angiographic studies

Several angiographic studies assessing effects of statins on plaque progression have been published. The main target was the assessment of the minimal lumen diameter or mean lumen diameter, differences between 0.03-0.08 mm were reported. It is questionable whether the angiography can precisely detect these negligible differences. Furthermore, these lumen changes are only indirect markers of plaque changes. The overview of angiographic studies is provided in Table 1.

	study	change of MLD	change of LDLc
simvastatin	SCAT[25]	- 0.07 mm / 3-5 years	- 30%
	MASS[26]	- 0.08 mm / 4 years	- 31.4%
lovastatin	CCAIT[27]	- 0.05 mm / 2 years	- 29%
pravastatin	REGRESS[28]	- 0.03 mm / 2 years	- 25%
	PLAC-1[29]	- 0.03 mm / 1 year	- 28
fluvastatin	LCAS[30]	- 0.028mm / 2.5 years	- 22.5%

Abbreviations: MLD = minimal lumen diameter, LDLc = low density lipoprotein cholesterol

Table 1. Angiographic studies with statins.

2.5 Studies with intravascular ultrasound - Methodology

IVUS can precisely measure lumen, vessel and plaque volumes and therefore is an ideal tool for performing follow-up studies assessing changes of these volumes during lipid lowering therapy. Two different IVUS designs can be used: Rotating element IVUS catheters operating at frequencies of 40 MHz, or electronic phased array catheters operating at a frequency of 20 MHz. Automatic motorized pullback is mandatory at a rate of 0.5 or 1.0 mm/s for reliable three-dimensional imaging. There are several important factors which influence the pullback quality[31]

1. Adequate battery power in battery controlled pullback device. Using a battery at the end of its life produces a non-continuous pullback with a decreasing speed.
2. Opening of the Y connector before starting the pullback. It causes small bleeding, but the movement of IVUS catheter is significantly smoother and thus more accurate.
3. Straightening of the IVUS catheter before pullback, otherwise the speed of the IVUS catheter is not continuous/constant-speed at the beginning of the acquisition
4. Even if the catheter is straightened, the pullback is the least accurate at the beginning of pullback and most accurate in the proximal part of image vessel. For this reason, it is recommended to start the IVUS pullback about 10 mm distal to the location of interest.

Patients suitable for a plaque regression study are usually admitted for stable angina pectoris and undergo diagnostic angiography in the majority of cases. Patients with normal findings on coronary angiography are excluded. For some research protocols, patients with a left main stenosis or a significant stenosis of all three coronary arteries may also be excluded because they will require revascularization and would not be suitable for a follow-up study. It is questionable whether patients with one significant stenosis should or should not be included. From our point of view, symptomatic patients with at least one significant stenosis should undergo revascularization and not be included in a medication-based plaque regression study.

The ideal situation would be to perform IVUS in all three coronary arteries and to follow all identified plaques. However, such a design would be time consuming and complicated for the analysis and therefore, in a majority of trials, only one vessel is investigated at a time.

The inclusion criterion is typically the identification of at least one location with the luminal stenosis > 20% by angiography, another useful criterion is may be plaque burden > 40% assessed by IVUS. In case of similar findings in more than one coronary artery during angiography, the artery with the longer plaque, or in case of several stenoses present in any single artery, the plaque with the most severe plaque burden should be selected for the IVUS analysis. The recommended segment length is greater than 30 mm with at least two clear landmarks (fiduciary points) in the proximal and distal parts of the analyzed segment. An obvious proximal landmark in the left coronary artery is the left main bifurcation. Further landmarks may be clearly defined side branches (conus branch or proximal atrial branch in the right coronary artery) or some recognizable calcifications. Despite the clear landmarks and identical conditions of the pullbacks during the baseline and follow-up, the baseline/follow-up pullback lengths represented by frame counts will not be identical in the majority of cases. Possible reasons for this situation are technical errors while performing of pullback (low battery power, not straightened IVUS catheter before pullback, tight Y connector), or a slightly different trajectory of the IVUS catheters due to different positions of guide wires inside the coronary artery. Differences between the baseline and follow-up in the number of frames may be up to 15%, which is considered acceptable. Consequently, volumes may have to be calculated using the mean length between landmarks from the two studies[31].

Several automatic border detection software applications were developed to decrease the necessity of manual tracing. However, according to our experiences, careful inspection of all acquired frames and providing manual correction of almost all frames is frequently necessary during baseline/follow-up trials. The presence of calcium further complicates adventitial border detection. Heavily calcified lesions should be avoided for these types of trials due to a high risk of inaccuracy of volume measurements. Using cross sectional analysis, a single deposit with an arc of calcium < 45 degrees or multiple small arcs of up to 180 degrees can be acceptable since they can be extrapolated. Another challenging part of a vessel when performing vessel wall border detection are regions with originating side branches. Several rules are recommended unless the branch is specifically modeled as such as described in the next paragraphs: The EEM contour should be interpolated to follow the main vessel cross-sections immediately proximal and distal to the side branch and the lumen contour should be drawn on top of the EEM contour at the mouth of the side branch[31].

The parameters, which may be calculated include total atheroma volume (TAV) counted as $\Sigma(EEM_{CSA}\text{-}Lumen_{CSA})$ and percent atheroma volume PAV counted as $(\Sigma(EEM_{CSA}\text{-}Lumen_{CSA}) / \Sigma EEM_{CSA}) \times 100$. Note that the presented simple calculation of TAV would not represent a true volume and would only be valid for comparisons if the inter-frame distance stays constant across all analyses. Therefore, TAV should be normalized with respect to the lesion length as described earlier: TAV / lesion length or normalized as $\Sigma(EEM_{CSA}\text{-}Lumen_{CSA})$ / (number of analyzed frames per patient) and multiplied by mean/median no. of analyzed frames in the population [31-33]. For expressing of changes between baseline and follow-up,- the absolute change of TAV or PAV (follow-up minus baseline) can be used and the percent change of TAV can be expressed as $(TAV_{follow\ up} - TAV_{baseline} / TAV_{baseline} \times 100)$[31]. The same approach to quantifying changes is possible for lumen volumes and vessel volumes.

Another set of interesting and important parameters is describes the vessel remodeling. For serial studies, it is recommended to calculate a remodeling index as (vessel $volume_{follow\ up}$ – vessel $volume_{baseline}$), in which a positive value means positive remodeling and conversely a negative value represents negative remodeling. Furthermore, vessels with the positive

remodeling should be subdivided into expansive (over compensatory) where ΔEEM / Δatheroma is > 1 or incomplete where ΔEEM / Δatheroma is between 0 and 1.0[31].
More sophisticated assessment of plaque behavior is enabled by 3D reconstruction of vessels, which is done by fusion of angiography and IVUS. This technique builds geometrically correct 3-D or 4-D (i.e., 3-D over all phases of the cardiac cycle) reconstructions of coronary arteries and computes quantitative indices of coronary lumen and wall morphology. The reconstructions may also serve as input for hemodynamic and morphologic analyses and allow for interactive visualization[34] (*Figure 1*).

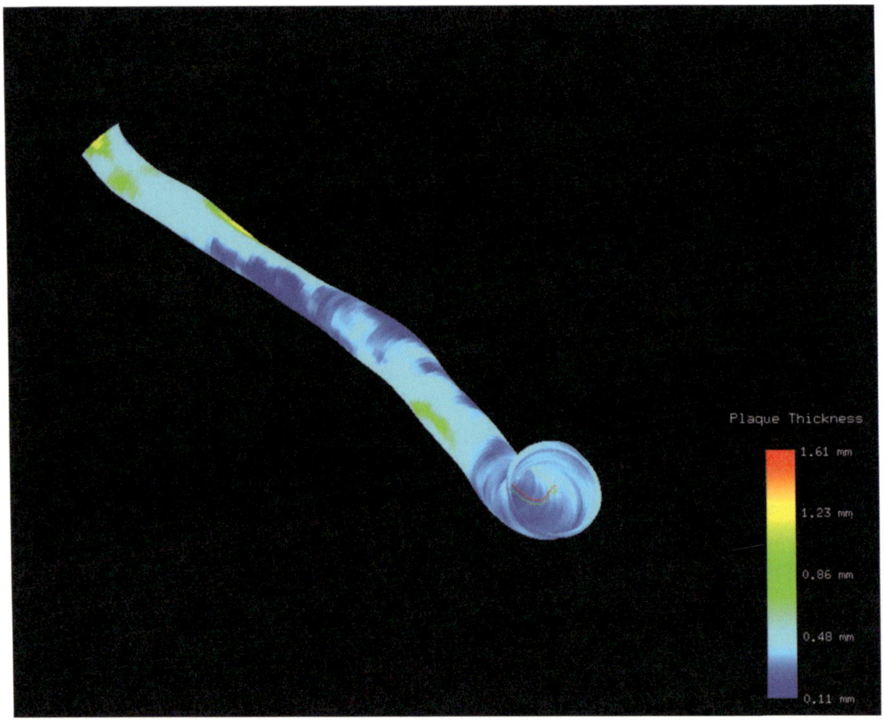

Fig. 1. Plaque thickness assessment with local plaque thickness indicated by color coding on the lumen surface.

In general, vessel curvature and torsion are derived from biplane (or a pair of single-plane) X-ray angiograms, and the cross-sectional information is obtained from IVUS. Thus, the resulting model accurately reflects the spatial geometry of the vessel and includes any accumulated plaque. Fusion leads to a 3-D or 4-D model, consisting of the lumen/plaque and media/adventitia contours oriented relative to the IVUS catheter. This may result in a surface mesh, which can include any branches segmented along with the main vessel to the extent visible in the IVUS (*Figure 2*). After proper meshing, this model is suitable for hemodynamic analyses.
Morphologic analyses are performed following the resampling of the cross sections orthogonal to the vessel centerline, to eliminate distortions from the position of the IVUS catheter within the vessel. The quantitative results may annotate this resampled contour model, which is then used for visualization and further analysis.

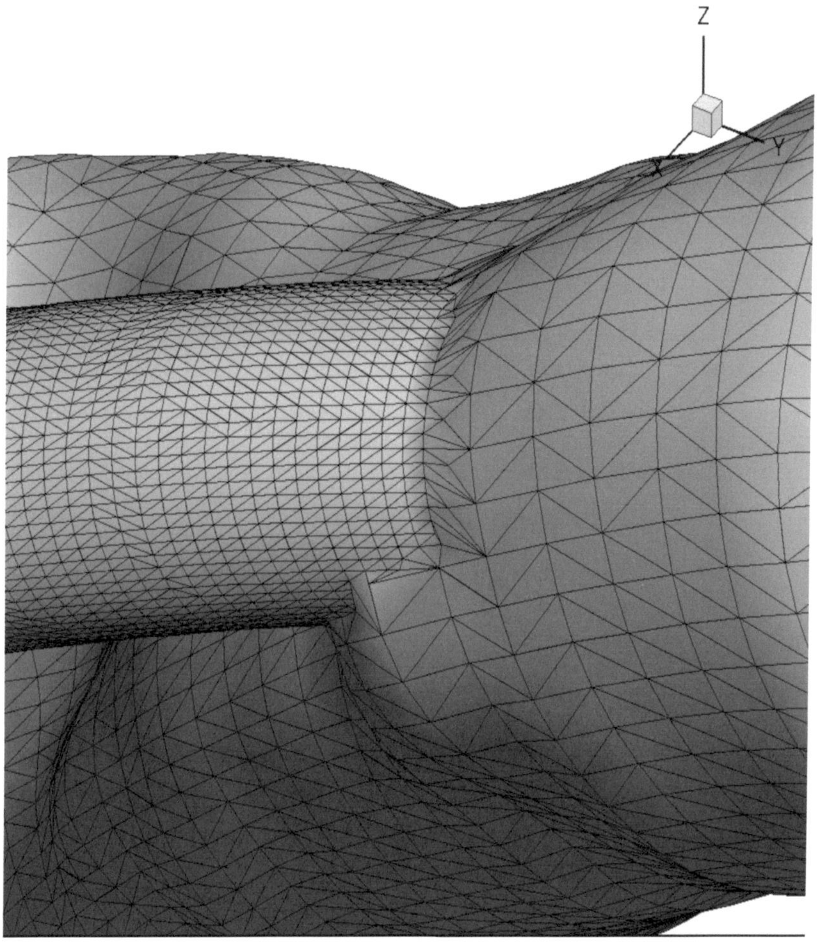

Fig. 2. Meshing of the luminal surface obtained from a geometrically-correct 3D reconstruction depicting a side branch.

The estimation of the absolute orientation of the IVUS frames in 3-D is a non-trivial issue and is usually resolved by using the angiographic lumen as a reference. The outline of the vessel lumen is visible in both angiographic projections when a small amount of contrast dye is injected. This is utilized to establish the orientation of the IVUS frames by finding their best fit with the angiographic outline. Using differential geometry, only the relative orientation changes from frame to frame can be established, the absolute orientation of the frame set yet needs to be determined at this stage. For this, a 3-D elliptical lumen outline is reconstructed from the angiograms and compared with the IVUS lumen outline, mapped into 3-D using an arbitrary initial orientation. This allows a non-iterative approach in which a single correction angle is calculated from an initial orientation and then applied to the entire frame set. The reconstructed vascular model provides 3-D locations for detected circumferential vertices (72 in our case) on both lumen/plaque and media/adventitia contours, oriented with respect to the IVUS catheter path. The blood flow through the coronary arteries is simulated and the wall shear stress distribution determined using computational fluid dynamics (CFD) methodology.

During the CFD, blood is treated as an incompressible, homogenous, and Newtonian fluid. Since the flow rate are difficult to be measured in each of the coronary arteries during data acquisition for each patient due to procedural limitations, a flow rate of 100 ml/min is sometimes assumed for all the coronary arterial segments employed in this analysis. Positive and negative wall shear stress values are determined at each circumferential lumen location and mapped onto the lumen vertices for each contour of the perpendicularly oriented 3-D model[35] (*Figure 3*).

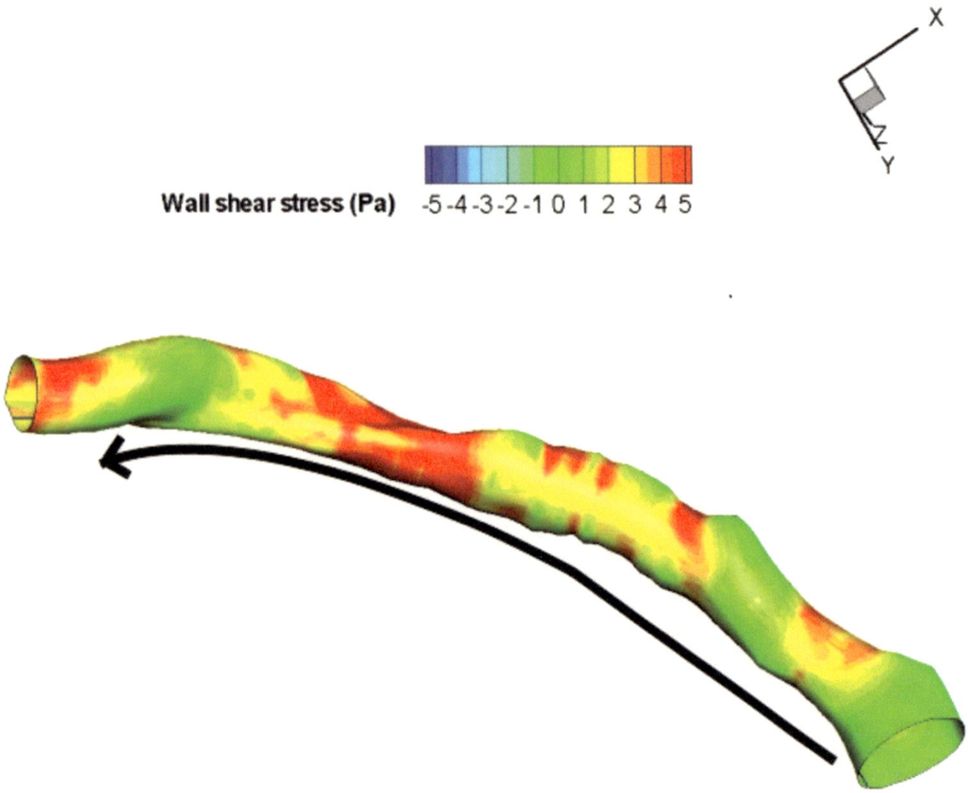

Fig. 3. Shear stress assessment on a 3-D reconstructed coronary artery (the arrow indicates the direction of blood flow).

2.6 Studies with intravascular ultrasound – Overview

Studies with intravascular ultrasound have shown that disease progression can be stopped (GAIN[1], REVERSAL[2]) or reversed (ASTEROID[3], ESTABLISH[4], COSMOS[5]) during lipid lowering therapy, as summarized in Table 2. The promising drug torcetrapib - inhibitor of cholesteryl ester transfer protein (CETP), which facilitates the transfer of cholesteryl ester from HDL cholesterol to LDL cholesterol and VLDL cholesterol did not decrease percent atheroma volume. Furthermore, it increased the mortality (cardiovascular and all cause mortality) in ILLUMINATE trial[36]. The reason was increasing of blood pressure together with decreasing of potassium level (aldosteron like action). However, new CETP inhibitor without these effects is tested in preclinical trials.

study	study design	number of patient	results	change of lipids
Takagi.[37]	pravastatin 10mg vs. dietary stabilization	25	decrease of plaque area in pravastatin group, no volumetric analysis	LDLc: -27% vs.-9% HDLc: +29% vs. +17%
Ishikawa [38]	pravastatin 10-20 mg	40	relative change of TAV 20%	LDLc : -23.5% HDLc : +9.3%
GAIN[1]	atorvastatin 20-80 mg vs. standard therapy,	131	relative change of TAV 2.5% vs. + 11.8%	LDLc: -42% vs. -16% HDLc: +9% vs. + 12%
REVERSAL[2]	80 mg atorvastatatin vs. 40 mg pravastatin	502	TAV: - $0.4mm^3$ vs. + $5.1mm^3$, relative change of TAV: + 4.1 vs. + 5.4% PAV: + 0.6% vs. + 1.9%	LDLc: -46.3% vs. -25.2 HDLc: +2.9 vs. +5.6%
ASTEROID[3]	rosuvastatin 40 mg	349	PAV: -0.98%, TAV in worst 10 mm segment: $-6.1mm^3$, 9.1% relative changes and - $14.7mm^3$ of normalized TAV	LDLc: -53.2% HDLc: +14.7%
COSMOS[5]	rosuvastatin 2.5-20mg	126	relative change of TAV: -5.1%	LDLc: -38.6% HDLc: +19.8%
ESTABLISH[4]*	atorvastatin vs. dietary treatment or cholesterol absorption inhibitors	70	TAV: - $8.3mm^3$ vs. + $4.2mm^3$ relative changes of TAV -13.1% vs. + 8.7	LDLc: -43.8% vs. -3.6% HDLc: +2.4% vs. +7.0%
JAPAN-ACS[39]	pitavastatin 4gm vs. atorvastatin 20mg	252	TAV: - $8,2mm^3$ and - 10,6 mm^3 PAV: -5,7% vs. - 6,3% patients with CAD and polyvascular extent of atherosclerosis had smaller regression compared to patients with CAD only[40]	LDLc -36.2% vs.- 35.8% HDLc +9.9% vs.+8%
Jensen[41]	simvastatin 40mg	40	TAV or PAV are not available, authors found plaque regression	LDLc: -13,6% HDLc: +7%

study	study design	number of patient	results	change of lipids
Nissen[42] ∇	recombinant ApoA-I Milano vs. placebo	57	PAV -1.1% vs + 0,14%	not available
REACH[43]	atorvatatin 10-20mg vs. usual care	58	TAV –1,4 mm^3 vs. +7,6 mm^3 PAV – 1,95 % vs. +1,6%	LDLc: –34% vs. 0% HDLc: -1% vs +1%
ILLUSTRATE[44]	torcetrapib♣+ atorvastatin vs-. atorvastatin	910	normalized TAV – 9.4 vs- - 6.3mm^3, p=0.02 PAV + 0.12% vs. + 0.19%, p=0.72	LDLc: –13.3% vs. +6.6% HDLc: +58.6% vs. +2.2%
ACTIVATE[32]	pactimibe∗ vs. placebo	???	normalized TAV: -1.3 mm^3 vs. – 5.6 mm^3 PAV: +0.8% vs. +0.6%	not available
Nakayama[45]	pioglitazon 15mg vs. standard therapy in diabetic patients	26	TAV - 6.7 vs. 2.3 mm3	not available
HEAVEN[46]	atorvastatin+ezetrol vs. standard care	89	PAV - 0.4% vs. + 1.4%, p=0.01	LDLc: -28.6% vs. – 1.9% HDLc: +4,5% vs. -1.3%
Clementi[47]	Atorvastatin 80mg + 30mg pioglitazone for 6 month, no control group	25	TAV -12.7	not available
Nasu[48]	Fluvastatin vs. control according to LDLc	80	TAV – 36.4 vs. + 11.2 mm^3, p<0.0001	LDL -47.7% vs. -1.1 HDL +2.2% vs. – 0.6%

* patiens with ACS, ∇ 2 weeks after ACS with repeated IVUS after two weeks, ♣ torcetrapib is an inhibitor for cholesteryl ester transfer protein , its development was stopped due to severe side effects (increase of blood pressure), ∗ ACAT inhibitor (acyl–coenzyme A:cholesterol acyltransferase, which esterifies cholesterol in a variety of cells and tissues, CAD coronary artery disease

Table 2. IVUS controlled progression / regression studies

The changes of plaque volume were also examined in trials focusing on plaque composition. Decrease of plaque volume was found in HEAVEN[46] (percent atheroma volume), IBIS 2[49] (total atheroma volume) and studies done by Clementi[47] (total atheroma volume) and Nasu[47] Only non-significant changes of plaque volume were found in studies done by Kawasaki[50], Hong[51].

The changes of plaques composition during lipid-lowering therapy are not clear, because aforesaid studies found different results. Decrease of fibrous (F) tissue and fibro-fatty (FF)

tissue and increase of necrotic core (NC) and calcification (DC) were found in HEAVEN and in IBIS 2 (non-darapladib arm) studies. Nasu found decrease of NC and FF and increase of F and DC tissues, Kawasaki published decrease of lipid and fibrous tissues, Clementi found increase of NC and Hong increase of F and FF and decrease of NC and DC.
However, there are a lot of substantial differences among these studies. They are comparing patients with or without lipid-lowering pretreatment, analyzing the whole examined segment or only the worst part of vessel and they are using different techniques for plaque composition assessment: VH-IVUS (Volcano Therapeutics), iMAP-IVUS (Boston Scientific), Integrated Backscatter IVUS and automated differential echogenicity[52].

2.7 Regresion of atherosclerosis as a surrogate study endpoint

Every new drug or new therapeutic approach must demonstrate a significant clinical benefit in terms of a reduction in cardiovascular morbidity and mortality. Due to the high standard of care in modern era, it becomes more and more difficult to find significant differences between new and previous treatments. The assessment of plaque volume changes can be used as an alternative end point instead of "hard" clinical endpoints, because both angiographic[53] and IVUS assessed plaque progression[54,55] correlate with coronary events. This strategy enables to decrease a number of patients and duration of study[56].

3. Conclusion

Studies with intravascular ultrasound confirmed the existence of atherosclerosis regression. This process can be started by high dose of lipid lowering drugs in combination with changing the life style, more recently also with ACAT inhibitors. To date, changes of plaque composition during development and regression of atherosclerosis have not been precisely described, and conflicting results continue being published in the literature.
Recent regression/progression studies performed with intravascular ultrasound have a well-defined methodology, which must be fully respected to obtain reliable and comparable results. In addition to plain 2D IVUS studies, more comprehensive studies can be performed with high-tech vessel analysis in terms of 3D/4D reconstruction with a full-range of descriptions of the observed atherosclerotic processes including volume measurements, assessments of plaque composition and computing functional aspects such as the luminal shear stress. This concept allows a more complex assessment of atherosclerosis development and can reveal additional relationships among the morphologic and functional factors.

4. References

[1] Schartl M, Bocksch W, Koschyk D, et al. Use of Intravascular Ultrasound to Compare Effects of Different Strategies of Lipid-Lowering Therapy on Plaque Volume and Composition in Patients With Coronary Artery Disease. *Circulation* 2001;104:387-392

[2] Nissen S, Tuzscu M, Schoenhagen P, et al. Effect of Intensive Compared With Moderate Lipid-Lowering Therapy on Progression of Coronary Atherosclertosis. *JAMA* 2004;291:1071-1080

[3] Nissen SE, Nicholls SJ, Sipahi I, Libby P, Raichlen JS, Ballantyne CM. Effect of very high-intensity statin therapy on regression of coronary atherosclerosis: The ASTEROID trial. JAMA 2006;295:1556-1565

[4] Okazaki S, Yokoyma T, Miyauchi K, Shimada K, Kurata T, Sato H. Early statin treatment in patients with acute coronary syndrome: Demonstration of beneficial effect on atherosclerotic lesion by serial volumetric intravascular ultrasound analysis during half a year after coronary event: The ESTABLISH study. *Circulation* 2004;110:1061-1068

[5] Takayama T, Hiro T, Yamahishi M, Daida H, Hirayama H, Saito S, Yamaguchi T, Matsuzaki M, for the COSMOS Investigators. Effect of rosuvastatin on coronary atheroma in stable coronary arthery disease. Multicenter coronary atherosclerosis study measuring effects of rosuvastatin using of intravascular ultrasound in Japanese subjects COSMOS. Circ J;2009:73:2110-2117

[6] Nair A, Klingensmith JD, Vince DG. Real-time plaque characterization and visualization with spectral analysis of intravascular ultrasound data. Stud Health Technol Inform. 2005;113:300-20

[7] Stary HC. The Histological Classification of Atherosclerotic lesions in Human Coronary Arteries. In: V.Fuster, R.Ross and E.J. Topol. Atheroslcerosis and Coronary Disease. *Lippincott-Raven Publishers, Philadelphia 1996: 272-28*

[8] Stary HC, Chandler AB, Dinsmore RE et al. A definition of advanced types of atherosclerotic lesions and histological classification of atherosclerosis: a report from the Comitee on Vascular Lesions of the Council of Arteriosclerosis, American Heart Association.Circulation 1995;92: 1355-1374

[9] Glagov S, Weisenberg E, Zarins C, et al. Compensatory enlargement of human atherosclerotic coronary arteries. *N Engl J Med* 1987;316:1371-1375

[10] Libby P. The molecular base of the acute coronary syndromes. *Circulation* 1995;91:2844-2850

[11] Virmani R, Narula J, Leon MB, Willerson JT. The Vulnerable atherosclerotic plaque. Strategies foir diagnosis and managemnent. Blackwell Publishing 2007.

[12] Burke AP, Farb A, Malcom GT, et al. Coronary risk factors and plaque morphology in men with coronary disease who died suddenly. *N Engl J Med* 1997;336:1276-1282

[13] Chatzizisis YS, Coskun AU, Jonas M, Edelman ER, Feldman CL, Stone PH. Role of endothelial shear stress in the natural history of coronary atherosclerosis and vascular remodeling. *JACC* 2007;49:2379

[14] Stone PH. Coskun AU, Kinlay S, Clark M, Sonka M, Wahle A, Illegbusi O, Yeghiazarians Y, Popma J, Orav J, Kuntz R, Feldman CL. Effect of endothelial shear stress on the progression of coronary artery disease, vascular remodeling, and in-stent restenosis in humans:in vivo 6-month follow-up study. *Circulation* 2003;108:438-444

[15] Wentzel JJ, Corti R, Fayad ZA et al. Does shear stress modulate both plaque progression and regression in the thoracic aorta? Human study using serial magnetic resonance imaging. J Am Coll Cardiol 2005;45:846-854

[16] Chatzizisis YS, Jonas M, Coskun AU, et al. Low endothelial shear stress (ESS) is responsible for the heterogenity and severity of coronary atherosclerotic plaques: an in-vivo IVUS natural history study (abstr). *Circulation* 2006;114:II23

[17] Coskun U. Voskuj A, Yeghiazarians Y, Inlay S,Clark M, Ilegbusi O, Wahle A, Sonka M, Popma J, Kuntz R, Feldman CL, Stone PH Reproducibility of Coronary Lumen, Plaque, and Vesel Wall Reconstruction and of Endothelial Shear Stress Measurements In Vivo in Humans. *Cathet and Cardiovasc Interv* 2003; 60:67–78

[18] Stone PH, Coskun AU, Kinlay S, Popma J, Sonka M, Wahle A, Yeghiazarians Y, Maynard Ch, Kuntz R, Feldman Ch. Regions of low endothelial shear stress are the sites where coronary plaque progress and vascular remodeling occurs in humans: an in vivo serial study. Eur. Heart J. 2007;28:705-710
[19] Wahle A, Lopez JJ, Olszewski ME, Vigmostad SC, Chandran KB, Rossen JD, Sonka M. Plaque Development, Vessel Curvature, and Wall Shear Stress in Coronary Arteries assessed by X-ray Angiography and Intravascular Ultrasound. *Medical Image Analysis* 2006;10:615-631
[20] Cheng C, Tempel D, van Haperen R , et al. Atherosclerotic lesion size and vulnerability are determined by patterns of fluid shear stress. *Circulation* 2006;113:2744-2753
[21] Helderman F, Segers D, de Crom R, Hierck BP, Poelmann RE, Evans PC, Krams R. Effect of shear stress on vascular inflammation and plaque development. Curr Opin Lipidol. 2007;18:527-33
[22] Resnicks N, Yahav H, Shay-Salit A, et al. Fluid shear stress and the vascular endothelium: for better and for worse. *Prog Biophys Mol Biol* 2003;81:177-199
[23] Stary HC. Macrophages, macrophage foam cells, and eccentric intimal thickening in the coronary arteries of young children. *Atherosclerosis* 1987;64:91-108
[24] Teo K, Burton J, Buller Ch, et al. Long term Effects of Cholesterol Lowering and Angiotensin-Converting Enzyme Inhibition on Coronary Atherosclerosis. The simvastatin/Enalaparil Coronary Atherosclerosis Trial (SCAT). *Circulation* 2000;102:1748-1754
[25] MASS investigators. Effect of simvastatin on coronary atheroma: the Multicentre Anti-Atheroma Study (MASS). *Lancet* 1994;344:633-638
[26] Waters D, Higginson L, Gladstone P, et al. Effects of cholesterol lowering on the progression of coronary atherosclerosis in women. A Canadian Coronary Atherosclerosis Intervention Trial (CCAIT) substudy. Circulation 1995;92:2404-10
[27] Jukema W, Bruschke A, van Boven A, et al. Effects of Lipid Lowering by Pravastatin on Progression and Regression of Coronary Artery Disease in Symptomatic Men With Normal to Moderately Elevated Serum Cholesterol Levels. The Regression Growth Evaluation Statin Study (REGRESS). *Circulation* 1995;91:2528-2540
[28] Pitt B, Mancini J, Ellis S, et al. Pravastatin Limitation of Atherosclerosis in the Coronary Arteries (PLAC I): Reduction in Atherosclerosis Progression and Clinical Events. *J Am Coll Cardiol* 1995;26:1133-1139
[29] Herd JA, Ballantyne CM, Farmer JA, et al. Effects of fluvastatin on coronary atherosclerosis in patients with mild to moderate cholesterol elevations (Lipoprotein and Coronary Atherosclerosis Study [LCAS]). Am J Cardiol 1997;80:278-286
[30] Mintz GS, Garcia-Gracia HM, Nicholls SJ, Weissman NJ, Bruining N, Crowe T, Tardif JC, Serruys PW. Clinical expert consensus document on standards for acquisition, measurement and reporting of intravascular ultrasound regression/progression studies. *Eurointervention* 2011;6:1123-1130
[31] Nissen SE, Tuzcu EM, Brewer HB, et al. Effect of ACAT inhibition on the progression of coronary atherosclerosis. *N Engl J Med.* 2006;354:1253-1263
[32] Gogas BD, Farooq V, Serruys PW, Garcia-Garcia HM. Assessment of coronary atherosclerosis by IVUS and IVUS-based imaging modalities: progression and

regression studies, tissue composition and beyond. *Int J Cardiovasc Imaging* 2011;27:225-237

[33] Wahle, A., Prause, GPM, DeJong, SC, Sonka, M. Geometrically correct 3-D reconstruction of intravascular ultrasound images by fusion with biplane angiography - methods and validation. *IEEE Transactions on Medical Imaging* 1999;18:686–699

[34] Wahle A , Lopez J, Olszewski M, Vigmostad S, Chandran K, Rossen J, Sonka M. Plaque development, vessel curvature, and wall shear stress in coronary arteries assessed by X-ray angiography and intravascular ultrasound. *Medical Image Analysis* 2006;10: 615–631

[35] Barter PJ, Caulfield M, Eriksson M, Grundy SM, Kastelein JJ, Komajda M, Lopez-Sendon J, Mosca L, Tardif JC, Waters DD, Shear CL, Revkin JH, Buhr KA, Fisher MR, Tall AR, Brewer B; ILLUMINATE Investigators. Effects of torcetrapib in patients at high risk for coronary events. *NEJM* 2007;357:2109-2022

[36] Takagi T, Yoshida K, Akasaka T, et al. Intravascular Ultrasound Analysis of Reduction in Progression of Coronary Narrowing by Treatment With Pravastatin. *Am J Cardiol* 1997;79:1673-1676.

[37] Ishikawa K, Tani S, Watanabe I, Matsumoto M, Furukawa K, Nomoto K, Nomoto K,Kushiro T, Nagao K, Kanmatsuse K .Efect of Pravastatin on Coronary Plaque Volume. *Am J Cardiol* 2003;92:975-977

[38] Hiro T, Kimura T, Morimoto T, Miyauchi K, Nakagawa Y, Yamagishi M, Ozaki Y, Kimura K, Saito S, Yamaguchi T, Daida H, Matsuzaki M, for the JAPAN-ACS Investigators. Effect of Intensive Statin Therapy on Regression of Coronary Atherosclerosis in Patients With Acute Coronary Syndrome. *J Am Coll Cardiol* 2009;54:293-302

[39] Hibi K, Kimura T, Kimura K, Morimoto T, Hiro T, Miyauchi K, Nakagawa Y, Yamagishi M, Ozaki Y, Saito S, Yamaguchi T, Daida H, Matsuyaki M; fot the JAPAN-ACS Investigators. Clinically evident polyvascular disease and regression of coronary atherosclerosis after intensive statin therapy in patients with acute corornary syndrome: Serial intravascular ultrasound from the Jaúanese assessment of pitavastatin and atorvastatin in acute coronary syndrome (JAPAN-ACS) trial. *Atherosclerosis* 2011 ahead of print

[40] Jensen L, MD, Thayssen P, Pedersen K, Stender S, Haghfelt T. Regression of Coronary Atherosclerosis by Simvastatin A Serial Intravascular Ultrasound Study. *Circulation* 2004;110:265-270

[41] Nissen S, Tsunoda T, Tuzcu M, Schoenhagen P, Cooper Ch, Yasin M, Eaton G, Lauer M, Sheldon S, Grines C, Halpern S, Crowe T, Blankenship J, Kerensky R. Effect of recombinant ApoA-I Milano on coronary atherosclerosis in patients with acure coronary syndromes. A randomized contrlled trial. *JAMA* 2003;290:2292-2300

[42] Yamada T, Azuma A, Sasaki S, Sawada T, Matsubara H, on behalf of REACH study group. Randomized evaluation of atorvastatin in pateints with coronary heart disease . A serial intravascular ultrasound study. *Circ J* 2007;71:1845-1850

[43] Nissen S, Tardif JD, Nicholls S, Revkin J, Shear Ch, Duggan W, Ruzyllo W, Bachinsky W, Lasala G, Tuzcu M, for the ILLUSTRATE Investigators. Effect of Torcetrapib on the Progression of Coronary Atherosclerosis. *N Engl J Med* 2007;356:1304-16

[44] Nakayamaa T, Komiyamab N,Yokoyamaa M, Namikawaa S, Kurodaa N, Kobayashia Y, Komuroa I. Pioglitazone induces regression of coronary atherosclerotic plaques in patients with type 2 diabetes mellitus or impaired glucose tolerance: A randomized prospective study using intravascular ultrasound. *Int J Cardiol.* 2010;138:157-65

[45] Kovarnik T, Mintz GS, Skalicka H, Kral A Horak J, Skulec R, Uhrova J, Martasek P, Downe RW, Wahle A, Sonka M, Mrazek V, Aschermann M, Linhart A Virtual histology evaluation of atherosclerosis regression during atorvastatin and ezetimibe administration - HEAVEN study. *Circulation Journal* 2011; ahead of print

[46] Clementi F, Luozzo M, Mango R, Luciani G, Trivisonno A, Pizzuto F, Martuscelli E, Mehta JL, Romeo F. Regression and shift in composition of coronary atherosclerosis plaques by pioglitazione: insight from an intravascular ultrasound analysis. J *Cardiovasc Med* 2009;10:231-237

[47] Nasu K, Tsuchikane E, Katoh O, Tanaka N, Kimura M,Ehara M,Kinoshita Y, Matsubara Matsuo T, Asakura K, Asakura Y, Terashima M,Takayama T, Honye J, Hirayama A, Saito S, Suzuki T. Effect of Fluvastatin on Progression of Coronary Atherosclerotic Plaque Evaluated by Virtual Histology Intravascular Ultrasound. JACC Cradiovasc Interv. 2009;2:689-969

[48] Serruys PW, García-García HM, Buszman P. Erne P, Verheye S, Aschermann M, Duckers H, Bleie O, Dudek D, Bøtker HE, von Birgelen C, Don D'Amico, MA, Hutchinson T, Zambanini A, Mastik F, van Es GA, van der Steen A, Vince G, Ganz, Hamm ChW, Wijns W, Zalewski A, for the Integrated Biomarker and Imaging Study-2 Investigators. Effects of the Direct Lipoprotein-Associated Phospholipase A2 Inhibitor Darapladib on Human Coronary Atherosclerotic Plaque. *Circulation* 2008;118:1172-1182

[49] Kawasaki M, Sano K, Okubo M, Yokoyama H, Ito Y, Murata I,Tsuchiya K, Minatoguchi S, Zhou X, Fujita H, Fujiwara H. Volumetric Quantitative Analysis of Tissue Characteristics of Coronary Plaques After Statin Therapy Using Three-Dimensional Integrated Backscatter Intravascular Ultrasound. J Am Coll Cardiol 2005;45: 1946–53

[50] Hong MK, Park DW, Lee ChW, Lee SW, Kim YH, Kang DH, et al. Effect of statin treatment on coronary plaques assessed by volumetric virtual histology intravascular ultrasound analysis. *J Am Coll Intv* 2009;2:679-688

[51] Garcia-Garcia HM, Gogas BD, Serruys PW, Bruining N. IVUS-based imaging modalities for tissue characterization: similarities and differences. *Int J Cardiovasc Imaging* 2011;27:215-224

[52] Azen SP, Mack WJ, Cashin-Hemphill L et al. Progression of coronary artery disease predicts clinical coronary events. Long-term follow-up from the Cholesterol Lowering Atherosclerosis Study. *Circulation* 1996;93:34-41

[53] von Birgelen C, Hartmann M, Mintz GS et al. Relationship between cardiovascular risk as predicted by established risk scores versus plaque progression as measured by serial intravascular ultrasound in left main coronary arteries. *Circulation* 2004;110:1579-1585

[54] Ricciardi MJ, Meyers S, Choi K, Pang JL, Goodreau L, Davidson CJ. Angiographically silent left main disease detected by intravascular ultrasound: a marker for future adverse cardiac events. Am Heart J 2003;146:507–12
[55] Bose D, von Birgelen C, Erbel R. Intravascular ultrasound for the evaluation of therapies targeting coronary atherosclerosis. J Am Coll Cardiol 2007;49:925-932

5

IVUS in the Assessment of Coronary Allograft Vasculopathy

Sudhir S. Kushwaha and Eugenia Raichlin
Mayo Clinic and University of Nebraska Medical Center
USA

1. Introduction

Cardiac allograft vasculopathy (CAV) is a unique form of accelerated atherosclerosis and remains the leading cause of late morbidity and mortality in heart transplant patients accounting for 30% mortality at 5 years (Miller et al., 1993), (Taylor et al., 2007).
Although the pathogenesis of CAV is not fully elucidated, it seems to result from a complex interplay between immunologic and nonimmunologic factors, with consequent repetitive vascular injury and a localized sustained inflammatory response (Costanzo et al., 1998), (Julius et al., 2000). CAV affects large epicardial vessels and the microcirculation which results in a progressive luminal narrowing (Gao et al., 1990) and reduces myocardial blood flow (Kushwaha et al., 1998). CAV may be present in intramyocardial vessels even if epicardial disease is not evident (Clausell et al., 1995). Autopsy findings have demonstrated the presence of CAV in nearly all specimens at two years and changes are seen as early as 6 weeks after cardiac transplant (Baldwin et al., 1987), (St. Goar et al., 1992).
Early CAV is clinically silent, and ischemia is usually not evident until the disease is far advanced (Ciliberto et al., 1993), (Collings et al., 1994, (Mairesse et al., 1995), (Smart et al., 1991), (Stark et al., 1991) and graft failure tends to develop as a late manifestation of the disease. Therefore, identification of the asymptomatic patient at early stages of the disease is an important strategy for the prevention of irreversible detrimental effects on the graft.

2. IVUS and allograft vasculopathy

2.1 Limitations of coronary angiogram

Noninvasive screening tests for CAV such as the exercise electrocardiogram, thallium scintigraphy, and exercise radionucleotide ventriculography have shown insufficient sensitivity and specificity for reliable detection of CAV (Smart, 1991). Traditionally, **coronary angiography** has been used for the diagnosis of CAV and, according to the amount of stenosis in the most severely affected vessel, CAV is usually classified as absent (0% stenosis), mild (up to 30% stenosis), moderate (30–70% stenosis), or severe (>70% stenosis).
However, coronary angiography, given that it basically provides images in the form of a lumenogram, has been shown to systematically underestimate the presence of coronary atherosclerosis in transplant recipients as validated in autopsy studies (St. Goar et al., 1992), (Dressler et al., 1992). No information on vessel wall structure and intimal thickening is provided by coronary angiography. Being a highly specific (97.8%) tool, the diffuse nature of

CAV limits the sensitivity of coronary angiography to 79.3% (Sharples et al., 2003), (St. Goar et al., 1992). As a result, one fifth of patients with CAV have false normal coronary angiography (Sharples et al., 2003). Moreover, the reported 50% negative predictive value (Cale et al. 2010) limits the clinical utility of routine angiographic surveillance for CAV in heart transplant recipients. Based on these limitations, at least one transplant center has abandoned coronary angiogram for routine monitoring of heart-transplant recipients (Clague et al., 2001).

Intravascular ultrasound (IVUS) is a safe and reproducible imaging technique (Batkoff et al., 1996) that is more sensitive than angiography and useful for the early diagnosis of CAV, morphometric and volumetric analysis, assessing plaque composition and vessel remodeling (Miller et al., 1995), (Pflugfelder et al., 1993), (St. Goar et al., 1992), (Yeung et al., 1995). Whereas angiographic disease is present in 10% to 20% of patients at 1 year and 50% by 5 years after transplantation (Gao et al., 1988), (Uretsky et al., 1987) the prevalence of abnormal intimal thickening is seen in 50% of patients by 1 year in IVUS imaging (Gao et al., 1988), (Tuzcu et al., 1996), (Yeung et al., 1995). Therefore, IVUS is now considered the "gold standard" for the evaluation of CAV (Kapadia et al., 2000).

2.2 Lesion morphology and quantitative analysis

IVUS reveals cross sectional coronary artery image, which in post-transplant patients typically have tri-laminar appearance (Figure 1) with bright inner layer (intima), an echo-fine middle layer (media) and a bright dense outer layer (adventitia); and allows the following measurements: (1) maximal intimal thickness (MIT) as the greatest distance from the intimal leading edge to media-adventitia border, (2) minimal intimal thickness as the shortest distance from the intimal leading edge to media-adventitia border, (3) minimal luminal diameter as the shortest distance between opposing intimal leading edges, (4) lumen area as the area within the boundaries of the intimal leading edge, (5) vessel area as the area within the media-adventitia border, (6) plaque cross-sectional area as the difference between vessel and lumen areas, (7) plaque index as (lumen area/vessel area) X 100, and (8) eccentric index: [(maximal plaque thickness - minimal plaque thickness)/ maximal plaque thickness] X 100 (Figure 2).

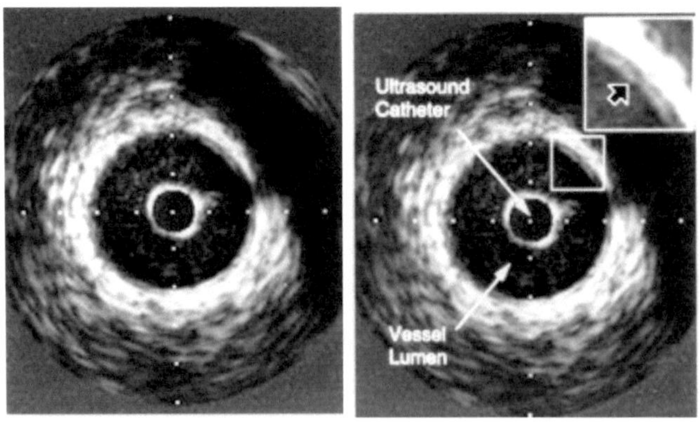

Adapter from Tuzcu et al., 1995

Inset shows the three layers of the vessel wall (black arrow). The thin echogenic inner layer corresponds to the intima, the thin echolucent middle layer to the media, and the echogenic outer layer to the adventitia

Fig. 1. Ultrasound image of a normal coronary artery

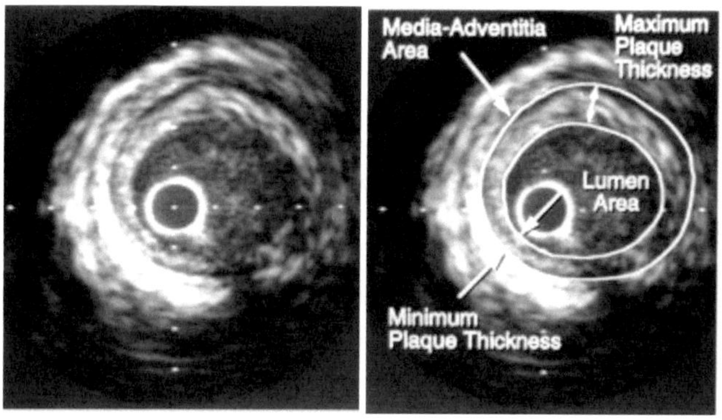

Adapted from Tuzcu et al., 1995

Fig. 2. Measurements of lumen and vessel wall dimensions in an ultrasound image

The maximal intimal thickness (MIT) assessed by 2D-IVUS is a commonly used measure to describe the severity of lesions and has been defined as a clinically useful surrogate for clinical outcome (Mehra et al., 1995a), (Rickenbacher et al., 1995a). The threshold of MIT > 0.5 mm is usually acceptable (Kapadia et al., 2000), but this categorical classification of MIT, a continuous variable, into normal or abnormal is inherently arbitrary. This definition, however, is based on information provided by histological and ultrasound studies. In an autopsy study, normal intimal thickness, not including media, ranged between 0.10 and 0.30 mm in individuals between 21 and 40 years of age (Sims et al., 2002), (Velican et al., 1985). Therefore, intimal thickness > 0.3 mm is considered to represent significant CAV. A classification of the vascular disease severity according to **intimal thickness** and degree of vessel circumference involved was proposed by the Stanford group (Table 1).
The thickness of the **media** is usually about 0.02-0.23 mm and is unchanged or decreased with the development of CAV. Thus, the thickness of the normal **intima plus media** in young and middle age individuals ranges from 0.45 to 0.50 mm. (Sims et al., 2002), (Velican et al., 1985).

	Class			
	I	II	III	IV
Severity	Minimal	Mild	Moderate	Severe
Intimal thickness	<0.3 mm	>0.3 mm	0.3–0.5 mm	>1.0 mm
			or	or
	<180°	>180°	>0.5 mm, <180°	>0.5 mm, >180°

Adapted from St. Goar, 1992

Table 1. Ultrasound classification of CAV in cardiac transplant recipients)

Despite this immense value of IVUS in the detection of CAV, there is controversy regarding the methodology and imaging protocols. Site selection and adequate sampling for quantitative analysis is crucial. Most studies have selectively visualized the LAD, making the assumption that CAV occurs uniformly throughout the coronary tree. It has been demonstrated, that multi-vessel imaging is definitely more sensitive in detecting transplant vasculopathy lesions compared to single-vessel imaging (Kapadia, 2000), and sampling of a single coronary artery for imaging may not be sufficient to adequately assess the prevalence of CAV. However, multi-vessel imaging is time consuming, adds to the cost of the procedure and, although procedural complications other than occasional spasm resolved with intracoronary nitroglycerin did not occur, the long-term safety of the multi-vessel imaging remains unknown. Thus, the limitations of single vessel imaging should be weighed against the potential benefits from adequate sampling of multi-vessel imaging.

2.3 Three-dimensional reconstruction (3D-IVUS)

2D-IVUS has limitation in spatial registration and the inability to assess the full extent of vascular disease (Tuzcu, 2005) which reduces its sensitivity to detect the changes of atherosclerotic burden in CAV. Three-dimensional (3D-IVUS) reconstruction allows rapid and accurate measurement of volume and plaque dimensions with full extent of atherosclerotic pathology. Automated pullback with a known pullback speed is necessary. The vessel, lumen and plaque volume can be calculated using the Simpson rule for images that are 1 mm apart. Since the histology literature does not commonly depend on volumetric indices, currently, there is no well-defined threshold for these measurements and the information is not readily obtainable. Because of its superior reproducibility, however, 3D-IVUS may be used to assess the progression of coronary artery disease and allow for more accurate evaluation of interventions aimed at preventing or attenuating coronary artery disease (Bae et al., 2006), (White et al., 2003).

2.4 Virtual Histology Intravascular Ultrasound (VH-IVUS)

Grayscale IVUS is able to visualize coronary atherosclerosis in vivo and allows rapid and accurate assessment of plaque area and distribution, lesion length, and coronary remodelling (Bae et al., 2006), (Kapadia et al., 2000), (White et al., 2003), but has a significant limitation in the evaluation of atherosclerotic plaque composition.

VH-IVUS is a novel technology to characterize the different types of plaque morphology in vivo which based on the spectral analysis of the radiofrequency ultrasound signals in a frequency domain (Nair et al., 2002), (Nasu et al., 2006), (Rodriguez-Granillo et al., 2005). It displays the reconstructed color coded tissue map of plaque composition overlaid on a grey-scale image and groups plaque components into 4 basic tissue types: fibrous tissue (green), fibro-fatty tissue (light green), necrotic core (red), and dense calcium (white). (Figure 3) This approach has not been validated with histological techniques in heart transplant patients, however in the non-transplant population the overall predictive accuracies were 90.4% for fibrous tissue, 92.8% for fibrolipidic, 89.5% necrotic core, and 90.9% for dense calcium (Nair et al, 2001), (Nair et al, 2002), (Nasu et al, 2006). In native coronaries morphological composition of atherosclerotic plaque is a useful determinant of the plaque vulnerability (Ehara et al., 2004), (Naghavi et al., 2003), (Valgimigli et al., 2007), and identified plaques with a high-risk of future clinical events (Bae et al., 2008), (Kawaguchi et al., 2007), (Kawamoto et al., 2007). After heart transplantation, simultaneous assessment of virtual histology with IVUS provides detailed information about plaque morphology and composition, may improve the risk stratification of heart transplant recipients (Konig et al., 2008) and add important information in the clinical evaluation of heart transplant recipients (Raichlin et al., 2009).

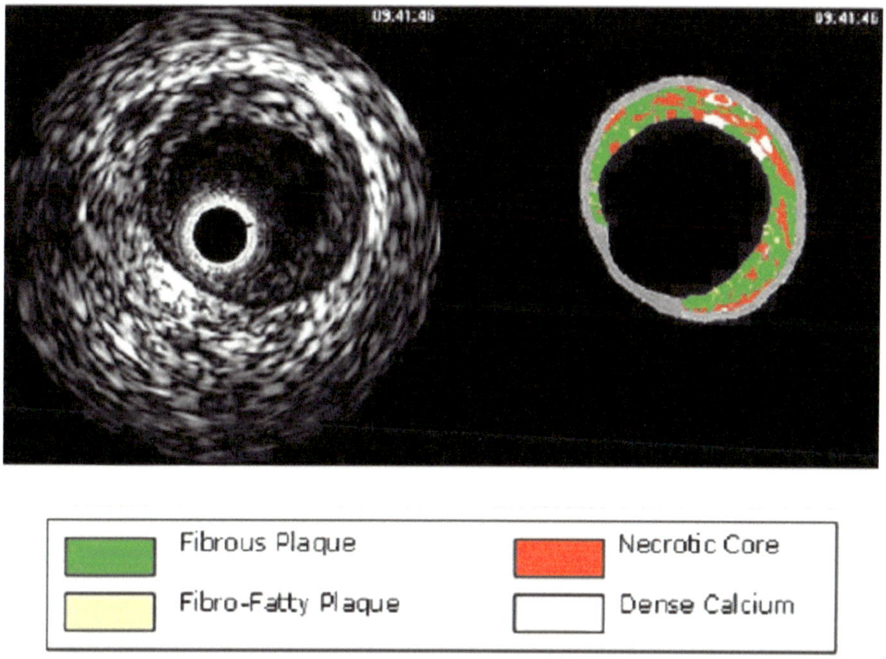

(Left) Gray scale IVUS cross-section imaging shows concentric plaque: a (PV/SL) of 6.79 and a PI of 32% was calculated

(Right) The corresponding VH-IVUS image depicts specific color-coded plaque components and demonstrates fibrous plaque of 47%, fibrofatty plaque of 20%, dense calcium of 14%, and necrotic core of 27%.PV/SL, plaque volume normalized for segment length; PI, plaque index

Adapted from Raichlin et al., 2007b

Fig. 3. Gray scale IVUS cross-section imaging shows concentric plaque with corresponding VH-IVUS image

2.5 Impact of IVUS in understanding coronary allograft vasculopathy

Morphologic studies performed with IVUS have led to important insights into the etiology and pathogenesis of CAV.

Coronary artery vasculopathy (CAV) is a multifactorial phenomenon with variable morphologic features. Previous histological ex-vivo studies described two microscopic types of coronary allograft lesions (Johnson, 1989). One type of coronary lesion is confined to the proximal region of epicardial arteries and indistinguishable from typical atherosclerosis of native vessels. The second type is characterized by the presence of vasculitis, involving the entire coronary arterial system and has been suggested to represent the immune mediated vessel injury (Higuchi et al., 1999). The ability to differentiate between the existence of classic atherosclerosis and transplant-specific immunologically mediated CAV holds both prognostic and therapeutic values and this

morphologic heterogeneity has been evident in gray scale (Tuzcu et al., 1996) and VH-IVUS study (Raichlin et al., 2009).
Typical atherosclerosis has been detected in 56% of donor hearts despite a mean donor age of thirty-two years (Tuzcu et al., 1995) and IVUS studies have demonstrated that atherosclerotic lesions located in proximal segments, involved the bifurcation sites with eccentric focal plaques, appeared similar to conventional atherosclerosis, were associated with fibrotic and fibro-fatty tissues in VH-IVUS (Konig et al., 2008), (Raichlin et al., 2009) positively correlated with the donor age and probably related to donor-derived coronary atherosclerosis (Kapadia et al., 1998), (Tuzcu et al., 1996).
On other hand de novo lesions assessed by IVUS were diffuse and circumferential, involved more commonly the mid and distal segments of the coronary arteries (Kapadia et al., 1998) and were associated with necrotic core and dense calcium burden ≥ 30%, which presumably reflects the inflammatory burden of the cardiac allograft atherosclerotic plaque (Raichlin et al., 2009). (Figure 4)
Previous studies have demonstrated that early immunological events surrounding engraftment lead to an inflammatory process in the vascular endothelium (Brunner-La Rocca et al., 1998), (Caforio et al., 2004), (Hornick et al., 1997), (Jimenez et al., 2001), (Narrod et al., 1989), (Opelz et al., 1997), (Vassalli et al., 2003), (Yamani et al., 2002). Although CAV may develop at any stage after transplantation, events during the first year, resulting most likely from initial and ongoing immunologically mediated injury to the vascular endothelium appear to be important in CAV pathogenesis (Kobashigawa et al., 2003) leading to more rapid progression in intimal thickening during the first year after transplantation (Kobashigawa et al., 1995), (Mehra et al., 1995d), (Rickenbacher et al., 1995a). A cross-sectional study demonstrated a mean absolute increase of 0.23 mm 10% in intimal thickening and intimal index respectively (Kobashigawa, 1995) during the first year of transplantation. After the first year, the intimal thickness and intimal area do not increase rapidly but new lesions continue to develop at previously normal sites (Kapadia SR et al., 1998). This underscores the importance for continued surveillance for transplant vasculopathy beyond first year after transplantation.
A relationship between immune events and an increase in systemic inflammatory markers following heart transplantation has been shown in several clinical studies (Eisenberg, 2000), (Labarrere, 2002) suggesting that chronic inflammation may be a central event in cardiac allograft vasculopathy. Experimental evidence demonstrated that acute cellular allograft rejection and CAV are closely related processes (Brunner-La Rocca et al., 1998), (Caforio et al., 2004), (Hornick et al., 1997), (Jimenez et al., 2001), (Narrod et al., 1989), (Opelz et al., 1997), (Vassalli et al., 2003), (Yamani et al., 2005) and elevated systemic levels of the inflammatory markers were predictive not only of cardiac allograft vasculopathy but also of allograft failure (Eisenberg & Pethig, 2000), (Hognestad et al., 2003), (Labarrere et al., 2002), (Raichlin et al., 2007b). An association between early recurrent cellular rejections and an increase in intimal thickening (Mehra et al., 1995a) and the presence of necrotic plaque (Raichlin et al., 2007b) has been revealed in 2D and VH-IVUS studies. Moreover, focal inflammation as assessed by VH-IVUS resulted in subsequent progression of CAV. Thus, VH-IVUS can be used for in-vivo identification of patients with increased burden of "inflammatory plaque" and the predicting the progression of CAV following heart transplantation (Raichlin et al., 2009). (Figure 5)

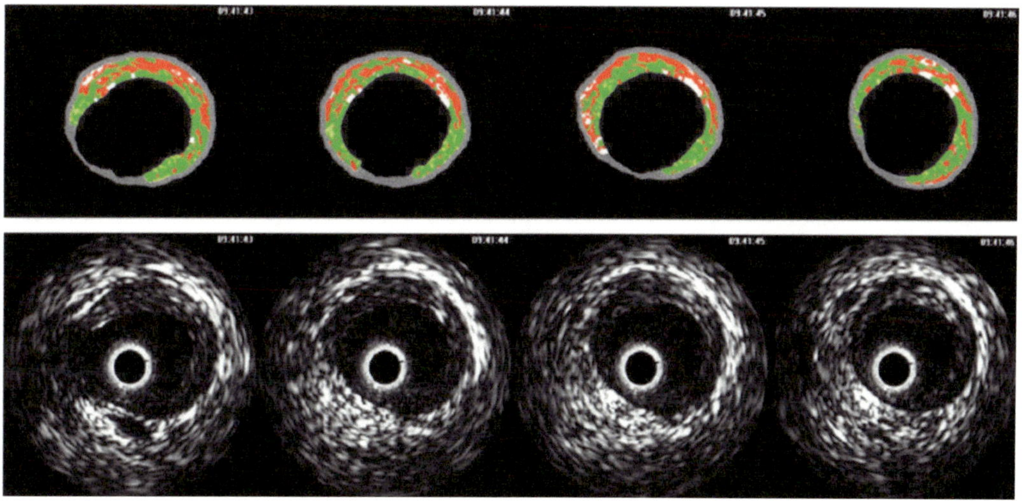

Adapted from Raichlin et al., 2009

Fig. 4. Grayscale intravascular ultrasound (IVUS) cross-section imaging (bottom) and corresponding virtual histology (VH)-IVUS images (top) from patients with VH-IVUS-derived inflammatory plaque

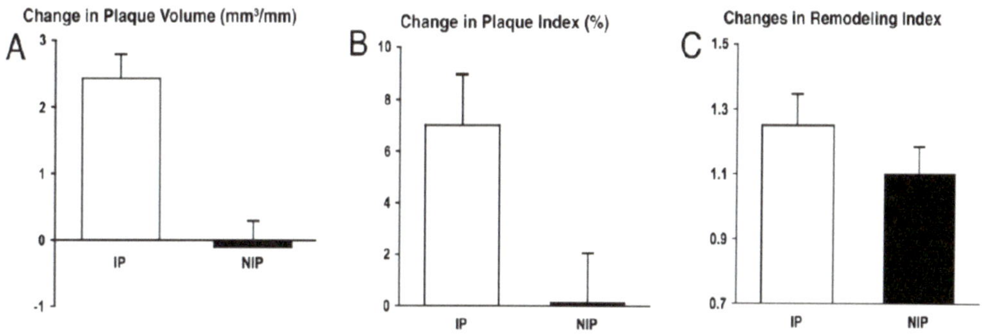

A Progression in plaque volume in VH-IVUS derived inflammatory plaque (IP) and noninflammatory plaque (NIP) groups
Change in Plaque Volume (mm3/mm) **IP** (n=21) 2.42 ± 1.78; **NIP** (n=17) -0.11±1.65; p=0.01
B Progression in plaque index in the in VH-IVUS derived inflammatory plaque (IP) and noninflammatory plaque (NIP) groups
Change in Plaque Index (%): **IP** (n=21) 7± 9; **NIP** (n=17) 0.1± 8; p=0.04
C Remodeling index in VH-IVUS derived inflammatory plaque (IP) and noninflammatory plaque (NIP) groups
Remodeling Index: **IP** (n=21) 1.24 ± 0.44, **NIP** (n=17) 1.09 ± 0.36; p=0.03

Adapted from Raichlin et al., 2009

Fig. 5. Progression in Plaque Volume, Plaque Index, and Remodeling Index in IP and NIP Groups

The natural history of donor lesions after transplantation is largely unknown. In the 2010 ISHLT registry older donor age is an independent risk factor for early CAV (Stehlik et al.,

1089). Several studies, however, have found no significant difference in the rate of intimal thickening between patients with donor hearts having pre-existing coronary artery disease and those without (Botas et al., 1995), (Li et al., 2006). From multiple variables only serum triglyceride level and pre-transplant body mass index were found to be significant predictors for the progression of donor atherosclerosis (Kapadia SR et al., 1998). A VH-IVUS study has demonstrated relatively slow progression of CAV in a group of patients with fibrous, presumably donor-derived plaque (Raichlin et al., 2009).(Figure 5) Several studies, however, have shown that the presence of donor lesions leads to the more frequent development of de novo transplant vasculopathy lesions (Botas et al., 1995), (Escobar et al., 1994), (Gao et al., 1997). The impact of donor and recipient gender on transplant vasculopathy has also been assessed. Male recipients of a female allograft had a higher degree of vascular intimal hyperplasia compared with either male or female recipients of a male allograft as detected by IVUS imaging 1 year after heart transplantation (Mehra et al., 1994).

Arterial remodeling has been studied in the transplant population in serial and cross-sectional IVUS study designs. In its early stages, CAV shows no decrease in luminal diameter due to vascular remodeling, thus limiting the ability of angiography to detect and diagnose early CAV (Nissen et al., 2001). Three year serial IVUS studies have shown that the rate of remodeling of donor lesions is different from CAV. Furthermore, the rate of remodeling is different depending on the time interval from transplantation (Ziada et al., 1997). Both compensatory local vessel enlargement (positive remodeling) and vascular constriction (negative remodeling) have been demonstrated and it is thought that inadequate compensatory enlargement probably contributes significantly to luminal obstruction (Pethig et al., 1998). In a study of 3D-VH-IVUS, the coronary arteries with "inflammatory plaque" showed positive remodeling compared to "non-inflammatory plaque" (Raichlin et al., 2009).(Figure 5) These data are consistent with previous findings from a non-transplant population, which showed that inflammation is associated with expansion of the internal elastic lamina and positive remodeling closely correlates with plaque vulnerability (Burke et al., 2004), (Rodriguez-Granillo et al., 2006).

IVUS imaging has also have been used to evaluate the impact of non-immunological factors in the development of transplant vasculopathy lesions. Total cholesterol, low-density lipoprotein cholesterol, triglyceride levels, obesity indexes, donor age greater than 35, and years following cardiac transplantation were independent predictors of the severity of cardiac allograft vasculopathy as determined by the severity of intimal thickening (Escobar et al.,, 1994), (Hauptman et al., 1995), (Mehra et al., 1995), (Rickenbacher et al., 1995b), (Valantine et al., 1995).

2.6 Clinical applications

Studies performed using IVUS have shown a strong association between the severity of the disease and the clinical outcome. Severe intimal thickening predicted both events (death, MI, and re-transplantation) and survival in patients after transplantation (Mehra et al., 1995b), (Mehra et al., 1995c) regardless of the presence of angiographic CAV (Rickenbacher et al., 1995b). Moreover, rapidly progressive vasculopathy, defined as an increase of ≥ 0.5 mm in intimal thickness within the first year after transplantation, was a powerful predictor of all-cause mortality, nonfatal MI, and the subsequent development of angiographic coronary obstructions independent of other confounding variables, including rejection episodes, age, gender, and conventional risk factors (Kobashigawa et al., 2005), (Tuzcu et al.,

2005). (Figure 6 and 7) Thus, the prognostic value of IVUS has significant clinical utility in the identification of a high-risk population and underscores the importance of serial IVUS examinations (Kapadia et al., 1999).

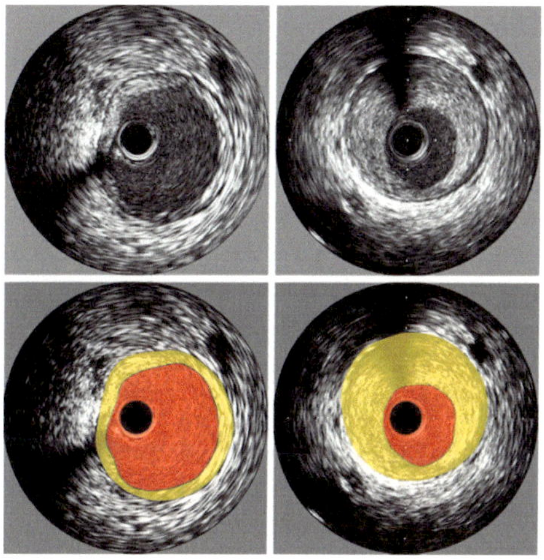

Adapted from Tuzcu et al., 2010

Fig. 6. Serial intravascular ultrasound examination at baseline (left side panel) and 1 year follow-up (right side panel) demonstrates significant plaque development at the first year. Transplant vasculopathy at the same site in a coronary vessel segment

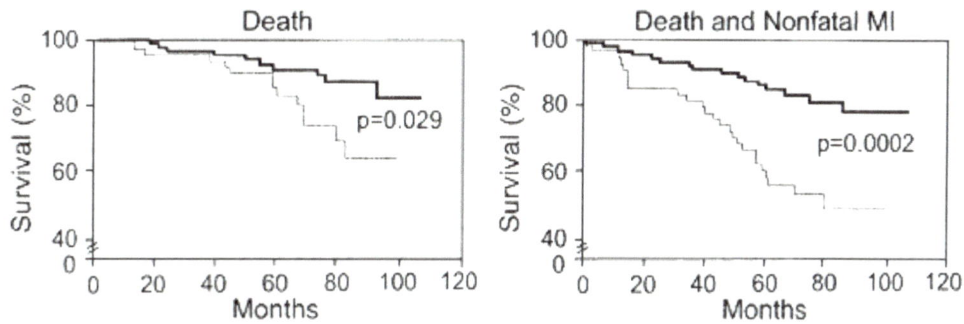

Adapted from Tuzcu et al., 2005

Fig. 7. Kaplan-Meier all-cause mortality **(left)** and death and myocardial infarction (MI) **(right)** rates of patients with and without rapidly progressive transplant vasculopathy. Thick lines - without rapid progression; thin lines - with rapid progression

IVUS also provides a sensitive tool to evaluate the effectiveness of different therapeutic and preventive modalities influencing CAV and various clinical protocols have incorporated IVUS findings as surrogate end-points for clinical events. Serial IVUS has been essential as a research tool in studies that assess emerging transplant vasculopathy therapies (Bae et al., 2006), (Eisen et al., 2003), (Fang et al., 2002), (Mehra et al., 1995c), (Raichlin et al., 2007a). The effects of early use of pravastatin on CAV have been assessed by IVUS imaging in a randomized study (Kobashigawa, 1995). 2D-IVUS measurements at baseline and 1 year after

transplantation showed less increase in MIT and maximal intimal index with pravastatin therapy. The incidence of coronary vasculopathy as determined by angiography and at autopsy also was lower (Kobashigawa, 1995).
The influence of angiotensin-converting enzyme inhibitors and calcium blockers on the development of CAV has also been assessed. Mehra et al., using IVUS, demonstrated that heart transplant recipients treated with either diltiazem or angiotensin-converting enzyme inhibitors, or both have significantly less intimal hyperplasia 1 year after cardiac transplantation than matched untreated control subjects (Mehra et al., 1995b), (Mehra et al., 1995c). Another IVUS study has demonstrated that a combination of a calcium channel blocker and an angiotensin-converting enzyme inhibitors is more effective in CAV prevention than the individual use of either drug alone. This effect was independent of mean arterial pressure, suggesting these drugs have a synergistic anti-proliferative effect beyond the anti-hypertensive efficacy (Erinc et al., 2005). Moreover, a 3D-IVUS study demonstrated that lower serum lipid levels and angiotensin-converting enzyme inhibitors use in patients after heart transplantation is associated with CAV plaque regression (Bae et al., 2006). The question of whether supplementation with antioxidant vitamins C and E retards the early progression of CAV has also been assessed by 2D-IVUS (Fang et al., 2002).
IVUS imaging has been used to evaluate the effect of immunosuppressive therapy on the development of CAV. A randomized, double-blind trial, comparing mycophenolate mofetil with azathioprine as adjuvant to cyclosporine, revealed that the change in mean MIT was less for the mycophenolate mofetil group than for the azathioprine group ($p = 0.056$) (Eisen et al., 2005).
The first clinical evidence that proliferation signal inhibitors (PSIs) could limit the development of CAV in heart transplant recipients was provided by an international multicenter randomized, double-blind study (Eisen et al., 2003) comparing everolimus with azathioprine as adjuvant to full dose of cyclosporin in 634 de-novo heart transplant patients. The results of the intravascular substudy with matched analysis of baseline and 1-year images were available for 211 patients. The average increase in intimal thickness was significantly larger with azathioprine than with everolimus. The 12 months of double-blind period of this study were followed by 12 month of open-labeled period (Vigano et al., 2007) in 149 patients and showed that continued treatment with everolimus limits the progression of intimal thickening and lowers the incidence of allograft vasculopathy at 24 months when compared with azathioprine.
Similar benefits have also been seen in patients treated with sirolimus. In an open-labeled study (Keogh, 2004) of 136 de-novo transplant patients randomized to sirolimus or azathioprine, IVUS showed that the use of sirolimus significantly reduced the progression in intimal and media proliferation by six months, whereas azathioprine therapy resulted in increased plaque volume and plaque burden over time. This effect was sustained at two years.
The first evidence of using sirolimus for primary immunosuppression after heart transplantation demonstrated that complete CNI withdrawal and replacement with SRL results in attenuation of CAV progression by reducing intimal hyperplasia as evidenced by 3D-IVUS. Treatment with azathioprine or mycophenolate mofetil did not significantly affect the results. A CNI-free regimen was more effective when initiated within the first two years following transplantation (Raichlin et al., 2007a).

3. Conclusion

Coronary angiography has a high specificity of 97.8% but only moderate sensitivity of 79.3% in CAV detection. The intimal changes in CAV are best detected by intravascular ultrasound, which has become the gold standard for the early diagnosis of CAV. The prognostic value of IVUS has significant clinical utility in identification a high-risk population and underscores the importance of serial IVUS examinations during annual routine screening of heart transplant recipients. 3D-IVUS with simultaneous assessment of virtual histology may add important information in the clinical evaluation of heart transplant recipients.

4. References

Bae, J.H., Rihal, C.S., Edwards, B.S., Kushwaha, S.S., Mathew, V., Prasad, A., et al. (2006). Association of Angiotensin-Converting Enzyme Inhibitors and Serum Lipids With Plaque Regression in Cardiac Allograft Vasculopathy. *Transplantation.* Oct 27;82(8):1108-11

Bae, J.H., Kwon, T.G., Hyun, D.W., Rihal, C.S., & Lerman, A. (2008). Predictors of Slow Flow During Primary Percutaneous Coronary Intervention: an Intavascular Ultrasound-Virtual Histology Study. *Heart.* 1:1

Baldwin, J.C., Oyer, P.E., Stinson, E.B., Starnes, V.A., Billingham, M.E., & Shumway, N.E. (1987). Comparison of cardiac rejection in heart and heart-lung transplantation. *J Heart Transplant.* 6(6):352-6

Batkoff, B.W., Linker, D.T. (1996). Safety of intracoronary ultrasound: data from a Multicenter European Registry. *Cathet Cardiovasc Diagn.* 38(3):238-41

Botas, J., Pinto, F.J., Chenzbraun, A., Liang, D., Schroeder, J.S., Oesterle, S.N., et al. (1995). Influence of preexistent donor coronary artery disease on the progression of transplant vasculopathy. An intravascular ultrasound study. *Circulation.* 92(5):1126-32

Brunner-La Rocca, H.P., Schneider, J., Kunzli, A., Turina, M., & Kiowski, W. (1998). Cardiac allograft rejection late after transplantation is a risk factor for graft coronary artery disease. *Transplantation.* Feb 27;65(4):538-43

Burke, A.P., Kolodgie, F.D., Zieske, A., Fowler, D.R., Weber, D.K., Varghese, P.J., et al. (2004). Morphologic findings of coronary atherosclerotic plaques in diabetics: a postmortem study. *Arterioscler Thromb Vasc Biol.* 24(7):1266-71

Caforio, A.L., Tona, F., Fortina, A.B., Angelini, A., Piaserico, S., Gambin,o A., et al. (2004). Immune and nonimmune predictors of cardiac allograft vasculopathy onset and severity: multivariate risk factor analysis and role of immunosuppression. *Am J Transplant.* Jun;4(6):962-70

Cale, R., Almeida, M., Rebocho, M.J., Aguiar, C., Sousa, P., Brito, J., et al. (2010). The value of routine intracoronary ultrasound to assess coronary artery disease in cardiac allograft recipients. *Rev Port Cardiol.* Feb;29(2):231-41

Ciliberto, G.R., Mangiavacchi, M., Banfi, F., Massa, D., Danzi, G., Cataldo, G., et al. (1993). Coronary artery disease after heart transplantation: non-invasive evaluation with exercise thallium scintigraphy. *Eur Heart J.* 14(2):226-9

Clague, J.R., Cox, I.D., Murday, A.J., Charokopos, N., & Madden, B.P. (2001). Low clinical utility of routine angiographic surveillance in the detection and management of cardiac allograft vasculopathy in transplant recipients. *Clin Cardiol.* 24(6):459-62

Clausell, N., Butany, J., Molossi, S., Lonn, E., Gladstone, P., Rabinovitch, M., et al. (1995). Abnormalities in intramyocardial arteries detected in cardiac transplant biopsy specimens and lack of correlation with abnormal intracoronary ultrasound or endothelial dysfunction in large epicardial coronary arteries. *J Am Coll Cardiol.* 26(1):110-9

Collings, C.A., Pinto, F.J., Valantine, H.A., Popylisen, S., Puryear, J.V., & Schnittger, I. (1994). Exercise echocardiography in heart transplant recipients: a comparison with angiography and intracoronary ultrasonography. *J Heart Lung Transplant.* 13(4):604-13

Costanzo, M.R., Naftel, D.C., Pritzker, M.R., Heilman, J.K., 3rd, Boehmer. J.P., Brozena, S.C., et al. (1998). Heart transplant coronary artery disease detected by coronary angiography: a multiinstitutional study of preoperative donor and recipient risk factors. Cardiac Transplant Research Database. *J Heart Lung Transplant.* Aug;17(8):744-53

Dressler, F.A., & Miller, L.W. (1992). Necropsy versus angiography: how accurate is angiography? *J Heart Lung Transplant.* 11(3 Pt 2):S56-9

Ehara, S., Kobayashi, Y., Yoshiyama ,M., Shimada, K., Shimada, Y., Fukuda, D., et al. (2004). Spotty calcification typifies the culprit plaque in patients with acute myocardial infarction: an intravascular ultrasound study. Circulation. 110(22):3424-9. Epub 2004 Nov 22

Eisen, H.J., Tuzcu, E.M., Dorent, R., Kobashigawa, J., Mancini, D., Valantine-von Kaeppler, H.A., et al. (2003). Everolimus for the prevention of allograft rejection and vasculopathy in cardiac-transplant recipients. *N Engl J Med.* Aug 28;349(9):847-58

Eisen, H.J., Kobashigawa, J., Keogh, A., Bourge, R., Renlund, D., Mentzer, R., et al. (2005). Three-year results of a randomized, double-blind, controlled trial of mycophenolate mofetil versus azathioprine in cardiac transplant recipients. *J Heart Lung Transplant.* 24(5):517-25

Eisenberg, M.S., Chen, H.J., Warshofsky, M.K., Sciacca, R.R., Wasserman, H.S., Schwartz, A., et al. (2000). Elevated levels of plasma C-reactive protein are associated with decreased graft survival in cardiac transplant recipients. *Circulation.* Oct 24;102(17):2100-4

Erinc, K., Yamani, M.H., Starling, R.C., Crowe, T., Hobbs, R., Bott-Silverman, C., et al. (2005). The effect of combined angiotensin-converting enzyme inhibition and calcium antagonism on allograft coronary vasculopathy validated by intravascular ultrasound. *J Heart Lung Transplant.* Aug;24(8):1033-8

Escobar, A., Ventura, H.O., Stapleton, D.D., Mehra, M.R., Ramee, S.R., Collins, T.J, et al. (1994). Cardiac allograft vasculopathy assessed by intravascular ultrasonography and nonimmunologic risk factors. *Am J Cardiol.* 74(10):1042-6

Fang, J.C., Kinlay, S., Beltrame, J., Hikiti, H., Wainstein, M., Behrendt, D., et al. (2002). Effect of vitamins C and E on progression of transplant-associated arteriosclerosis: a randomised trial. *Lancet.* 359(9312):1108-13

Gao, S.Z., Alderman, E.L., Schroeder, J.S., Silverman, J.F., & Hunt, S.A. (1988). Accelerated coronary vascular disease in the heart transplant patient: coronary arteriographic findings. *J Am Coll Cardiol.* 12(2):334-40

Gao, S.Z., Alderman, E.L., Schroeder, J.S., Hunt, S.A., Wiederhold, V., & Stinson EB. (1990). Progressive coronary luminal narrowing after cardiac transplantation. *Circulation.* 82(5 Suppl):IV269-75

Gao, H.Z., Hunt, S.A., Alderman, E.L., Liang, D., Yeung, A.C., & Schroeder, J,S. (1997). Relation of donor age and preexisting coronary artery disease on angiography and intracoronary ultrasound to later development of accelerated allograft coronary artery disease. *J Am Coll Cardiol.* 29(3):623-9

Hauptman, P.J., Davis, S.F., Miller, L., & Yeung, A.C. (1995). The role of nonimmune risk factors in the development and progression of graft arteriosclerosis: preliminary insights from a multicenter intravascular ultrasound study. Multicenter Intravascular Ultrasound Transplant Study Group. *J Heart Lung Transplant.* 14(6 Pt 2):S238-42

Higuchi, M.L., Benvenuti, L.A., Demarchi, L.M., Libby ,P. (1999). Histological evidence of concomitant intramyocardial and epicardial vasculitis in necropsied heart allografts: a possible relationship with graft coronary arteriosclerosis. *Transplantation.* 67(12):1569-76

Hognestad, A., Endresen, K., Wergeland, R., Stokke, O., Geiran, O., Holm T., et al. (2003). Plasma C-reactive protein as a marker of cardiac allograft vasculopathy in heart transplant recipients. *J Am Coll Cardiol.* Aug 6;42(3):477-82

Hornick, P., Smith, J., Pomerance, A., Mitchell, A., Banner, N., Rose, M., et al. (1997). Influence of acute rejection episodes, HLA matching, and donor/recipient phenotype on the development of 'early' transplant-associated coronary artery disease. *Circulation.* Nov 4;96(9 Suppl):II-148-53

Jimenez, J., Kapadia, S.R., Yamani, M.H., Platt, L., Hobbs, R.E., Rincon, G., et al. (2001). Cellular rejection and rate of progression of transplant vasculopathy: a 3-year serial intravascular ultrasound study. *J Heart Lung Transplant.* Apr;20(4):393-8

Johnson, D.E., Gao, S.Z., Schroeder, J.S., DeCampli, W.M., & Billingham, M.E. (1989). The spectrum of coronary artery pathologic findings in human cardiac allografts. *J Heart Lung Transplant.* 8(5):349-59

Julius, B.K., Attenhofer Jost, C.H., Sutsch, G., Brunner, H.P., Kuenzli, A., Vogt, P.R., et al. (2000). Incidence, progression and functional significance of cardiac allograft vasculopathy after heart transplantation. *Transplantation.* 69(5):847-53

Kapadia, S.R., Ziada, K.M., Young, J.B., Hobbs, R.E., Guetta, V., Magyar , W.A., Nissen, S.E., & Tuzcu, E.M. (1998). Natural history of donor transmitted atherosclerosis in transplant patients: serial intravascular ultrasound study *J Am Coll Cardiol.* 31:856

Kapadia, S.R., Nissen, S.E., Ziada, K.M., Guetta, V., Crowe, T.D., Hobbs, R.E., et al. (1998). Development of transplantation vasculopathy and progression of donor-transmitted atherosclerosis: comparison by serial intravascular ultrasound imaging. *Circulation.* 98(24):2672-8

Kapadia, S.R., Nissen, S.E., Tuzcu, E.M. (1999). Impact of intravascular ultrasound in understanding transplant coronary artery disease. *Curr Opin Cardiol.* 14(2):140-50

Kapadia, S.R., Ziada, K.M., L'Allier, P.L., Crowe, T.D., Rincon, G., Hobbs, R.E., et al. (2000). Intravascular ultrasound imaging after cardiac transplantation: advantage of multi-vessel imaging. *J Heart Lung Transplant.* 19(2):167-72

Kawaguchi, R., Oshima, S., Jingu, M., Tsurugaya, H., Toyama, T., Hoshizaki, H., et al. (2007). Usefulness of virtual histology intravascular ultrasound to predict distal embolization for ST-segment elevation myocardial infarction. *J Am Coll Cardiol.* 50(17):1641-6

Kawamoto, T., Okura, H., Koyama, Y., Toda, I., Taguchi, H., Tamita, K., et al. (2007). The relationship between coronary plaque characteristics and small embolic particles during coronary stent implantation. *J Am Coll Cardiol.* 50(17):1635-40

Keogh, A., Richardson, M., Ruygrok, P., Spratt, P., Galbraith, A., O'Driscol, G., et al. (2004). Sirolimus in de novo heart transplant recipients reduces acute rejection and prevents coronary artery disease at 2 years: a randomized clinical trial. *Circulation.* Oct 26;110(17):2694-700

Kobashigawa, J.A., Katznelson, S., Laks, H., Johnson, J.A., Yeatman, L., Wang, X.M., et al. (1995). Effect of pravastatin on outcomes after cardiac transplantation. *N Engl J Med.* 333(10):621-7

Kobashigawa, J.A. (2003). First-year intravascular ultrasound results as a surrogate marker for outcomes after heart transplantation. *J Heart Lung Transplant.* 22(7):711-4

Kobashigawa, J.A., Tobis, J.M., Starling, R.C., Tuzcu, E.M., Smith, A.L., Valantine, H.A., et al. (2005). Multicenter intravascular ultrasound validation study among heart transplant recipients: outcomes after five years. *J Am Coll Cardiol.* May 3;45(9):1532-7

Konig, A, Kilian, E., Sohn, H.Y., Rieber, J., Schiele, T.M., Siebert, U., et al. (2008). Assessment and characterization of time-related differences in plaque composition by intravascular ultrasound-derived radiofrequency analysis in heart transplant recipients. *J Heart Lung Transplant.* 27(3):302-9

Kushwaha, S.S., Narula, J., Narula, N., Zervos, G., Semigran, M.J., Fischman, A.J., et al. (1998). Pattern of changes over time in myocardial blood flow and microvascular dilator capacity in patients with normally functioning cardiac allografts. *Am J Cardiol.* 82(11):1377-81

Labarrere, C.A., Lee, J.B., Nelson, D.R, Al-Hassani, M., Miller, S.J., & Pitts, D.E. (2002). C-reactive protein, arterial endothelial activation, and development of transplant coronary artery disease: a prospective study. *Lancet.* 2002 Nov 9;360(9344):1462-7

Li, H., Tanaka, K., Anzai, H., Oeser, B., Lai, D., Kobashigawa, J.A., et al. (2006). Influence of pre-existing donor atherosclerosis on the development of cardiac allograft vasculopathy and outcomes in heart transplant recipients. *J Am Coll Cardiol.* 47(12):2470-6. Epub 006 May 26

Mairesse, G.H., Marwick, T.H., Melin, J.A., Hanet, C., Jacquet, L., Dion, R., et al. (1995). Use of exercise electrocardiography, technetium-99m-MIBI perfusion tomography, and two-dimensional echocardiography for coronary disease surveillance in a low-prevalence population of heart transplant recipients. *J Heart Lung Transplant.* 14(2):222-9

Mehra, M.R., Stapleton, D.D., Ventura, H.O., Escobar, A., Cassidy, C.A., Smart, F.W., et al. (1994). Influence of donor and recipient gender on cardiac allograft vasculopathy. An intravascular ultrasound study. *Circulation.* 90(5 Pt 2):II78-82

Mehra, M.R., Ventura, H.O., Chambers, R., Collins, T.J, Ramee, S.R., Kates, M.A., et al. (1995). Predictive model to assess risk for cardiac allograft vasculopathy: an intravascular ultrasound study. *J Am Coll Cardiol.* 26(6):1537-44

Mehra, M.R., Ventura, H.O., Smart, F.W., Stapleton, D.D. (1995). Impact of converting enzyme inhibitors and calcium entry blockers on cardiac allograft vasculopathy: from bench to bedside. J Heart Lung Transplant. 14(6 Pt 2):S246-9

Mehra, M.R., Ventura, H.O., Smart, F.W., Collins, T.J., Ramee, S.R., & Stapleton, D.D. (1995). An intravascular ultrasound study of the influence of angiotensin-converting enzyme inhibitors and calcium entry blockers on the development of cardiac allograft vasculopathy. *Am J Cardiol.* 75(12):853-4

Mehra, M.R., Ventura, H.O., Stapleton, D.D., Smart, F.W., Collins, T.C., & Ramee, S.R. (1995). Presence of severe intimal thickening by intravascular ultrasonography predicts cardiac events in cardiac allograft vasculopathy. *J Heart Lung Transplant.* 14(4):632-9

Mehra, M.R., Ventura, H.O., Stapleton, D.D., & Smart, F.W. (1995). The prognostic significance of intimal proliferation in cardiac allograft vasculopathy: a paradigm shift. *J Heart Lung Transplant.* 14(6 Pt 2):S207-11

Miller, L.W., Schlant, R.C., Kobashigawa, .J, Kubo, S., & Renlund, D.G. (1993). 24th Bethesda conference: Cardiac transplantation. Task Force 5: Complications. *J Am Coll Cardiol.* 22(1):41-54

Miller, L.W. (1995). Role of intracoronary ultrasound for the diagnosis of cardiac allograft vasculopathy. *Transplant Proc.* 27(3):1989-92

Naghavi, M., Libby, P., Falk, E., Casscells, S.W., Litovsky, S., Rumberger, J., et al. (2003). From vulnerable plaque to vulnerable patient: a call for new definitions and risk assessment strategies: Part II. *Circulation.* 108(15):1772-8

Nair, A., Kuban, B.D., Obuchowski, N., & Vince, D.G. (2001). Assessing spectral algorithms to predict atherosclerotic plaque composition with normalized and raw intravascular ultrasound data. *Ultrasound Med Biol.* 27(10):1319-31

Nair, A., Kuban, B.D., Tuzcu, E.M., Schoenhagen, P., Nissen, S.E., & Vince, D.G. (2002). Coronary plaque classification with intravascular ultrasound radiofrequency data analysis. *Circulation.* 106(17):2200-6

Narrod, J., Kormos, R., Armitage, J., Hardesty, R., Ladowski, J., & Griffith, B. (1989). Acute rejection and coronary artery disease in long-term survivors of heart transplantation. *J Heart Transplant.* Sep-Oct;8(5):418-20; discussion 20-1

Nasu, K., Tsuchikane, E., Katoh, O., Vince, D.G., Virmani, R., Surmely, J.F., et al. (2006). Accuracy of in vivo coronary plaque morphology assessment: a validation study of in vivo virtual histology compared with in vitro histopathology. *J Am Coll Cardiol.* 47(12):2405-12. Epub 006 May 30

Nissen, S. (2001). Coronary angiography and intravascular ultrasound. Am J Cardiol. 87(4A):15A-20A.

Opelz, G. (1997). Critical evaluation of the association of acute with chronic graft rejection in kidney and heart transplant recipients. The Collaborative Transplant Study. *Transplant Proc.* Feb-Mar;29(1-2):73-6

Pethig, K., Heublein, B., Kutschka, I., & Haverich, A. (2000). Systemic inflammatory response in cardiac allograft vasculopathy: high-sensitive C-reactive protein is associated with progressive luminal obstruction. *Circulation.* Nov 7;102(19 Suppl 3):III233-6

Pethig, K., Heublein, B., Wahlers, T., & Haverich, A. (1998). Mechanism of luminal narrowing in cardiac allograft vasculopathy: inadequate vascular remodeling rather than intimal hyperplasia is the major predictor of coronary artery stenosis. Working Group on Cardiac Allograft Vasculopathy. *Am Heart J.* 135(4):628-33

Pflugfelder, P.W., Boughner, D.R., Rudas, L., & Kostuk, W.J. (1993). Enhanced detection of cardiac allograft arterial disease with intracoronary ultrasonographic imaging. *Am Heart J.* 125(6):1583-91

Raichlin, E., Bae, J.H., Khalpey, Z., Edwards, B.S., Kremers, W.K., Clavell, A.L., et al. (2007). Conversion to sirolimus as primary immunosuppression attenuates the progression of allograft vasculopathy after cardiac transplantation. *Circulation.* Dec;116(23):2726-33

Raichlin, E.R., McConnell, J.P., Lerman, A., Kremers, W.K, Edwards, B.S., Kushwaha, S.S, et al. (2007). Systemic inflammation and metabolic syndrome in cardiac allograft vasculopathy. *J Heart Lung Transplant.* 26(8):826-33

Raichlin, E., Bae, J.H., Kushwaha, S.S., Lennon, R.J,, Prasad. A,, Rihal, C.S., et al. (2009). Inflammatory burden of cardiac allograft coronary atherosclerotic plaque is associated with early recurrent cellular rejection and predicts a higher risk of vasculopathy progression. *J Am Coll Cardiol.* 53(15):1279-86

Rickenbacher, P.R., Pinto, F.J., Chenzbraun, A., Botas, J., Lewis, N.P., Alderman, E.L., et al. (1995). Incidence and severity of transplant coronary artery disease early and up to 15 years after transplantation as detected by intravascular ultrasound. *J Am Coll Cardiol.* 25(1):171-7

Rickenbacher, P.R., Pinto, F.J., Lewis, N.P., Hunt, S.A., Alderman, E.L., Schroeder, J.S., et al. (1995). Prognostic importance of intimal thickness as measured by intracoronary ultrasound after cardiac transplantation. *Circulation.* 92(12):3445-52

Rodriguez-Granillo, G.A., Garcia-Garcia, H.M., Mc Fadden, E.P., Valgimigli, M., Aoki, J., de Feyter, P., et al. (2005). In vivo intravascular ultrasound-derived thin-cap fibroatheroma detection using ultrasound radiofrequency data analysis. *J Am Coll Cardiol.* 46(11):2038-42. Epub 05 Nov 9

Rodriguez-Granillo, G.A., Serruys, P.W., Garcia-Garcia, H.M., Aoki, J., Valgimigli, M., van Mieghem, C.A, et al. (2006). Coronary artery remodelling is related to plaque composition. *Heart.* 92(3):388-91

Sharples, L.D., Jackson, C.H., Parameshwar, J., Wallwork, J., & Large, S.R. (2003). Diagnostic accuracy of coronary angiography and risk factors for post-heart-transplant cardiac allograft vasculopathy. *Transplantation.* Aug 27;76(4):679-82

Sims, F.H., Gavin, J.B., Edgar, S., Koelmeyer, T.D., Sims, F.H., Gavin, J.B., et al. (2002). Comparison of the endothelial surface and subjacent elastic lamina of anterior descending coronary arteries at the location of atheromatous lesions with internal thoracic arteries of the same subjects: a scanning electron microscopic study. *Pathology.* 34(5):433-41

Stark, R.P., McGinn, A.L., & Wilson, R.F. (1991). Chest pain in cardiac-transplant recipients. Evidence of sensory reinnervation after cardiac transplantation. *N Engl J Med.* 324(25):1791-4

Stehlik, J., Edwards, L.B., Kucheryavaya, A.Y., Aurora, P., Christie, J.D,, Kirk, R., et al. (2010). The Registry of the International Society for Heart and Lung Transplantation: twenty-seventh official adult heart transplant report--2010. *J Heart Lung Transplant.* 29(10):1089-103

Taylor, D.O., Edwards, L.B., Boucek, M.M., Trulock, E.P., Aurora, P., Christie, J., et al. (2007). Registry of the International Society for Heart and Lung Transplantation: twenty-fourth official adult heart transplant report--2007. *J Heart Lung Transplant.* 26(8):769-81

Tuzcu, E.M., Hobbs, R.E., Rincon, G., Bott-Silverman, C., De Franco, A.C., Robinson, K., et al. (1995). Occult and frequent transmission of atherosclerotic coronary disease with cardiac transplantation. Insights from intravascular ultrasound. *Circulation.* 91(6):1706-13

Tuzcu, E.M., De Franco, A.C., Goormastic, M., Hobbs, R.E., Rincon, G, Bott-Silverman, C., et al. (1996). Dichotomous pattern of coronary atherosclerosis 1 to 9 years after transplantation: insights from systematic intravascular ultrasound imaging. *J Am Coll Cardiol.* 27(4):839-46

Tuzcu, E.M., Kapadia, S.R., Sachar, R., Ziada, K.M., Crowe, T.D., Feng, J., et al. (2005). Intravascular ultrasound evidence of angiographically silent progression in coronary atherosclerosis predicts long-term morbidity and mortality after cardiac transplantation. *J Am Coll Cardiol.* May 3;45(9):1538-42

Tuzcu, E.M., Bayturan, O., & Kapadia, S. (2010). Invasive imaging: Coronary intravascular ultrasound: a closer view. *Heart.* 96(16):1318-24

Uretsky, B.F., Murali, S., Reddy, P.S., Rabin, B., Lee, A., Griffith, B.P., et al. (1987). Development of coronary artery disease in cardiac transplant patients receiving immunosuppressive therapy with cyclosporine and prednisone. *Circulation.* 76(4):827-34

Valantine, H.A. (1995). Role of lipids in allograft vascular disease: a multicenter study of intimal thickening detected by intravascular ultrasound. *J Heart Lung Transplant.* 14(6 Pt 2):S234-7

Valgimigli, M., Rodriguez-Granillo, G.A., Garcia-Garcia, H.M., Vaina, S., De Jaegere, P., De Feyter, P., et al. (2007). Plaque composition in the left main stem mimics the distal but not the proximal tract of the left coronary artery: influence of clinical presentation, length of the left main trunk, lipid profile, and systemic levels of C-reactive protein. *J Am Coll Cardiol.* 49(1):23-31. Epub 2006 Dec 13

Vassalli, G., Gallino, A., Weis, M., von Scheidt, W., Kappenberger, L., von Segesser, L.K., et al. (2003). Alloimmunity and nonimmunologic risk factors in cardiac allograft vasculopathy. *Eur Heart J.* Jul;24(13):1180-8

Velican, C., & Velican, D. (1985). Study of coronary intimal thickening. Atherosclerosis. 56(3):331-44

Vigano, M., Tuzcu, M., Benza, R., Boissonnat, P., Haverich, A., Hil,l J., et al. (2007). Prevention of acute rejection and allograft vasculopathy by everolimus in cardiac transplants recipients: a 24-month analysis. *J Heart Lung Transplant.* Jun;26(6):584-92

White, J.A., Pflugfelder, P.W., Boughner, D.R., & Kostuk, W.J. (2003). Validation of a three-dimensional intravascular ultrasound imaging technique to assess atherosclerotic burden: potential for improved assessment of cardiac allograft coronary artery disease. *Can J Cardiol.* Sep;19(10):1147-53

Yamanim, M.H., Haji, S.A., Starling, R.C., Tuzcu, E.M., Ratliff, N.B., Cook, D.J., et al. (2002). Myocardial ischemic-fibrotic injury after human heart transplantation is associated with increased progression of vasculopathy, decreased cellular rejection and poor long-term outcome. *J Am Coll Cardiol.* Mar 20;39(6):970-7

Yamani, M.H., Erinc, S.K., McNeill, A., Ratliff, N.B., Sendrey, D., Zhou, L., et al. (2005). The impact of donor gender on cardiac peri-transplantation ischemia injury. *Journal of Heart and Lung Transplantation.* Nov;24(11):1741-4

Yeung, A.C., Davis, S.F., Hauptman, P.J., Kobashigawa, J.A., Miller, L.W., Valantine, H.A., et al. (1995). Incidence and progression of transplant coronary artery disease over 1 year: results of a multicenter trial with use of intravascular ultrasound. Multicenter Intravascular Ultrasound Transplant Study Group. *J Heart Lung Transplant.* 14(6 Pt 2):S215-20

Ziada, K.M .K.S., Crowe, T.D., Binak, E., Motwani, J.G., Young, J.B., Nissen, S.E., & Tuzcu, E.M. (1997). Three year ultrasound follow-up of donor transmitted atherosclerosis in transplant recipients. *Circulation.* 96(suppl 1):I65;353

6

Intravascular Ultrasound (IVUS) and Clinical Applications

T. Ozcan
*Mersin University, Faculty of Medicine,
Department of Cardiology, Mersin
Turkey*

1. Introduction

1.1 Intravascular ultrasound (IVUS) and clinical applications

Atherosclerosis is a chronic disease potentially involving the whole vascular system that causes a spectrum of clinical manifestations ranging from stable angina to acute myocardial infarction or stroke. The continuous accumulation of lipids, inflammatory and/or fibrous elements in the arterial wall leads to progressive lumen narrowing. Acute coronary syndromes (acute myocardial infarction, unstable angina) have a complex and dynamic pathogenesis with coronary plaque rupture. Some plaques lead to clinical events whereas many others remain asymptomatic for life, different imaging modalities have been applied to define the atherosclerotic burden and the anatomical characteristics of unstable or vulnerable lesions.

The vascular response to endothelial dysfonction is a well-orchestrated inflammatory response triggered by the accumulation of macrophages within the vessel wall. The formation of such vulnerable plaques prone to rupture underlies the majority of cases of acute myocardial infarction. The complex molecular and cellular inflammatory cascade is orchestrated by the recruitment of T lymphocytes and macrophages and their paracrine effects on endothelial and smooth muscle cells (1). Molecular imaging in atherosclerosis has evolved into an important clinical and research tool that allows in vivo visualization of inflammation and other biological processes. Several recent examples demonstrate the ability to detect high-risk plaques in patients, and assess the effects of pharmacotherapeutics in atherosclerosis (2).

Intravascular ultrasound (IVUS) performed with an ultrasound machine that has been especially adapted to intravascular imaging. The machine can be permanently affixed in the catheterization lab or can be portable and moved from one catheterization room to another as needed. The IVUS catheter is attached to the ultrasound machine through an interface that ensures sterility of the catheter. Intravascular ultrasound is an exciting technology that allows in-vivo visualization of vascular anatomy by utilizing a miniature transducer. The IVUS catheter can be advanced into different vascular structures including peripheral arteries, coronary arteries, and intracardiac chambers. Intracoronary ultrasound has become particularly useful in further delineating plaque morphology and distribution, and providing a rationale to guide transcatheter coronary interventions (3). The reflected ultrasound from the intima is displayed as a single concentric echo. All of the ultrasound, however, is not reflected

by the intima; some will penetrate through to the media. Since the media is composed primarily of homogeneous smooth muscle cells, ultrasound passes through with minimal reflection and appears as a dark zone devoid of echoes. The adventitia, is highly reflective because it has numerous collagen fibers laid down in parallel, thereby producing multiple interfaces from which to reflect sound. The adventitia will appear very bright. As a result, the normal coronary anatomy produces alternating bright and dark echoes:
1-A bright echo from the intima, 2-A dark zone from the media, 3-Multiple bright echoes from the adventitia
This pattern is called the normal "three layer appearance" of a coronary artery (4). The three-layer appearance is actually a simplified view since the IVUS resolution (approximately 120 microns) is not sufficient to detect the truly nondiseased intima (one or two cell layers thick or approximately 50 microns). The tomographic cross-sectional view of the artery is ideal to discern concentric from eccentric plaque distribution. This feature makes IVUS far more accurate than angiography for assessing plaque eccentricity (3). Because of the limitations of angiography, hazy angiographic sites could represent an irregular plaque/distorted lumen, a napkin-ring lesion, thrombus, or a dissection. IVUS is particularly useful in this situation because it immediately distinguishes between plaque and lumen irregularities, dissection, or discrete stenosis (5).
IVUS has also demonstrated that apparently normal areas by angiography are often markedly abnormal. One of the areas that IVUS can be useful is Slow coronary flow (SCF). Slow coronary flow is characterized with the late opacification of the epicardial coronary arteries without occlusive disease (6,7). It was first described by Tambe et al. in 1972 (10). In 1973, Kemp et al. suggested it to be a variant of "syndrome X" (11). However, SCF differs in a distinct manner in which is a phenomenon characterized by delayed opacification of epicardial coronary arteries in the absence of epicardial occlusive disease. The exact etiology, pathogenesis and long term outcome of SCF patients is still unknown. Endothelial and vasomotor dysfunction, microvascular dysfunction, and occlusive disease of small coronary arteries were suggested in its etiology (8-17). The carotid artery intima-media thickness (CIMT) is the best known sonographic marker for early atherosclerotic vascular wall lesions (18). Previous cross-sectional studies in different populations have shown that, increase in CIMT is associated with cardiovascular event prevalence (19-25). Additionally, CIMT increase was strongly and significantly correlated with myocardial infarction and stroke incidence (26). Angiography depicts only 2D silhouette of the lumen, whereas IVUS allows tomographic assessment of lumen area, plaque size, distribution, and composition. In young subjects, normal intimal thickness is typical 0.15 mm (27). Intravascular ultrasound (IVUS) can detect intimal thickening of the coronary arteries and is suitable for detection of early atherosclerosis that cannot be detected by conventional angiography (28-30).
In additon Intravascular ultrasound (IVUS) is useful during stent implantation to assess lesion severity, length, and morphology before stent implantation; to optimize stent expansion, extension, and apposition; and to identify and treat possible complications after stent implantation (31). Most of the evidence from the era of bare-metal stents indicates that IVUS guidance offers incremental information leading to lower rates of angiographic restenosis and repeat revascularization (32). In the current era of drug-eluting stents (DES) with ensuing low restenosis rates, the relationship between IVUS-guided DES implantation and clinical outcomes is less well established.

In cases of coronary dissection, IVUS can distinguish atherosclerotic plaques from intramural hematoma and also detect the media dissection, false and true lumen and, if present, the intimal flap. Treatment of spontaneous dissection in particular is often especially challenging, since it commonly affects young individuals with little or no atherosclerotic burden. Ther-apy has traditionally been guided by clinical and angiographic findings. However, in small series of patients IVUS has been proven useful in the context of interventional treatment (33).

There are some controversies between the results of the studies which compared the CIMT values of SCF patients and normal subject. A previous study shows that patients with SCF have a significantly increased carotid IMT compared with those with normal coronary flow (34). But recent studies do not support this result (35). The investigated these values with comparing the IVUS and TIMI frame counts. Measurements of CIMT using ultrasound assess the extent and the severity of systemic atherosclerosis. Today, CIMT, measured with high-resolution B-mode ultrasound, is the standard for noninvasive surrogate measurements of atherosclerosis. It has been shown that a direct relation exits between CIMT and clinical cardiovascular disease (19-22). Due to these data, CIMT assessment can be used to document regression or progression of atherosclerosis (19-36) Besides, at least two large epidemiologic studies proposed that increased CIMT values are associated prospectively with increased risk of coronary artery disease (24,25,37). Several studies, CIMT was significantly increased in SCF patients. This would mean the increased risk of coronary, cerebral and peripheral vascular diseases in these patients. However these risks are still not studied enough, and are unknown in this special group of patients. It was shown another study diffuse or regional calcification and intimal thickening in coronary arteries in most of the patients with SCF, despite the absence of angiographically detectable coronary focal stenosis or plaques in them. These results suggest that epicardial coronary arteries were affected as a part of diffuse atherosclerotic disease of all arterial system in this specific group of patients. IVUS imaging can detect early intimal thickening, which cannot be detected by conventional angiography (28-30,38). Some previous studies have shown the evidence of diffuse atherosclerosis despite angiographically normal coronary arteries in syndrome-X patients by intravascular ultrasound (28-30). Pekdemir et al. showed that most patients with SCF had longitudinally extended massive calcification throughout the epicardial coronary arteries. Cin et al. demonstrated that the patients with SCF had diffuse intimal thickening, widespread calcification along the coronary vessel wall, and atheroma which did not cause luminal irregularities in the coronary angiography (39,40). In the present study, according to the findings of IVUS, the speculate that SCF may be a form or preliminary phase of diffuse atherosclerotic process that involve epicardial coronary arteries. However, in a previous study, Chilian et al. (41) have observed enhanced vasocon-strictor response in the monkeys with atherosclerosis and they speculated that the early pathophysiological consequences of atherosclerosis might extend into the microcirculation, which may be another mechanism for SCF. Erdogan et al. (42) suggest that coronary flow reserve (CFR) is impaired in patients with SCF. Impairment of endothelial function and reduced CFR, which reflects coronary microvascular function, has been shown to be early manifestation of atherosclerosis. Mangieri et al. (12) and Kurtoglu et al. [11] have observed remarkable progress in restoring coronary flow when they studied dypyridamole in this group of patients. They concluded the theory that the pathophysiology underlying this disorder is closely related to the microvasculature and has a dynamic character. Near these results, some other studies have shown the evidence of diffuse epicardial atherosclerosis despite angiographically normal coronary arteries (28-30,43). All these data, however, do not clearly delineate the borders of this disorder neither does it imply any interaction between micro and macrovasculature of the heart. In the present study, the correlation of TIMI frame count and the CIMT and coronary intima-media thickness suggest the atherosclerosis would be the pathophysiological mechanism of the disease. However, it is impossible to conclude any suggestion about microvascular pathology. The occurrence of myocardial ischemia was only sporadically demonstrated in these patients. It is concluded that most of these patients continue to experience regular and/or worsening chest pain despite reassurance that they do not have obstructed coronary arteries (44).

Prior to IVUS, only the lumen of a vessel could be visualized in vivo with angiography or angioscopy. IVUS extends our capability to visualize and assess the size of the vessel, should it be devoid of atherosclerotic disease. Prior to a discussion of the applications of IVUS, it is important to appreciate the added information provided by this procedure when compared with conventional angiography for the assessment of coronary artery disease. Today intravascular ultrasound (IVUS) offers qualitative details on plaque composition, like hard and soft components, that are helpful to assess unstable lesions. As a result, the appropriate indications and clinical cases provide impotant information.

2. References

[1] Andersson, J., Libby, P., *et al.* Adaptive immunity and atherosclerosis. Clin Immunol. 134 (1), 33-46 (2010).

[2] Jaffer, F. A., Libby, P. *et al.* Molecular Imaging of Cardiovascular Disease. Circulation. 116 (9), 1052-1061 (2007).

[3] Yock, P, Fitzgerald, P, Popp, R. Intravascular ultrasound. Sci Am Science Med 1995; 2:68.

[4] Fitzgerald, PJ, St Goar, FG, Connolly, AJ, et al. Intravascular ultrasound imaging of coronary arteries: is three layers the norm? Circulation 1992; 86:154.

[5] Ziada, KM, Tuzcu, EM, De Franco, AC, et al. Intravascular ultrasound assessment of the prevalence and causes of angiographic "haziness" following high-pressure coronary stenting. Am J Cardiol 1997; 80:116.

[6] Lierde JV, Vrolix M, Sionis D, De Geest H, Piessens J. Lack of evidence for small vessel disease in a patient with "slow dye progres sion" in the coronary arteries. Cathet Cardiovasc Diagn 1991;23:117–20

[7] Yigit F, Sezgin AT, Demircan S, et al. Slow coronary flow is associated with carotid artery dilatation. Tohoku J Exp Med 2006;209:41–8.

[8] Tambe AA, Demany MA, Zimmerman HA, Mascarenhas E. Angina pectoris and slow flow velocity of dye in coronary arteries—a new angiographic finding. Am Heart J 1972;84:66–71.

[9] Kemp Jr HG, Vokonas PS, Cohn PF, Gorlin R. The anginal syndrome associated with normal coronary arteriograms. Report of a 6-year experience. Am J Med 1973;54:735–42.

[10] Vrints C, Herman AG. Role of the endothelium in the regulation of coronary artery tone. Acta Cardiol 1991;46:399–418.

[11] Mosseri M, Yarom R, Gotsman MS, Hasin Y. Histologic evidence for small vessel coronary artery disease in patients with angina pectoris and patent large coronary arteries. Circulation 1986;74:964–72.

[12] Mangieri E, Macchiarelli G, Ciavolella M, et al. Slow coronary flow: clinical and histopathological features in patients with otherwise normal epicardial coronary arteries. Cathet Cardiovasc Diagn 1996;37:375-81.
[13] Kurtoglu N, Akcay A, Dindar I. Usefulness of oral dipyridamole therapy for angiographic slow coronary artery flow. Am J Cardiol 2001;87:777-9.
[14] MotzW,Vogt M, Rabenau O, et al. Evidence of endothelial dysfunction in coronary resistance vessels, in patients with angina pectoris and normal coronary angiograms. Am J Cardiol 1991;68:996-1003.
[15] Quyyumi AA, Cannon III RO, Panza JA, Diodati JG, Epstein SE. Endothelial dysfunction in patients with chest pain and normal coronary arteries. Circulation 1992;86:1864-71.
[16] Egashira K, InouT, HirookaY, et al. Evidence of impaired endotheliumdependent coronary vasodilatation in patients with angina pectoris and normal coronary angiograms. N Engl J Med 1993;328:1659-64.
[17] Zeiher AM, Krause T, Schachinger V, Minners J, Moser E. Impaired endothelium dependent vasodilation of the coronary resistance vessels is associated with exercise-induced myocardial ischaemia. Circulation 1995;91:2345-52.
[18] Kaslival RR, Bansal M, Bhargava K, Gupta H, Tandon S. Carotid intima-media thickness and brachial-ankle pulse wave velocity in patients with and without coronary artery disease. Indian Heart J 2004;56(2):117-22.
[19] For the ARIC Study Group. Arterial wall thickness is associated with prevelant cardiovascular disease in middle-aged adults. Stroke 1995;26:386-91.
[20] Kronmal RA, Smith VE, O'Leary DH, et al. Carotid artery measures are strongly associated with left ventricular mass in older adults (a report from the Cardiovascular Health Study). Am J Cardiol 1996;77:628-33.
[21] Mattace Raso F, Rosato M, Talerico A, Cotronei P, Mattace R. Intimalmedial thickness of the common carotid arteries and lower limbs atherosclerosis in the elderly. Minerva Cardioangiol 1999;47:321-7.
[22] Mannami T, Baba S, Ogata J. Strong and significant relationships between aggregation of major coronary risk factors and the acceleration of carotid atherosclerosis in the general population of a Japanese city. Arch Intern Med 2000;160:2297-303.
[23] Hodis HN, Mack WJ, LaBree L, et al. The role of carotid arterial intimamedia thickness in predicting clinical coronary events. Ann Intern Med 1998;128:262-9.
[24] Chambless L, Heiss G, Folsom AR, et al. Association of coronary heart disease incidence with carotid arterial wall thickness and major risk factors: the atherosclerosis risk in communities (ARIC) study. Am J Epidemiol 1997;146:483-94.
[25] NewmanAB, Naydeck B, Sutton-Tyrell K, et al. Coronary artery calcification in older adults with minimal clinical or subclinical cardiovascular disease. J Am Geriatr Soc 2000;48:256-63.
[26] For the Cardiovascular Health Study Collaborative Research Group. Carotid artery intima and media thickness as a risk factor for myocardial infarction and stroke in older adults. N Eng J Med 1999;340:14-22.
[27] Steven E. Nissen, Paul Yock. Intravascular ultraound: novel pathophhysiological insight and current clinical applications. Circulation 2001;103:604-16.
[28] Nakatani S, Yamagishi M, Tamai J, et al. Assessment of coronary artery distensibility by intravascular ultrasound application of simultaneous measurements of luminal area and pressure. Circulation 1995;91:2904-10.

[29] Mintz GS, Painter JA, Pichard AD, et al. Atherosclerosis in angiographically "normal" coronary artery reference segments: an intravascular ultrasound study with clinical correlations. J Am Coll Cardiol 1995;25:1479–85.

[30] Tuzcu EM, Kapadia SR, Tutar E, et al. High prevalence of coronary atherosclerosis in asymptomatic teenagers and young adults evidence from intravascular ultrasound. Circulation 2001;103:2705–10.

[31] Mintz GS, Nissen SE, Anderson WD, et al. American College of Cardiology clinical expert consensus document on standards for acquisition, measurement and reporting of intravascular ultrasound studies (IVUS). A report of the American College of Cardiology Task Force on Clinical Expert Consensus Documents. J Am Coll Cardiol 2001; 37:1478 -92.

[32] Parise H, Maehara A, Stone GW, Leon MB, Mintz GS. Metaanalysis of randomized studies comparing intravascular ultrasound versus angiographic guidance of percutaneous coronary intervention in the pre-drug-eluting stent era. Am J Cardiol 2011;107:374–82.

[33] Arnold JR, West NE, van Gaal WJ, Karamitsos TD, Banning AP. The role of intravascular ultrasound in the management of spontaneous coronary artery dissection. Cardiovasc Ultrasound.2008; 6: 24.

[34] Tanriverdi H, Evrengul H. Carotid intima.-media thickness in coronary slow flow: relationship with plasma homocysteine levels. Coron Artery Dis 2006;17(4):331-7.

[35] Yigit F, Sezgin AT, Demircan S, et al. Slow coronary flow is associated with carotid artery dilatation. Tohoku J Exp Med 2006;2091:41–8.

[36] Ishizu T, Ishimitsu T, Kamiya H, et al. The correlation of irregularities in carotid arterial intima-media thickness with coronary artery disease. Heart Vessels 2002;17(1):1–6.

[37] Cerne A, Kranjec I. Atherosclerotic burden in coronary and peripheral arteries in patients with first clinical manifestation of coronary artery disease. Heart Vessels 2002;16(6):217–26.

[38] Kawano S, Yamagishi M, Hao H, Yutani C, Miyatake K.Wall composition in intravascular ultrasound layered appearance of human coronary artery. Heart Vessels 1996;11(3):152–9.

[39] Pekdemir H, Polat G, CinVG, et al. Elevated plasma endothelin-1 levels in coronary sinus during rapid right atrial pacing in patients with slow coronary flow. Int J Cardiol 2004;97:35–41.

[40] Cin VG, Pekdemir H, Camsarı A, et al. Diffuse intimal thickening of coronary arteries in slow coronary flow. Jpn Heart J 2003;44:907–19.

[41] ChillianWM,Dellsperger KC, Layne SM, et al. Effects of atherosclerosis on the coronary microcirculation. Am J Physiol 1990;258:529–39.

[42] Erdogan D, Caliskan M, Gullu H, et al. Coronary flow reserve is impaired in patients with slow coronary flow. Atherosclerosis 2007;191:168–74.

[43] Nissen SE, Gurley JC, Grines CL, et al. Intravascular ultrasound assessment of lumen size andwall morphology in normal subjects and patients with coronary artery disease. Circulation 1991;84:1087–99.

[44] Przybojewski JZ, Becker PH. Angina pectoris and acute myocardial infarction due to "slow-flow phenomenon" in nonatherosclerotic coronary arteries: a case report. Angiology 1986;37:751–61.

Part 2

Interventional Applications

Clinical Applications of Intravascular Ultrasound

Dermot Phelan, Sajjad Matiullah and Faisal Sharif
University College Hospital Galway
Ireland

1. Introduction

Intravascular Ultrasound (IVUS) is an invasive grey scale tomographic imaging modality providing cross-sectional images of the vessel wall. The reflected or scattered ultrasound signal received at the transducer is converted to a voltage. This voltage is known as radiofrequency data or backscattered signal. The time delay and amplitude of these emitting pulses provides 256 such backscattered signals or A-scans to produce one image. For IVUS imaging, high ultrasound frequencies typically centred between 25-50 MHz are used. The size of conventional IVUS catheter is 2.9 and 3.5 Fr and has a typical pullback speed of 0.5 mm/s and a frame rate of 30 images per second. At 30 MHz the wavelength is 50 μm, which yields a spatial resolution of >150μm allowing detail evaluation of the blood vessel wall.
IVUS imaging is complementary to coronary angiography and allows the simultaneous assessment of lumen and components of the vessel wall. In the IVUS image the catheter is in the centre of the image surrounded by vessel lumen, the three layers of the vessel and surrounding structures (Figure 1). It can assess plaque geometry including plaque burden and size, luminal area, longitudinal extent of the disease, circumferential extent of the

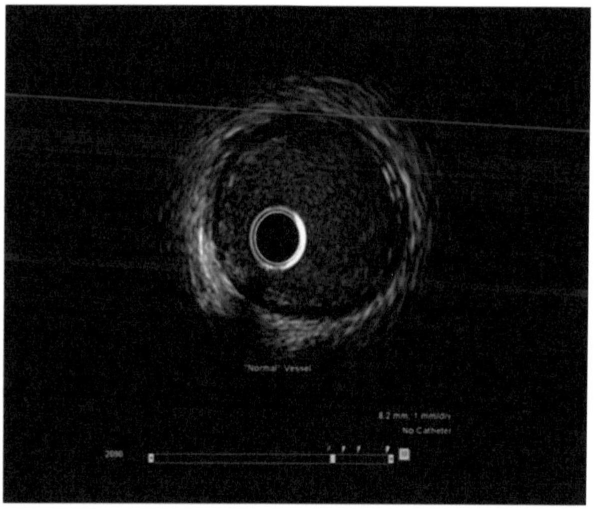

Fig. 1. IVUS of normal coronary artery

plaque, arterial remodelling and plaque vulnerability. Therefore IVUS provides detailed insight to the anatomy of plaque burden and allows the interventional cardiologist to adapt an optimal strategy for percutaneous coronary intervention (PCI) and subsequently assess the success of this strategy. In this chapter we will describe the potential applications of IVUS for every day use in the catheterization laboratory.

2. Clinical applications of IVUS

2.1 Assessment of vessel size for stent selection and ischemia evaluation

Standard coronary angiography is intrinsically limited to evaluate three-dimensional anatomical coronary cross sectional area due to planar silhoutte imaging. In addition, the plaque burden, its delineation and constituents cannot be assessed by coronary angiography. With angiography, the severity of stenosis is assessed by minimal lumen diameter at the lesion site, in comparison with an adjacent normal appearing reference. However, it is well documented that atherosclerosis is diffuse in nature and may appear normal in a small calibre coronary artery with concentric plaque (Figure 2)(Grondin, Dyrda et al. 1974; Roberts and Jones 1979). IVUS provides a complete 360 degrees tomographic view that allows accurate lumen measurements. In fact direct comparison of atherosclerotic disease by angiography and IVUS are frequently discrepant often as a result of eccentric plaque.(Figure 2) IVUS studies have clearly demonstrated that there is no correlation between the size of the atheroma and the size of the lumen(Topol and Nissen 1995) . This difference can be explained by positive (expansive) remodelling where lumen size is maintained due to plaque accumulation within in the vessel wall and resulting vessel wall expansion. It is claimed that these positive plaques are more unstable and vulnerable to rupture than negative (constrictive) plaques and also responsible for in-stent restenosis (ISR) following coronary intervention.(Schoenhagen, Ziada et al. 2000).

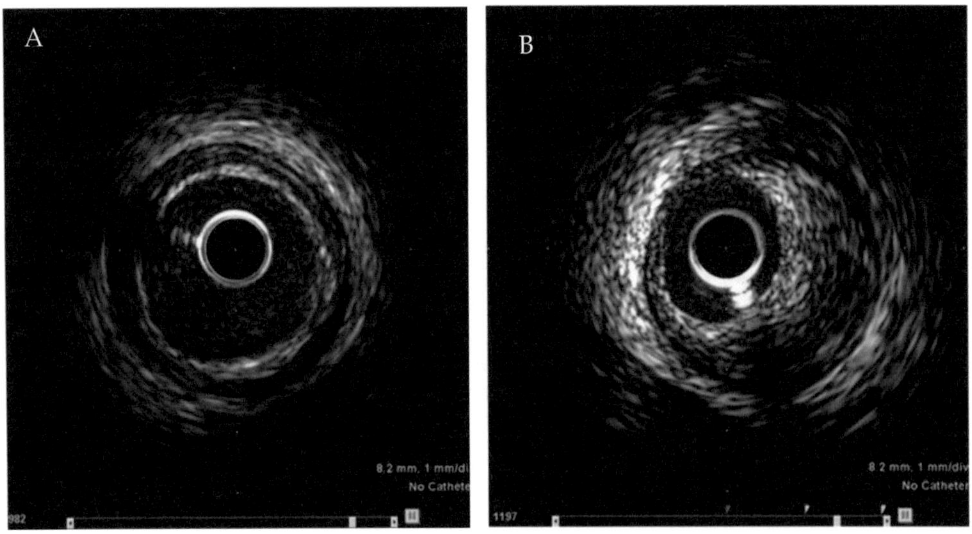

Fig. 2. IVUS images of A) concentric plaque and B) eccentric plaque

In addition to accurate stent sizing, IVUS can be used to evaluate lesion lumen area to predict the presence or absence of myocardial ischemia and/or significant coronary stenosis. There was strong correlation between lesion lumen area of < 4.0 mm2 on IVUS and positive stress myocardial perfusion SPECT in seventy native coronary lesions (Nishioka, Amanullah et al. 1999). In another study, IVUS guided deferral of coronary intervention of 248 lesions with luminal area of >4 mm^2 resulted in clinical rates of 4.4% and target lesion revascularisation (TLR) of 2.8% at 12 month follow up. (Abizaid, Mintz et al. 1998).

2.2 Assessment of restenosis

Following coronary intervention, the formation of neointimal hyperplasia is mainly responsible for ISR (Figure 3). There is strong correlation with between late lumen loss and the degree of in-stent neointimal growth (r=0.98) (de Jaegere, Mudra et al. 1998; Hoffmann, Mintz et al. 1998). Although drug eluting stents (DES) has significantly reduced the incidence of neointimal proliferation, the rate of ISR still remains around 10-15%.

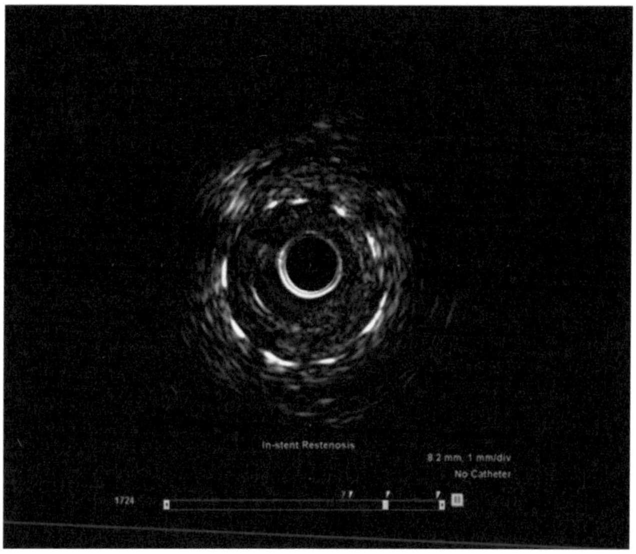

Fig. 3. IVUS image of in-stent restenosis

One of the main factors for ISR is stent **underexpansion** (Figure 4). IVUS can detect vessel stent subtleties not apparent by coronary angiography. In addition to assessing plaque geometry, IVUS can be used to achieve complete stent apposition and adequate geometric expansion within the stented segment. IVUS studies have demonstrated that incomplete stent and vessel wall apposition, residual stenosis and irregular eccentric lumen in the stented segment was present in almost 88% of the patients despite achieving an optimal angiographic result (Nakamura, Colombo et al. 1994) . Clinical trials have shown that patients who have their coronary intervention guided by IVUS have larger post procedure stent areas and significant reductions in TLR as compared to angiography-guided PCI alone (de Jaegere, Mudra et al. 1998; Schiele, Meneveau et al. 1998; Fitzgerald, Oshima et al. 2000; Sonoda, Morino et al. 2004; Hong, Mintz et al. 2006) In addition to detecting stent underexpansion, IVUS can also assist in achieving optimal stent expansion, exclude stent edge dissections and plaque protrusion (Hong, Jeong et al. 2008).

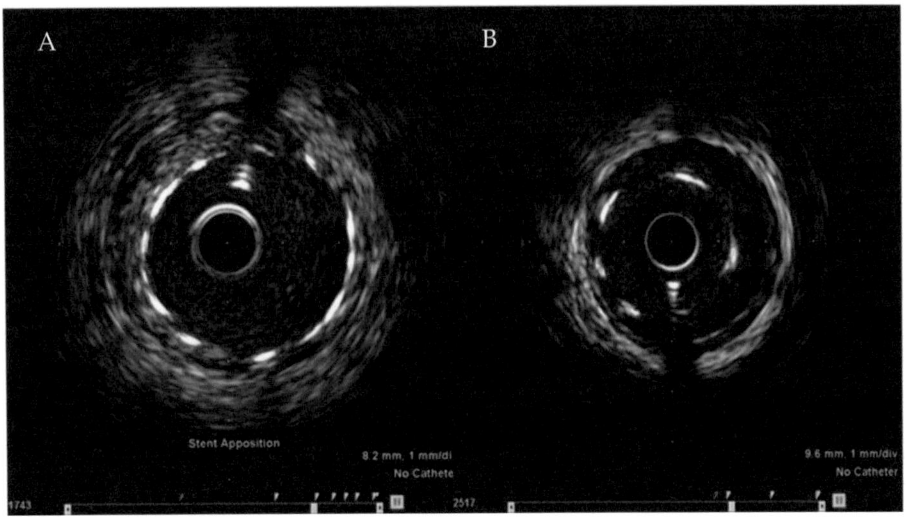

Fig. 4. IVUS demonstrating A) stent well apposed to vessel wall and B) stent mal-apposition

2.3 Guidance for left main stem intervention

Coronary interventions of unprotected left main coronary artery (UPLM) with bare metal stents in the 1990s were associated with high rates of revascularization (25% to 30%) due to restenosis (Black, Cortina et al. 2001; Park, Hong et al. 2001; Takagi, Stankovic et al. 2002). Although the use of DES for UPLM PCI have significantly reduced the rate of revascularization as compared with bare metal stents (BMS), the long term outcomes remain less favourable. Most of the poor outcomes following UPLM PCI relates to distal bifurcation intervention, which is a technically complex procedure. The current American College of Cardiology (ACC)/American Heart association (AHA) practice guidelines for PCI categorize UPLM stenting as a class IIb indication or IIa indication in selected patients without co-existing multivessel disease. At present there is a paucity of randomized control trial data comparing Coronary artery bypass grafting (CABG) to PCI in patients with UPLM. The best available evidence comes from the SYNTAX trial (SYNergy between Percutaneous Coronary Intervention with TAXus and Cardiac Surgery), which randomly assigned 1800 patients with either UPLM (n=705) or multivessel CAD not involving the left main stem (n=1095) (Ong, Serruys et al. 2006) . The major adverse cardiac or cerebrovascular events were not significantly different between the CABG and PCI groups (13.7 vs 15.8%). However, the rate of revascularization was significantly higher in those treated with PCI (11.8 vs 6.5 %). One of the main limitations of the SYNTAX trial was felt to be the lack of use of IVUS for UPLM in the PCI group.

While the European Society of Cardiology guidelines give IVUS-guided stenting of the UPLM a Class IIb recommendation we feel IVUS interrogation of the UPLM pre and post intervention should be used in all cases. Not least because IVUS interrogation has been demonstrated to, frequently prove angiographic assessment of the UPLM as inaccurate. This obviously may have significant impact on patient management resulting in either erroneous treatment of a lesion which may appear severe angiographically but in fact has minimal plaque burden or failure to treat lesions which are mis-labelled as mild-to-moderate (Mintz and Maehara 2009).

Moreover, IVUS is an ideal method for confirming the presence of significant left main disease and also for guiding selection of stent size, assessing the presence and extent of calcification and especially evaluating the distal left main vessel and its branches. IVUS assessment pre and post left main intervention is very important to evaluate larger lumen area of the ostial and midshaft left main and adequate post dilatation post stenting. In comparison to native coronary vessels, a minimal luminal area of <6.0 mm2 is a commonly used threshold for significant left main disease (Sano, Mintz et al. 2007). While there are no randomized trials to inform practice in this area, registry data has shown a trend toward reduced mortality in IVUS guided UPLM PCI.(Park, Kim et al. 2009)

2.4 Guidance for Chronic Total Occlusion (CTO) intervention

CTOs are the most complex lesions that are considered for percutaneous coronary revascularization. PCI of CTO results in symptomatic improvement, improved left ventricle function and reduction in adverse remodelling. In addition recanalization of CTO leads to long-term survival benefit and avoidance of bypass surgery (Melchior, Doriot et al. 1987; Ivanhoe, Weintraub et al. 1992; Chung, Nakamura et al. 2003; Cheng, Selvanayagam et al. 2008). The number of CTO interventions has risen gradually due to better operator experience, technical improvements, and newer procedural techniques (these include contra-lateral coronary injection, "parallel" wire techniques, subintimal tracking and re-entry (STAR), retrograde approach with control antegrade retrograde tracking (CART), reverse CART). Despite these advances, the success rate of CTO interventions remains low (<60%)(Di Mario, Werner et al. 2007), largely due to difficulty crossing the occlusion with the guidewire and entering the true distal lumen beyond the occlusion (Safian, McCabe et al. 1988; Kinoshita, Katoh et al. 1995). In most instances of failed CTO intervention, the guidewire enters the false lumen (subintimal space) at the site of occlusion, often making it impossible to re-enter the true lumen (Figure 5). CTO interventions can be performed via an antegrade approach or retrograde approach using septal collaterals (Surmely, Tsuchikane et al. 2006).

IVUS studies provide insights into the anatomy of the CTO lesion. In one report IVUS demonstrated presence of calcium mostly across the side branch take-off, especially in abrupt-origin CTOs (Fujii, Mintz et al. 2006). This anatomical variance can explain the preferential entry of the guidewire into the side branch at the point of occlusion. The use of IVUS for CTO interventions can be extremely useful especially in ensuring that the guidewire is positioned within the coronary lumen (true or false), and also helps to identify the optimal entry point within the CTO cap(Ochiai, Ogata et al. 2006). IVUS can help to avoid subintimal stenting during CTO intervention as this has been reported to result in stent thrombosis and stent mal-apposition due to the formation of multiple aneurysms (Erlich, Strauss et al. 2006; Tsujita, Maehara et al. 2009). IVUS imaging for CTO can also detect vessel wall haematoma, dissection and small perforations that are not detected by routine coronary angiography. Further advances in IVUS technology especially the development of 'forward facing IVUS' will significantly improve our anatomical understanding of the chronically occluded lumen. Although IVUS guided intervention of chronic occlusions may enhance procedural outcome, the current use of this technology for CTO intervention is limited only to experienced operators.

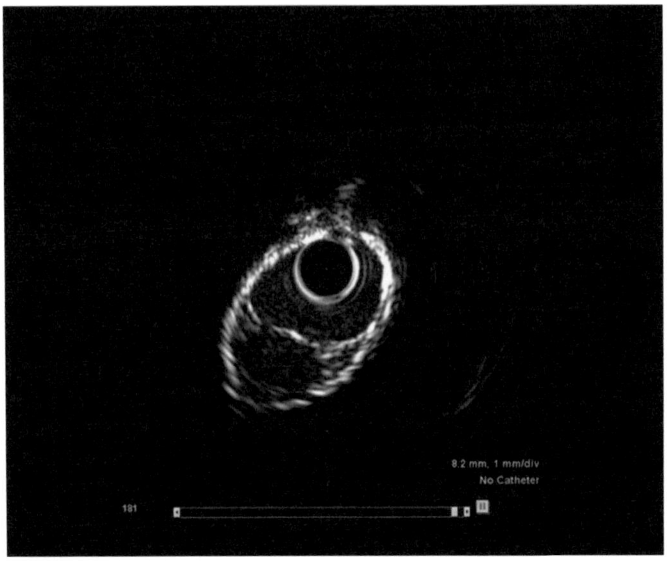

Fig. 5. IVUS image of false lumen

2.5 Guidance for bifurcation lesion intervention

PCI of bifurcation lesions have been associated with lower procedural success rate and worse clinical outcome than when used to treated non-bifurcation lesions. This is largely related to the complexity of the bifurcation lesions, significant anatomical variation of the bifurcation lesion, and lack of standard guidelines for the treatment of bifurcation lesions. The current therapeutic strategies for bifurcation lesions have mainly stemmed from personal clinical experience of the operators. (Suzuki, Angiolillo et al. 2007). In recent years there has been better understanding of bifurcation lesions especially with use of DES, acceptance of provisional stenting (acceptance of a suboptimal result in a small side branch SB), specific treatment of bifurcation lesions with a two-stent strategy and increasing use of final kissing balloon. The use of IVUS for bifurcation lesions can provide valuable information especially in anatomical evaluation of plaque burden, plaque location, angle assessment, lumen size of main branch [MB] and [SB]. In addition post PCI, IVUS can assist in evaluation of plaque shift, change in carina angle, dissection, and above all optimal stent deployment (Costa, Mintz et al. 2005). We feel that IVUS guided optimization of the bifurcation lesion post intervention, especially the ostium of a large side branch will enhance long term outcome of these technically challenging subset of lesions.

2.6 Vulnerable plaque assessment

The composition of atherosclerotic plaque is heterogeneous by nature and contains 1) fibrocellular components (extracellular matrix and smooth muscle cells), 2) lipid-cellular components (crystalline cholesterol and cholesterol esters mixed with macrophages), 3) thrombotic components (platelets and fibrin) and 4) calcium (Figure 6) (Fuster, Badimon et al. 1992; Fuster, Badimon et al. 1992; Stary 2000; Virmani, Kolodgie et al. 2000). Vulnerable plaques that result in rupture have been now well described as thin cap fibroatheroma (TCFA).

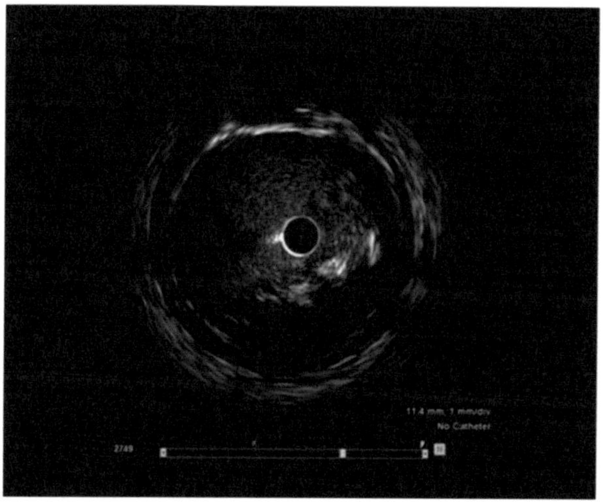

Fig. 6. IVUS image of atherosclerotic plaque

Ultrasound provides some information about the morphological features of atherosclerotic plaque. The American College of Cardiology Clinical Expert Consensus Document for IVUS imaging has described that a vulnerable plaque can appear as an 'echolucent' plaque (Mintz, Nissen et al. 2001). Frequently these echolucent plaques have a prominent echogenic border at the lumen-intima interface. This may correspond to the TCFA. However, it should be emphasized that the fibrous cap of TCFA is <65 μm and therefore could not be detected using this modality. Imaging IVUS provides limited insight into the chemical composition of the plaque and is dependent on simple interpretation of acoustic reflections. Lipid-laden echolucent plaques can be detected with a sensitivity of between 78% and 95% and specificity of 30% (Mallery, Tobis et al. 1990; Potkin, Bartorelli et al. 1990). Furthermore, reduced echogenicity may also be observed in large necrotic zones, intramural hemorrhage or a thrombus.

Echodense plaques have an intermediate echogenicity between echolucent and highly echogenic calcified plaques. The echodensity of plaques correlate well with plaque fibrosis in histological studies. The identification of echolucent plaques is subjective and no prospective clinical trials are available. In an IVUS based study, echolucent plaque was identified in 31 patients from a total of 144 patients. Of these 31 patients, 23 patients (74%) presented with unstable angina. Plaque rupture was confirmed by injecting contrast with subsequent filling of the plaque cavity on IVUS (Ge, Haude et al. 1995). In another study, IVUS images of 114 coronary lesions with <50% stenosis were recorded and followed up for two years.(Yamagishi, Terashima et al. 2000). The patients who developed Acute coronary syndrome during the follow up were identified and events correlated with large echolucent zones in the eccentric plaques at the time of their first IVUS study. These plaques had histological features similar to vulnerable plaques and were associated with increased risk of instability. In addition, IVUS can also identify vulnerable plaques at high risk of rupture in vessels with adaptive remodelling (von Birgelen, Klinkhart et al. 2001).

IVUS has excellent blood penetration and in the absence of calcium is able to visualize and calculate plaque area, volume and eccentricity. The use of IVUS to identify TCFA and lipid pool is at present limited. It suffers from signal attenuation and geometric effects that result in different backscatter signal properties from similar tissues due to differences in tissue orientation and position relative to the imaging transducer. Ultra- high frequency catheters can be employed to achieve high resolution and visualize subluminal fibrous cap, while low-resolution components can be used for better penetration of the plaque to assess plaque components.

The conventional IVUS image undergoes considerable processing such as envelope detection, time-gain compensation, and logarithmic compression to create real time imaging. However, this processing significantly reduces the ability to characterize the imaged tissue, the echogenicity of the imaged tissue is difficult to repeat and interpret quantitatively. The reflected unprocessed ultrasound signal in the form of A-scan or individual backscattered signals (256 A scans for an image) is called the radiofrequency data and it is the analysis of these individual A-scans that holds potential for tissue characterization. This imaging modality is known as IVUS virtual histology (IVUS -VH) or IVUS radiofrequency (IVUS-RF).

Ex-vivo studies have demonstrated that raw backscattered ultrasound signal allows a more detailed analysis of the vessel components with scope to identify different tissue morphology (Moore, Spencer et al. 1998). IVUS-VH uses spectral analysis of radiofrequency data to construct tissue maps that classify plaque into four major components (fibrous [labeled green], fibrolipidic [labeled greenish-yellow], necrotic core [labeled red] and calcium [labeled white]) which were correlated with a specific spectrum of the radiofrequency signal and assigned color codes (Nair, Kuban et al. 2001). In a clinical study, IVUS-VH was used to investigate the presence of IVUS-derived thin cap fibroatheroma (IDTCFA) in non-culprit, non-obstructive (<50%) lesions in 55 patients who presented with acute coronary syndrome (Rodriguez-Granillo, Garcia-Garcia et al. 2005). The axial resolution of the IVUS-VH is between 100 to 150 µm and therefore in this study the authors assumed that the absence of visible atheroma tissue overlying a necrotic core would suggest a cap thickness of below 100 to 150 µm and used the absence of such tissue to define a thin fibrous cap. In this study, IDTCFA was defined and identified as a lesion with a necrotic core ≥10% without evident overlying fibrous tissue and percent atheroma volume (PAV) ≥40%. In this study significantly higher prevalence of IDTCFA was observed in patients with Acute coronary syndrome in comparison with controls [(3.0 IQR 0.0 to 5.0 vs. 1.0 IQR 1.0 to 2.8) $p=0.018$]. The large multicenter PROSPECT trial (700 patients with Acute coronary syndrome) looked at long-term outcomes of non-culprit lesions (based on IVUS-VH) at the time of Percutaneous coronary intervention of the culprit lesions. The investigators reported that only 11 percent of the patients had high event rate (i.e. 17%) in association with thin-capped fibroatheromas with minimal luminal area (MLA) ≤4 mm^2 and plaque burden ≥70%. Although high-risk focal sites can be detected with IVUS-VH, the predictive power (significantly higher numbers of vulnerable plaques than clinical events) of vulnerable plaque to cause a clinical event remains low.

IVUS-RF data acquisition and real time processing with three dimensional imaging and spectral analysis is a potential tool to assess vulnerable plaque *in vivo*. This imaging tool provides detailed volumetric assessment of the histological components of the plaque *in vivo* and therefore may represent a unique technique to identify the vulnerable plaque in future.

3. Conclusion

Over the past decade there has been a significant technological advance in cardiovascular imaging that has changed the way we assess coronary atherosclerosis and approach coronary intervention. IVUS is a validated clinical tool that allows precise evaluation of angiographically stenotic lesions helping guide the cardiologist's approach to revascualisation and assess complications and sub-optimal results post-procedure. In addition it provides important information regarding non-critical but vulnerable plaque which is not appreciable by traditional coronary angiography. In an era of more complex and ambitious coronary intervention IVUS is a vitally important addition to the interventionalist's armamentarium. In this chapter we have briefly described the various potential uses of IVUS and their clinical application.

4. References

Abizaid, A., G. S. Mintz, et al. (1998). "Clinical, intravascular ultrasound, and quantitative angiographic determinants of the coronary flow reserve before and after percutaneous transluminal coronary angioplasty." *Am J Cardiol* 82(4): 423-8.

Black, A., R. Cortina, et al. (2001). "Unprotected left main coronary artery stenting: correlates of midterm survival and impact of patient selection." *J Am Coll Cardiol* 37(3): 832-8.

Cheng, A. S., J. B. Selvanayagam, et al. (2008). "Percutaneous treatment of chronic total coronary occlusions improves regional hyperemic myocardial blood flow and contractility: insights from quantitative cardiovascular magnetic resonance imaging." *JACC Cardiovasc Interv* 1(1): 44-53.

Chung, C. M., S. Nakamura, et al. (2003). "Effect of recanalization of chronic total occlusions on global and regional left ventricular function in patients with or without previous myocardial infarction." *Catheter Cardiovasc Interv* 60(3): 368-74.

Costa, R. A., G. S. Mintz, et al. (2005). "Bifurcation coronary lesions treated with the "crush" technique: an intravascular ultrasound analysis." *J Am Coll Cardiol* 46(4): 599-605.

de Jaegere, P., H. Mudra, et al. (1998). "Intravascular ultrasound-guided optimized stent deployment. Immediate and 6 months clinical and angiographic results from the Multicenter Ultrasound Stenting in Coronaries Study (MUSIC Study)." *Eur Heart J* 19(8): 1214-23.

Di Mario, C., G. S. Werner, et al. (2007). "European perspective in the recanalisation of Chronic Total Occlusions (CTO): consensus document from the EuroCTO Club." *EuroIntervention* 3(1): 30-43.

Erlich, I., B. H. Strauss, et al. (2006). "Stent thrombosis following the STAR technique in a complex RCA chronic total occlusion." *Catheter Cardiovasc Interv* 68(5): 708-12.

Fitzgerald, P. J., A. Oshima, et al. (2000). "Final results of the Can Routine Ultrasound Influence Stent Expansion (CRUISE) study." *Circulation* 102(5): 523-30.

Fujii, K., G. S. Mintz, et al. (2006). "Intravascular ultrasound profile analysis of ruptured coronary plaques." *Am J Cardiol* 98(4): 429-35.

Fuster, V., L. Badimon, et al. (1992). "The pathogenesis of coronary artery disease and the acute coronary syndromes (1)." *N Engl J Med* 326(4): 242-50.

Fuster, V., L. Badimon, et al. (1992). "The pathogenesis of coronary artery disease and the acute coronary syndromes (2)." *N Engl J Med* 326(5): 310-8.

Ge, J., M. Haude, et al. (1995). "Silent healing of spontaneous plaque disruption demonstrated by intracoronary ultrasound." *Eur Heart J* 16(8): 1149-51.

Grondin, C. M., I. Dyrda, et al. (1974). "Discrepancies between cineangiographic and postmortem findings in patients with coronary artery disease and recent myocardial revascularization." *Circulation* 49(4): 703-8.

Hoffmann, R., G. S. Mintz, et al. (1998). "Intimal hyperplasia thickness at follow-up is independent of stent size: a serial intravascular ultrasound study." *Am J Cardiol* 82(10): 1168-72.

Hong, M. K., G. S. Mintz, et al. (2006). "Intravascular ultrasound predictors of angiographic restenosis after sirolimus-eluting stent implantation." *Eur Heart J* 27(11): 1305-10.

Hong, Y. J., M. H. Jeong, et al. (2008). "Plaque prolapse after stent implantation in patients with acute myocardial infarction: an intravascular ultrasound analysis." *JACC Cardiovasc Imaging* 1(4): 489-97.

Ivanhoe, R. J., W. S. Weintraub, et al. (1992). "Percutaneous transluminal coronary angioplasty of chronic total occlusions. Primary success, restenosis, and long-term clinical follow-up." *Circulation* 85(1): 106-15.

Kinoshita, I., O. Katoh, et al. (1995). "Coronary angioplasty of chronic total occlusions with bridging collateral vessels: immediate and follow-up outcome from a large single-center experience." *J Am Coll Cardiol* 26(2): 409-15.

Mallery, J. A., J. M. Tobis, et al. (1990). "Assessment of normal and atherosclerotic arterial wall thickness with an intravascular ultrasound imaging catheter." *Am Heart J* 119(6): 1392-400.

Melchior, J. P., P. A. Doriot, et al. (1987). "Improvement of left ventricular contraction and relaxation synchronism after recanalization of chronic total coronary occlusion by angioplasty." *J Am Coll Cardiol* 9(4): 763-8.

Mintz, G. S. and A. Maehara (2009). "Serial intravascular ultrasound assessment of atherosclerosis progression and regression. State-of-the-art and limitations." *Circ J* 73(9): 1557-60.

Mintz, G. S., S. E. Nissen, et al. (2001). "American College of Cardiology Clinical Expert Consensus Document on Standards for Acquisition, Measurement and Reporting of Intravascular Ultrasound Studies (IVUS). A report of the American College of Cardiology Task Force on Clinical Expert Consensus Documents." *J Am Coll Cardiol* 37(5): 1478-92.

Moore, M. P., T. Spencer, et al. (1998). "Characterisation of coronary atherosclerotic morphology by spectral analysis of radiofrequency signal: in vitro intravascular ultrasound study with histological and radiological validation." *Heart* 79(5): 459-67.

Nair, A., B. D. Kuban, et al. (2001). "Assessing spectral algorithms to predict atherosclerotic plaque composition with normalized and raw intravascular ultrasound data." *Ultrasound Med Biol* 27(10): 1319-31.

Nakamura, S., A. Colombo, et al. (1994). "Intracoronary ultrasound observations during stent implantation." *Circulation* 89(5): 2026-34.

Nishioka, T., A. M. Amanullah, et al. (1999). "Clinical validation of intravascular ultrasound imaging for assessment of coronary stenosis severity: comparison with stress myocardial perfusion imaging." *J Am Coll Cardiol* 33(7): 1870-8.

Ochiai, M., N. Ogata, et al. (2006). "Intravascular ultrasound guided wiring for chronic total occlusions." *Indian Heart J* 58(1): 15-20.

Ong, A. T., P. W. Serruys, et al. (2006). "The SYNergy between percutaneous coronary intervention with TAXus and cardiac surgery (SYNTAX) study: design, rationale, and run-in phase." *Am Heart J* 151(6): 1194-204.

Park, S. J., M. K. Hong, et al. (2001). "Elective stenting of unprotected left main coronary artery stenosis: effect of debulking before stenting and intravascular ultrasound guidance." *J Am Coll Cardiol* 38(4): 1054-60.
Park, S. J., Y. H. Kim, et al. (2009). "Impact of intravascular ultrasound guidance on long-term mortality in stenting for unprotected left main coronary artery stenosis." *Circ Cardiovasc Interv* 2(3): 167-77.
Potkin, B. N., A. L. Bartorelli, et al. (1990). "Coronary artery imaging with intravascular high-frequency ultrasound." *Circulation* 81(5): 1575-85.
Roberts, W. C. and A. A. Jones (1979). "Quantitation of coronary arterial narrowing at necropsy in sudden coronary death: analysis of 31 patients and comparison with 25 control subjects." *Am J Cardiol* 44(1): 39-45.
Rodriguez-Granillo, G. A., H. M. Garcia-Garcia, et al. (2005). "In vivo intravascular ultrasound-derived thin-cap fibroatheroma detection using ultrasound radiofrequency data analysis." *J Am Coll Cardiol* 46(11): 2038-42.
Safian, R. D., C. H. McCabe, et al. (1988). "Initial success and long-term follow-up of percutaneous transluminal coronary angioplasty in chronic total occlusions versus conventional stenoses." *Am J Cardiol* 61(14): 23G-28G.
Sano, K., G. S. Mintz, et al. (2007). "Assessing intermediate left main coronary lesions using intravascular ultrasound." *Am Heart J* 154(5): 983-8.
Schiele, F., N. Meneveau, et al. (1998). "Impact of intravascular ultrasound guidance in stent deployment on 6-month restenosis rate: a multicenter, randomized study comparing two strategies--with and without intravascular ultrasound guidance. RESIST Study Group. REStenosis after Ivus guided STenting." *J Am Coll Cardiol* 32(2): 320-8.
Schoenhagen, P., K. M. Ziada, et al. (2000). "Extent and direction of arterial remodeling in stable versus unstable coronary syndromes : an intravascular ultrasound study." *Circulation* 101(6): 598-603.
Sonoda, S., Y. Morino, et al. (2004). "Impact of final stent dimensions on long-term results following sirolimus-eluting stent implantation: serial intravascular ultrasound analysis from the sirius trial." *J Am Coll Cardiol* 43(11): 1959-63.
Stary, H. C. (2000). "Natural history and histological classification of atherosclerotic lesions: an update." *Arterioscler Thromb Vasc Biol* 20(5): 1177-8.
Surmely, J. F., E. Tsuchikane, et al. (2006). "New concept for CTO recanalization using controlled antegrade and retrograde subintimal tracking: the CART technique." *J Invasive Cardiol* 18(7): 334-8.
Suzuki, N., D. J. Angiolillo, et al. (2007). "Percutaneous coronary intervention of bifurcation coronary disease." *Minerva Cardioangiol* 55(1): 57-71.
Takagi, T., G. Stankovic, et al. (2002). "Results and long-term predictors of adverse clinical events after elective percutaneous interventions on unprotected left main coronary artery." *Circulation* 106(6): 698-702.
Topol, E. J. and S. E. Nissen (1995). "Our preoccupation with coronary luminology. The dissociation between clinical and angiographic findings in ischemic heart disease." *Circulation* 92(8): 2333-42.
Tsujita, K., A. Maehara, et al. (2009). "Cross-sectional and longitudinal positive remodeling after subintimal drug-eluting stent implantation: multiple late coronary aneurysms,

stent fractures, and a newly formed stent gap between previously overlapped stents." *JACC Cardiovasc Interv* 2(2): 156-8.

Virmani, R., F. D. Kolodgie, et al. (2000). "Lessons from sudden coronary death: a comprehensive morphological classification scheme for atherosclerotic lesions." *Arterioscler Thromb Vasc Biol* 20(5): 1262-75.

Von Birgelen, C., W. Klinkhart, et al. (2001). "Plaque distribution and vascular remodeling of ruptured and nonruptured coronary plaques in the same vessel: an intravascular ultrasound study in vivo." *J Am Coll Cardiol* 37(7): 1864-70.

Yamagishi, M., M. Terashima, et al. (2000). "Morphology of vulnerable coronary plaque: insights from follow-up of patients examined by intravascular ultrasound before an acute coronary syndrome." *J Am Coll Cardiol* 35(1): 106-11.

Wu, X., Maehara A, et al. (2010). "Virtual histology intravascular ultrasound analysis of non-culprit attenuated plaques detected by grayscale intravascular ultrasound in patients with acute coronary syndromes." *J Am Coll Cardiol* 105(1):48-53.

Gregg W. Stone., Akiko Maehara, et al. (2011). " A Prospective Natural-History Study of Coronary Atherosclerosis". *N Engl J Med* 364:226-35.

8

IVUS Guided PCI

T. Kovarnik and J. Horak
2nd Department of Medicine - Department of Cardiovascular Medicine, First Faculty of Medicine, Charles University in Prague and General University Hospital in Prague, Czech Republic

1. Introduction

Intravascular ultrasound is a clinical tool that has been used in a complimentary manner to contrast angiography in order to enhance the procedure success rate and patient outcomes. Particularly, there are some specific situations where IVUS can be very useful and information from IVUS overcome angiography limitations. These situations can be divided into three parts:

- pre-interventional
- during intervention
- post-interventional

Pre-interventional use of IVUS can help with assessment of hemodynamic significance of stenosis (in this place must be emphasized, that IVUS can estimate hemodynamic significance only non directly, but with acceptable correlation with fractional flow reserve and nuclear stress test), precise anatomic analysis (type of bifurcation, plaque burden in ostial part of side branch or left main) and can help with device selection: precise measurement of diameters in reference segments for better sizing of balloon or stent, type of lesion preparation such as dilatation with cutting balloon or atherectomy devices in bulky lesions, drug eluting stent for lesions with high probability of small in stent area achievement.

IVUS can be used during intervention for assessment of lesion preparation (proper position of wire; especially it's relation to stent struts, effect of predilatation, assessment of side branch ostium) for guiding in more complicated intervention (left main stenting, navigation of wires during PCI of chronic total occlusion, trifurcation PCI).

Post-interventional use of IVUS can answer questions about result adequacy (stent expansion, stent apposition), angiographic filling defects ("hazy lesions") after PCI (edge dissection, thrombus formation, inadequate stent expansion, prominent calcification) and diagnosis of complications (dissection, geographic mismatch, plaque protrusion inside the stent, inadequate stent expansion or apposition). IVUS can in most cases also reveal the reasons behind development of complications after PCI such is in stent thrombosis (mainly inadequate stent expansion or edge troubles such as dissection, or uncovered lesion) or unexpected early in stent restenosis (inadequate stent expansion).

IVUS is a mandatory tool in the cardiac catheterization laboratory today. Like all medical equipments it should be used by an experienced investigator for better understanding of PCI mechanisms, prevention and solution of complications. Nowadays it is possible to use many semi-automatic softwares for border detection, but all of them must be corrected manually to avoid serious mistakes and misunderstanding. The best way how to do that is just routine use of IVUS.

1.1 Limitation of angiography

Angiography is a gold standard for assessment of atherosclerotic impairment of coronary arteries and for guiding of coronary intervention. On the other hand it has many limitations. Widely accepted decision making point for diagnosis of flow-limiting lesion is lumen diameter less than 50% of the reference segment. However, it has been proven that there is no correlation between angiography assessment and functional measurement by fractional flow reserve (FFR) in intermediate lesions between 40-70%[1].

Based on autopsy studies we know, that atherosclerosis is more often diffuse than focal process affecting coronary arteries. These findings are in good correlation with intravascular ultrasound. The reference segment, which is angiographically normal often contains atherosclerotic plaques visible on IVUS. From this point of view we are comparing less affected segments with more affected ones during angiography and thus underestimate stenosis significance[2,3]. Other challenging issues are assessment of ostial lesions and bifurcations.

2. Quantitative lesion assessment

2.1 Technique

The most important parameter for quantitative lesion assessment is minimal lumen area (MLA), which has the best correlation with presence of ischemia (see below).Common misunderstanding comes from the assessment of relative severity of stenosis in percentage of "normal" reference diameter. Angiographic stenosis assessment is based on comparison of lumen diameter in reference segment and lumen diameter in the lesion. The most corresponding IVUS parameter is lumen area stenosis (LAS), which is calculated as minimal lumen area in reference segment - minimal lumen area in lesion / minimal lumen are in reference segment. More frequently used description of stenosis is plaque burden (PB), computed as external elastic membrane area - lumen area / external elastic membrane area[4]. We must interrogate each frame and look for the smallest lumen area, use routinely nitrates before IVUS probe insertion for avoiding spasms. In case of uncertainty in lumen measurement, especially in present of soft plaque it is recommended to flush guiding catheter by saline for clearing of picture. Using of automatic pullback devices is not necessary for quantitative lesion assessment, but allows us to perform longitudinal diameters or volumetric analysis. Manual pullback is better for analysis of a precise part of plaque, where we can stop IVUS probe to obtain more frames from the region of interest. For imaging of aorto-ostial lesions it is necessary to retract the guiding catheter back into the aorta and verify that the path of the IVUS probe is still coaxial with the ostium of the vessel[5].

2.2 Indication for coronary intervention

The main indication for coronary intervention is lesion producing myocardial ischemia, which can be detect either non-invasively by stress myocardial perfusion imaging (SPECT) or invasively by measurement of pressure gradient across stenosis (fraction flow reserve, FFR). IVUS measurement correlates with both of them (table one).

Author	Description	Methods	No of patients	Results
Briguori[6]	angiographic stenosis 40-70%	IVUS vs. FFR	43	*FFR < 0.75 correlates with:* - MLA ≤ 4 mm² - MLD ≤ 1.8 mm - PB > 70% - Lesion length > 10 mm
Abizaid[7]	patients indicated for PCI	IVUS vs. CFR	73	*CFR ≥2 correlates with:* - MLA ≥ 4 mm² - MLD ≥ 2 mm
Nishioka[8]	consecutive IVUS examinations	IVUS vs. myocardial SPECT	79	*Positive scan correlates with:* - MLA ≤ 4 mm² - PB > 73% - LAS >59%
Takagi[9]	consecutive IVUS examinations	IVUS vs. FFR	42	*FFR <0.75 correlates with:* - MLA ≤ 3 mm² - LAS > 60%
Lee[10]	vessels smaller than 3 mm	IVUS vs. FFR	94	*FFR < 0.75 correlates with:* - MLA ≤ 2.0 mm2 - PB ≥ 80% - Lesion lenght ≥ 20 mm
Abizaid[11]	IVUS deferred PCI	IVUS	300	*Safe deferral of PCI correlates with:* - MLA ≥ 4 mm² - MLD ≥ 2 mm
Jasti[12]	ambiguous left main stenosis	IVUS vs. FFR	55	*FFR < 0.75 correlates with:* - MLA ≤ 5.9 mm² - MLD ≤ 2.8 mm
Abizaid[13]	patients with borderline left main stenosis	IVUS	122	*MACE predictor :* - MLD ≤ 3.0 mm
Kang [14]	Consecutive patients	IVUS vs. FFR	201	*FFR <0.80 correlates with:* - MLA 2.4 mm² - PB ≥79%
Ben Dor[15]	patients with intermediate lesion during QCA	IVUS vs. FFR	84	*FFR < 0.8 correlates with:* - MLA 2.4 mm² mm for vessels 2.5-3.0 mm - MLA 2.7 mm² for vessels 3.0-3.5 mm - MLA 3.6 mm² for vessels >3.5 mm
Ahn[16]	consecutive patients with SPECT and IVUS	IVUS vs. SPECT	150	*Positive scan correlates with:* - MLA 2.1 mm²
PROSPECT[17]	clinical follow-up after ACS	IVUS and MACE	700	*Predictors for MACE:* - PB > 70% - MLA < 4 mm² - TCFA

Abbreviations: CFR - coronary flow reserve, MACE – major cardiac adverse event, MLA – minimal lumen area, MLD – minimal lumen diameter, PB - plaque burden, PCI- percutaneous coronary interventions, QCA – quantitative coronary angiography, SPECT – single photon emission computed tomography, TCFA thin cap fibroatheroma

Table 1. Studies with IVUS evaluation of hemodynamic significance

Based on older studies the following recommendations for IVUS detection of significant stenosis were established:
Main epicardial artery:
- MLA < 4 mm^2
- MLD < 2 mm

Left main:
- MLA < 6 mm^2
- MLD 3 mm

However, recently published studies do not support these cut-off values. Instead of clear cut-off points there are number of different recommended values, which do not seem to be useful for routine practice. Based on these findings we must conclude that IVUS is not suitable for assessment of haemodynamic significance of intermediate lesions. IVUS can be only used for exclusion of haemodynamicly significant lesion with MLA more than 4 mm^2 for main epicardial arteries and more than 6 mm^2 for left main. The haemodynamic significance of each lesion is caused not only by lumen area, but also by amount of viable myocardium supplied by this vessel and by presence or absence of collaterales. These facts simply cannot be examined solely by a morphologic modality like IVUS. On the other hand the PROSPECT trial[17] with clinical endpoints confirmed, that large plaque compromising lumen to 4 mm^2 and less, especially together with higher content of necrotic tissue is a risk factor for future events. These issues will be matter of further studies.
There are no data about IVUS criteria for hemodynamic significance in saphenous vein graft, but it is recommend to use a cut-off point MLA 4 mm^2 for graft supplying one coronary artery and MLA 6 mm^2 for graft supplying two arteries.
The precise assessment of hemodynamic significance is a crucial point, because the rate of ischemic events is 5-10% / year in significant lesion and less than 1%/ year in non-ischemic lesion. Performing PCI in non-ischemic lesion increase risk of event to 2-3% / year[18] and furthermore increases risk of periprocedural ischemia or myocardial necrosis during PCI.
Very old IVUS-skeptic sentence "If you want to stent, do IVUS" was quite recently supported by the work of Nam et al.[19]. Authors randomized 167 patients with intermediate coronary lesion between FFR guided (cut-off for PCI was FFR <0.8) and IVUS guided (cut-off MLA< 4.0 mm^2) coronary intervention. PCI was performed in 33.7% lesion in FFR arm and in 91.5% in IVUS arm. This difference was highly statisticaly significant ($p<0.001$). On the other hand we ourselves have a different experience with IVUS assessment in borderline lesions. We estimate that we are performing PCI in 40-50% of borderline lesions based on IVUS criteria, which is closer to FRR guided arm in this study. The finding of 91.5% frequency of MLA < 4 mm^2 in lesion between 40-70% is in our eyes unrealistic.

2.3 Assessment of left main (LM)

Left main stenosis is a very important predictor for future cardiac events[20]. Angiographic assessment of LM is often complicated for overlapping branches and short or no reference segment and can lead to inappropriate estimates of lesion severity[21]. IVUS is more sensitive for left main atherosclerosis than angiography[22]. Suter et al.[23] found that in half of the patients with an inconclusive angiogram IVUS detects a significant stenosis. There is no difference for left main assessment during pullback from left anterior descending artery (LAD) or left circumflex artery (LCX)[24]. On the other hand for accurate assessment of ostial part of LAD and LCX is necessary to perform two pullbacks from both daughter vessels, because oblique view can overestimates lumen area[25]. The main target in left main bifurcation (like in other bifurcation) is to make a decision between one or two stent strategy. Pullback from just one daughter artery can answer the question whether the ostium of second branch is affected or not. For a more precise evaluation of minimal lumen area it is necessary to perform pullback from both daughter branches.

The precise coaxial position of guiding catheter is important for measurement or ostial left main stenosis, other than coaxial position of guiding catheter overestimates the lumen area. This type of inappropriate measurement can be detected by elliptical instead of spherical shape of ostial left main.

The ostium of LM can be influenced not only by atherosclerosis but also by external compression between enlarged pulmonary artery and aorta. This compression occur during systolic phase and lumen is enlarged during diastolic phase (*figure 1,2*). This finding can be seen in patients with severe pulmonary artery hypertension

According to our experience we recommend to perform all PCI´s of LM with IVUS guidance. This is supported by results of MAIN-COMPARE registry, where IVUS guidance of left main PCI was superior to angiographic guidance[26].

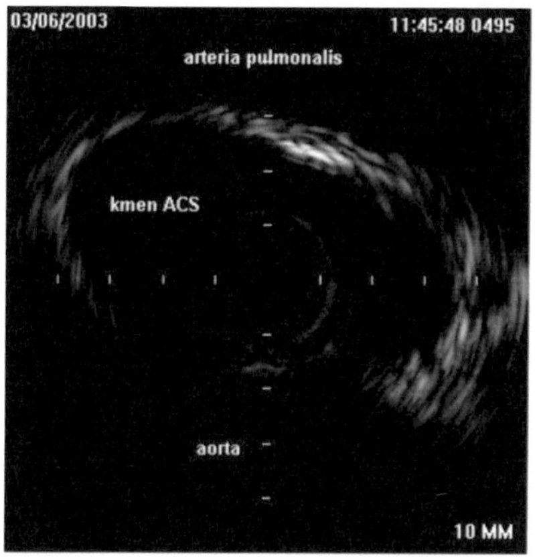

Fig. 1. External compression of left main during systolic phase of cardiac cycle. "Kmen ACS" means left main coronary artery.

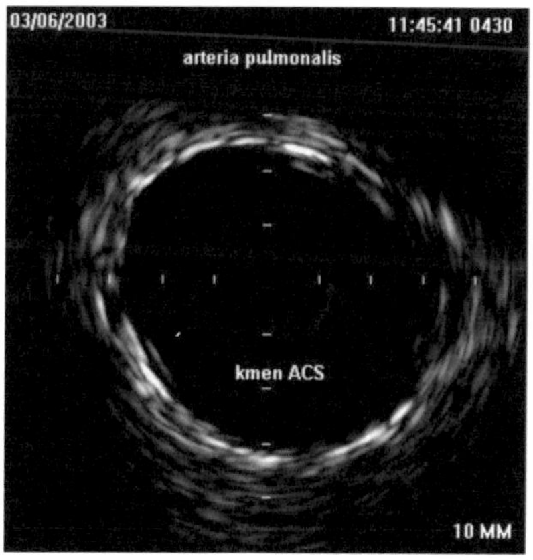

Fig. 2. No evidence of left main compression during diastolic phase of cardiac cycle.

3. Lesion morphology

3.1 IVUS in lesion with angiographic filling defect "hazy lesions"

The main finding in so called hazy lesions is a defect in the contrast filling of coronary artery. The reasons for this include:

- eccentric calcification (*figure 3*)
- significant stenosis
- dissection (*figure 4*)
- thrombosis (*figure 5*)
- plaque rupture (*figure 6*)
- "flow phenomenon" (inadequate filling of big arteries during dye injection).

Thrombus is the most dangerous cause and many hazy lesions are treated like thrombus-containing lesions with administration of IIbIIIa glycoprotein inhibitors, use of embolic protection devices or covered stents. However, real presence of intracoronary thrombosis is 50-60% of all hazy lesions[27]. Sensitivity of IVUS for thrombus is low (about 50%), so from IVUS picture we simply cannot rule out the presence of thrombus (the highest sensitivity for thrombus has optical coherence tomography), but IVUS can confirm other causes and mainly causes which are not indicated fore PCI. This strategy decreases frequency of PCI in hazy lesions to 15-20%[28-30]

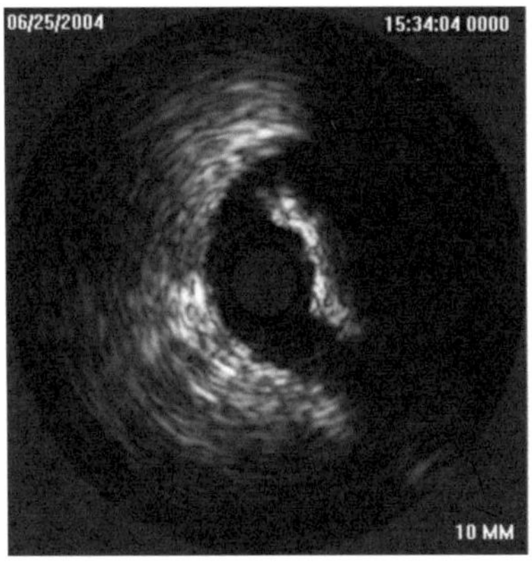

Fig. 3. Eccentric calcification.

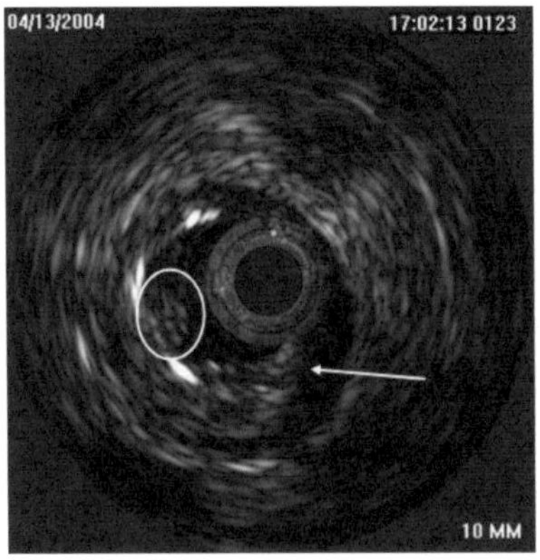

Fig. 4. Dissection with visible tear (arrow) and small thrombus (in circle).

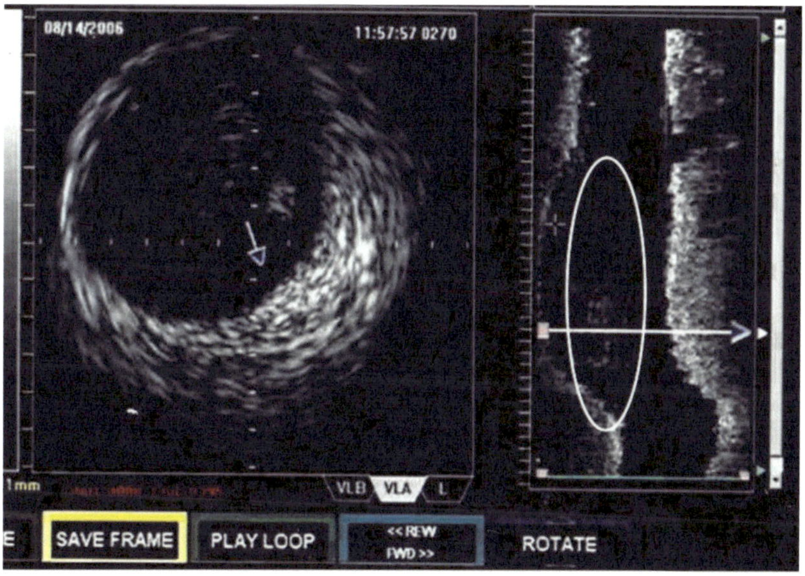

Fig. 5. Huge thrombus located on very small plaque causing acute coronary syndrome. Left side is cross sectional view, right side is longitudinal view (thrombus is located in the circle).

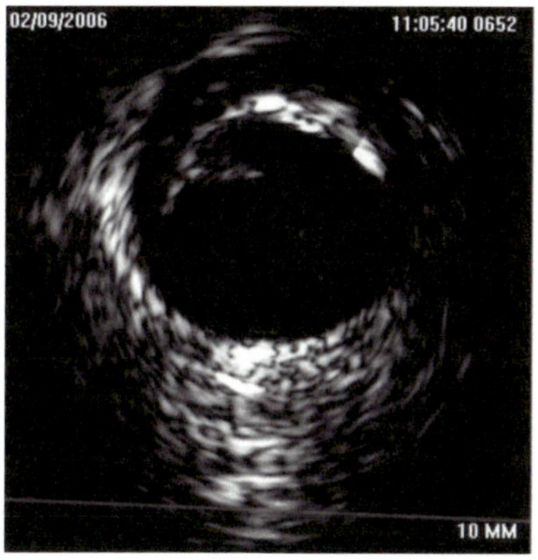

Fig. 6. Plague rupture with visible cavity after embolization of plaque mass. Patient with acute myocardial infarction.

3.2 Aneurysms

True aneurysm is defined as both an external elastic membrane (EEM) and lumen area 50% larger than the proximal reference segment with intact three layers of vessel wall (*figure 7*). Lesions which seem to be the aneurysms from angiographic assessment are an true aneurysm in 37% of such findings. The rest are normal segments adjacent to plaque (53%), complex atherosclerotic plaque (16%) and pseudoaneurysm (4%)[31]. Coronary pseudoaneurysm is due to rupture of vessel wall and in IVUS picture the three layers of vessel are not present, the shape of pseudoaneurysm is often irregular. From a practical point of view, pseudoaneurysms are seen only after coronary interventions causing trauma of vessel wall.

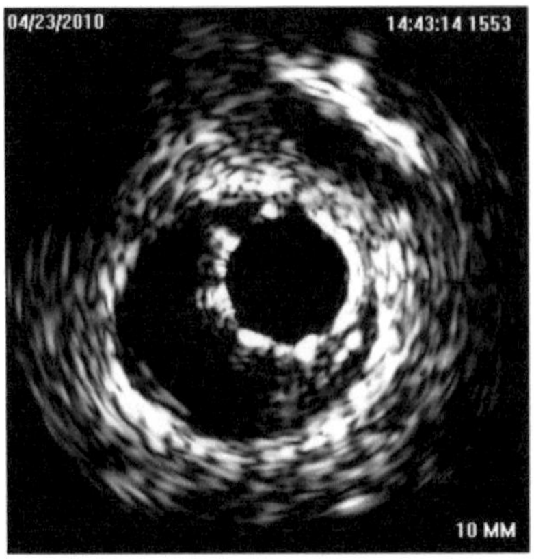

Fig. 7. Stent located in coronary aneurysm.

3.3 True versus false lumen

False lumen is created by dissection, either spontaneous or iatrogenic during coronary intervention (wire insertion or after balloon/stent dilatation). Dissections are treated by stent implantation and a flow non limiting dissection can be let to spontaneous healing. Stent insertion to the true lumen is a crucial point for proper treatment of dissection. True lumen can be identified by three-layered appearance and by origin of side branches. False lumen contains more echogenic blood flow[5] (*figure 8*).

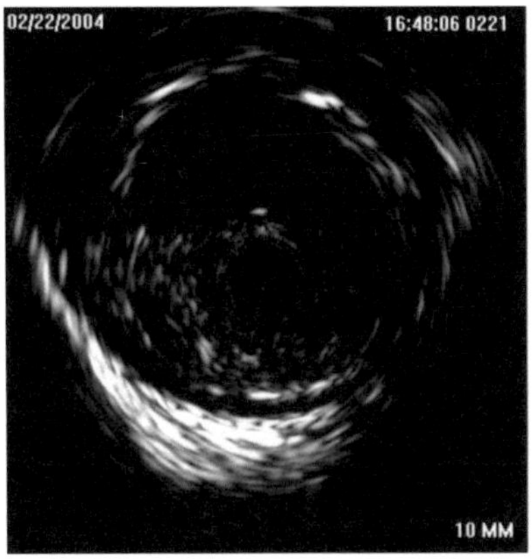

Fig. 8. Dissection with IVUS probe located in the false lumen with staying blood.

4. Balloon angioplasty

4.1 The mechanism of balloon PCI

The main mechanism of lumen enlargement during balloon dilatation is a plaque rupture, which enables lumen dilatation[32]. This finding was also confirmed by IVUS during *in vivo* studies, mainly in eccentric plaques (which are mainly present in coronary arteries). Another mechanism of lumen enlargement during balloon angioplasty is plaque compression and plaque redistribution, which are the main mechanism in concentric plaques[33].

4.2 IVUS guided plain balloon PCI

Several studies have been conducted in this field. Their results are summarized in table 2.

study	target	restenosis	MACE	comments
CLOUT[34] 102 pts.	using larger balloon than angiographicly measured vessel diameter	not declared	1.9%*	plaques compensated by positive remodeling allow use of aggressive dilatation without risk of significant dissections
Haase[35] 144 pts.	IVUS guided balloon dilatation	21%$^{+}$	12^{+}%	use of larger balloon than angiographic lumen diameter is safe and with low risk for restenosis
Schroeder[36] 252 pts.	IVUS guided balloon dilatation	19%$^{+}$	14^{+}%	small dissection are not flow limiting IVUS decreases number of implanted stents low restenosis comparable with BMS
Abizaid[37] 284 pts.	IVUS guided balloon dilatation and stent only in case of unsatisfactory result	8%$^{+}$- PCI 16% - stent	8%$^{+}$ - PCI 11%- stent	„stent like" effect after IVUS guided balloon dilatation has similar rate restenosis like a BMS
BEST[38] 254 pts.	IVUS guided aggressive PCI (stent only when necessary) vs. routine stenting	16.8%$^{♣}$ aggressive PCI 18.1% stent	16%$^{♣}$ - aggressive PCI 20% -stent	IVUS guided aggressive PCI with provisional stenting is safe and with the same results like routine stenting
SIPS[39] 269 pts.	IVUS vs. angio guided PCI	29%$^{♣}$ IVUS, 35% angio	30%$^{\nabla}$ IVUS 37% angio	same restenosis rate. Lower TLR in IVUS group
Gaster[40] 108 pts.	IVUS guided vs. angio guided (IVUS controlled) PCI	not declared	22%$^{\bullet}$ IVUS 41% angio	lower MACE in IVUS guided group, better C/E[3] ratio in IVUS group
Meuller[41] C/E analysis of SIPS study	IVUS guided vs. angio guided PCI	not declared	19.8%$^{\nabla}$ IVUS 31.1% angio	lower MACE in IVUS guided group, better C/E[4] ratio in v IVUS group
Colombo[42*] 130 pts.	IVUS guided intervention in lesions longer than 15 mm	25%$^{♣}$ IVUS 39% angio ($p < 0.05$)	22%$^{♣}$ IVUS 38% angio ($p < 0.05$)	Lower restenosis, MACE and number of stents in IVUS group

$^{+}$ 12 months MACE, $^{♣}$ 6 months MACE, $^{\bullet}$ 2,5 year, C/E cost/effectiveness ratio , $^{\nabla}$ 2 years, TLR: target lesion revascularization, BMS: bare metal stents

* non randomized study, control group is composed by similar lesions

Table 2. IVUS guided coronary intervention

The table 3 summarizes the strategy for choosing balloon diameter, acute complications and frequency of stenting in aforesaid studies.

study	B/A ratio	equation for balloon diameter	occurrence of acute severe dissection	stenting
CLOUT[34]	1.3 * 0.8-1**	mean MLDref + mean MVDref / 2	5%	not declared
Haase[35]	0.8-1 **	EEM in lesion	11%	0%
Schroeder[36]	1.4 * 0.88**	(2xEEM ref_{prox} + 2x$EEMref_{dist}$ + 2xEEM lesion)/ 6	12%	2%
Abizaid[37]	1.34 *	($EEMmax_{lesion}$ + EEM min_{lesion}) / 2	28%	53%
BEST[38]	1.25 *	(EEM ref_{prox} + $EEMref_{dist}$) / 2	18%	44% (in IVUS group)
SIPS[39]	1.23 IVUS* 1.03 angio	MLDref + MVDref / 2 (in smallest ref. segment)	3% IVUS, 3.2% angio	49.5% angio, 49.7% IVUS
Gaster[40]	not declared	($MLAref_{prox}$ + $MLAref_{dist}$) / 2	not declared	85% angio, 87% IVUS
Meuller[41]	not declared	not declared	not declared	49.5% angio, 49.7% IVUS
Colombo[42] °	1.23 **	EEM in lesion	4.6%	51.5%

Abbreviations: ref – reference segment, ref_{prox} - reference proximal segment, ref_{dist} – reference distal segment, * angiographic, ** IVUS, B/A - balloon artery ratio, mean MLA_{ref} – mean lumen in reference segments, QCA = quantitative coronary angiography - $EEMmax_{lesion}$ – maximal EEM in lesions, EEM min_{lesion} – minimal EEM in lesions, ° long lesion intervention

Table 3. Different strategies for choosing of balloon diameter.

The most frequent formula for choosing of balloon diameter is ($EEMref_{prox}$ + $EEMref_{dist}$) / 2 coming form BEST study or just $EEMref_{dist}$, which is adapted form the study SIPS.
IVUS criteria for optimal result after balloon dilatation are listed in table 4.

study	criteria
CLOUT[34]	MLA ≥ 65% mean MLA_{ref}, no signs of flow limiting disection
Haase[35]	increasing of MLA by at least 20% of EEM, no signs of flow limiting disection
Abizaid[37]	MLA ≥ 65% mean MLA_{ref}, or MLA ≥ 6mm², no signs of flow limiting disection
BEST[38]	residual stenosis < 30% (IVUS and angio), MLA > 6mm², no signs of flow limiting disection
SIPS[39]	MLA ≥ 65% mean MLA_{ref}, no signs of flow limiting disection
Mueller[41]	residual stenosis ≤ 35%, MLA > 65% meanMLA_{ref}, no signs of flow limiting disection
Colombo[42]*	MLA ≥ 50% EEM_{lesion}, MLA ≥ 5.5 mm²

Abbreviations: mean MLA_{ref} - mean minimal lumen area in reference segment, QCA - quantitative coronary angiography, * long lesion intervention

Table 4. IVUS criteria of optimal result after balloon dilatation.

Based on these studies with IVUS guided balloon dilatation we can summarize:

1. Using of larger balloons (balloon/artery ratio more than 1 according to angiographic assessment) is safe and without increased risk for acute severe complications. In hospital MACE were 1.4-3.9%. Occurrence of significant dissection varies in large range, probably for different definition of this kind of complication. However, all authors declare low risk for sever acute dissection.
2. The rate of in stent restenosis is consistently low in all studies. It means that it is safe to avoid stent implantation after fulfilling of IVUS criteria for adequate results after balloon dilation. Surprisingly, higher in stent restenosis and higher MACE were found in some studies in patients with stent implantation compared to plain balloon dilatation. The reason for this finding is probably for bias; according to the study design stents were implanted to lesions with non satisfactory results after balloon dilatation or for treatment of complications after balloon dilatation. Higher occurrence of in stent restenosis and MACE is expected in these types of lesions.
3. The dark side of IVUS guided balloon angioplasty is a prolonged procedural time (5-13 minutes), increased X-ray time (2-3.6 minutes) and higher amount of contrast dye (12-34 ml)[38-41]
4. Routine IVUS guided intervention can be beneficial from financial point of view. Optimal decision making decreases number of implanted stent and frequency of in stent restenosis and avoids peri-procedural complications from non-indicated coronary interventions[40,41].
5. IVUS guided intervention should be used for avoiding stent implantation in patients unsuitable for dual antiplatelet therapy.

5. Bare-metal stent implantation

5.1 Mechanism of lumen enlargement during stent implantation

The most important mechanisms are plaque redistribution (inside stent) and plaque extrusion (outside stent) to the reference segments (more frequently to the distal one)[43]. Plaque redistribution and extrusion play role during restenosis in edge segment of stent[44]. Less important factors are plaque compression, plaque embolization and vessel enlargement (more in vessel with negative remodeling before PCI)[43].

Final stent diameter is a result of interplay between pressure during implantation and vessel wall resistance. Declared stent diameters for different pressures during dilatation do not correlate with real stent diameter after implantation. These numbers for stent diameter come from *in vitro* tests in water and do not reflect real situation in the vessel. Costa et al.[45] compared 200 drug eluting stent diameters from IVUS measurement immediately after implantation and declared stent diameter for nominal pressure. At least 90% of minimal lumen diameter for nominal pressure was reached only in 4% of stents. In stent area can be decreased immediately after implantation also by protrusion of plaque material through the struts[46] (*figure9*).

It is important to distinguish between stent expansion and stent apposition. Expansion means ratio between minimal stent area (MSA) and lumen area in reference segment. Inadequate expansion (*figure 10*) can be improved by high pressure postdilatation. Apposition reflects contact between stent struts and vessel wall. Inadequate apposition (*figure 11*) can be solved by low pressure dilatation with a bigger balloon.

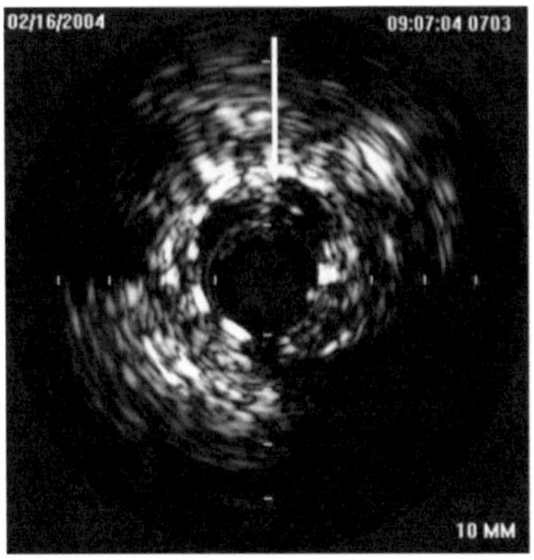

Fig. 9. Plaque protrusion through the struts to the lumen.

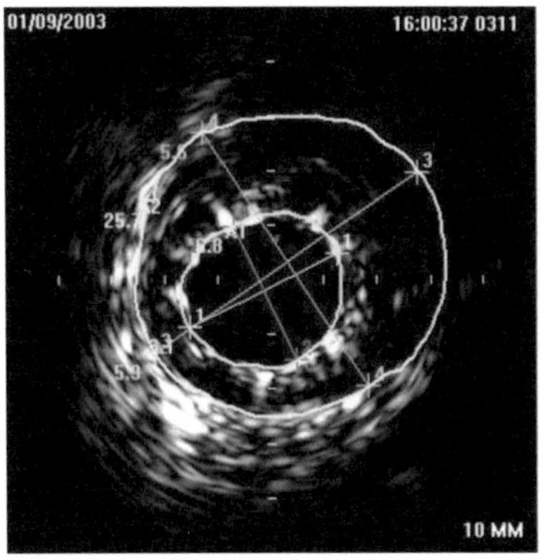

Fig. 10. Inadequate stent expansion.

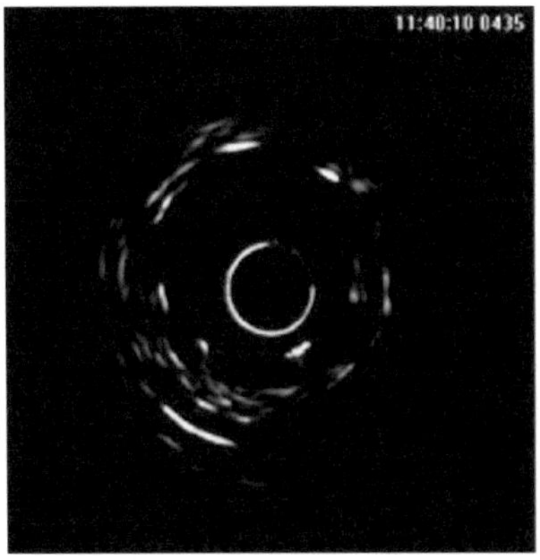

Fig. 11. Inadequate stent aposition

5.2 High pressure stent dilatation

The first implantations of Palmaz-Schatz and Gianturco-Roubin stents were complicated by high occurrence of subacute stent thrombosis. Colombo and coworkers started IVUS guided high pressure dilatation, which (together with dual antiagregation) decreased the rate of subacute stent thrombosis to 0.9%[47]. Routine use of high pressure dilatation (up to 20 atm.) improves stent expansion and apposition without increasing acute complications[48]. Choi et al.[49] found, that only 54% of angiographically adequatly expanded stents fulfill IVUS criteria for optimal stent expansion. Authors performed high pressure postdilatation and final MACE was only 11% in 6 months. This study confirms minimal stent area (MSA) as the most important risk factor of restenosis (*figure 12*).

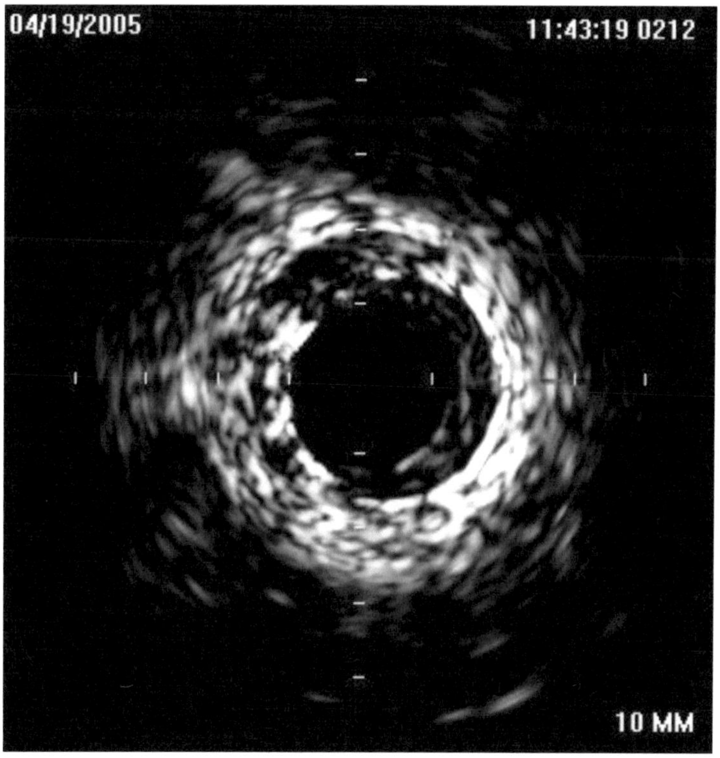

Fig. 12. In stent restenosis

5.3 IVUS guided stent implantation

There are many studies focusing on impact of IVUS guidance on stent implantation. They are summarized in table 5.

Different criteria for optimal stent expansion were used in published trials, details are summarized in table 6.

study name	study goal	restenosis	MACE	comments
MUSIC[50] 161 pts.	restenosis during IVUS guided stent implantation	9.7%	12.1% +	the second lowest restenosis rate in studies with BMS
Blasini[51] 105 pts.	IVUS vs. angio* guided stent implantation	20.9% IVUS 29.9% angio (p=0.033) **	not analyzed	Restenosis 13.5% in stent fulfilling IVUS criteria

study name	study goal	restenosis	MACE	comments
RESIST[52] study 155 pts.	IVUS vs. angio guided (IVUS controlled) stent implantation	22.5% IVUS 28.8% angio (p=0.25)	not declared	IVUS guidance does not decrease rate of in stent restenosis
OPTICUS[53] 550 pts.	IVUS vs. angio guided stent implantation	24.5% IVUS 22.5% angio (p=0.68)	17.9%[♣] IVUS 15.3% angio (p=0.4)	IVUS guiding do not decrease neither rate of in stent restenosis nor MACE
CRUISE[54] 499 pts.	IVUS vs. angio guided (IVUS controlled) stent implantation	not declared	TVR 8.5%[•] in IVUS group 15.3% in angio group (p=0.019)	IVUS guided stenting leads to lower TVR
Choi[49] 278 pts.	IVUS vs. angio guided stent implantation	not declared	12%[+]IVUS 19% angio (p=0,11)	IVUS leads to lower periprocedural complications with a trend for lower TVR in IVUS group(p=0.08)
AVID[55] 800 pts.	IVUS vs. angio guided stent implantation	not declared	18% IVUS 19% angio	IVUS leads to larger lumen, but without any effect on 30 days and 12 months MACE
TULIP[56] 150 pts.	IVUS vs. angio guided stenting of long lesions	23%[+] IVUS 46% angio (p=0.008)	6%[+] IVUS 20% angio (p=0.01)	Better clinical and angiographic results in IVUS group despite more implanted stents
PRESTO[57] 796 pts with IVUS vs. 8274 with angio	IVUS vs. angio guided stenting	not declared	TVR 13.8% IVUS 12.2% angio (p=0.9)	Larger MLD in IVUS group, but without difference in MACE. Criteria for adequate IVUS stent expansion was let only on operators discretion
DIPOL[58] 163 pts.	IVUS vs. angio guided stenting	10% IVUS 27% angio	7.3% IVUS 16% angio	Best results for IVUS guided in randomized trial
Gaster[55,60] 108 pts	IVUS vs. angio guided stenting	16% IVUS 25% angio	22% IVUS 41% angio	IVUS guiding is cost saving

* non randomized trial, angio group is a historic control, ** IVUS criteria was fulfilled in 49.5% patients and in these ones was restenosis 13.5%, + 6 months, ♣ 12 months, • 9 months, TVR - target vessel revascularization

Table 5. Trials assessing IVUS guided stent implantation.

study	criteria for optimal expanded stent
Katritsis[61]	full stent apposition, MSA ≥ 90% $meanMLA_{ref}$, symmetrical expansion (min SD/maxSD > 0.7) (correlation with FFR 0.94)
Fearon[62]	MSA 7 mm^2 (correlates with FFR 0.96)
Hanekamp[63]	full stent apposition, MSA ≥ 90% $meanMLA_{ref}$, or MSA ≥ 100% $minMLA_{ref}$, symetrical expansion (minSD/maxSD > 0.7), (correlation with FFR 0.94)
Gorge[48]	symmetrical stent expansion, MSD ≥ 3 mm, full apposition
Choi[49]	complete stent apposition, MSA ≥ 80% $distalMLA_{ref}$, symmetrical expansion (minSD/maxSD > 0.8)
Colombo[47]	full stent apposition , MSA ≥ $minMLA_{ref}$, MLA > 60% MLA_{ref} in edge regions
Ahmed[44]	complete stent apposition, MSA ≥ 80% $meanMLA_{ref}$ or MSA 7.5 mm^2
MUSIC[50]*	- complete stent apposition, MSA ≥ 90 $meanMLA_{ref}$ or ≥ 100 $minMLA_{ref}$ - in case of > 9 mm^2: MSA ≥ 80% $meanMLA_{ref}$ or ≥ 90% $minMLA_{ref}$ MSA in proximal part of stent ≥ 90% $proxMLA_{ref}$ symmetrical expansion (minSD/maxSD > 0.7)
Blasini[51]	full stent apposition, MSA > 8 mm^2, or MSA ≥ 90% $meanMLA_{ref}$, complete coverage of dissection
RESIST[52]	MSA ≥ 80% $meanMLA_{ref}$
OPTICUS[53]	MUSIC criteria, residual stenosis les than 10% (angiographically)
CRUISE[54]	residual stenosis < 10% (angiographically)
AVID[55]	full stent apposition, residual stenosis < 10%, no signs of dissection
TULIP[56]	complete stent apposition, MSD ≥ 80% $meanMLD_{ref}$, MSA ≥ 90% $distalMLA_{ref}$

Abbreviations: SD - stent diameter, $meanMLA_{ref}$ - mean minimal lumen area in reference segments, $minMLA_{ref}$ minimal - minimal lumen area i reference segments, MSD – minimal stent diameter, MSA – minimal stent area

* all criteria were fulfilled in 81% patients and these patients were treated only with acetylosalycilic acid and rate of subacute stent thrombosis was 1.3%

Table 6. Different criteria for optimal stent expansion.

The main goal for IVUS guidance of stent implantation is a larger minimal stent diameter and minimal stent area. Further improvement is seen in strut apposition. Minimal stent area is the most important risk factor for development of in stent restenosis (ISR). The cut-off point for risk of ISR is 8mm2 in vessel ≥ 3 mm and 6 mm2 in vessel < 3mm[64]. The rate of in stent restenosis according to achievement of different IVUS parameters is summarized in table 7.

criteria	restenosis rate
MSA > 9 mm^2	11%
MSA > 9 mm^2 a MSA ≥ 80% $meanMLA_{ref}$	12.5%
MSA ≥ 55% $meanEEM_{ref}$	17%
MSA ≥ 90% $meanMLA_{ref}$	21%
MSA ≥ 90% distal MLA_{ref}	22%

Abbrevation: MSA – minimal stent area

Table 7. Risk of ISR and achievement of different IVUS parameters.

The lowest rate of ISR is in stents with MSA > $9mm^2$. However, for achievement of this MSA it is necessary to use a 3.5mm stent (with ideal stent area $9.6mm^2$), because 3mm stent has an ideal stent area $7.1mm^2$. MSA 8 mm^2 as a sufficient post-stenting area was confirmed by Hoffmann et al[65]. They found a mean MSA in stent with ISR $7.1mm^2$ and $8.1mm^2$ in stents without development of ISR. This cut-off MSA is also a predictor for development of ISR in long stents[66]. Further predictors for ISR are:

- length of stents[67]
- strong calcification[68]
- bulky plaque compensated by positive vessel remodelation[69-72] (*figure 13*)
- plaque protrusion through the stent struts[73]

MSA is the most important factor for development of in stent thrombosis (IST)[74]. The incidence of this feared complication is less than 0.5%[74].

Parise et al.[75] published recently a meta-analysis of all randomized studies comparing IVUS guided vs. angio guided stenting in pre-drug-eluting stent era. They concluded that IVUS guided stenting significantly lowered the 6-month angiographic restenosis rates, 12-month revascularization and MACE rate. They did not find any effect of IVUS guidance on death or myocardial infarction.

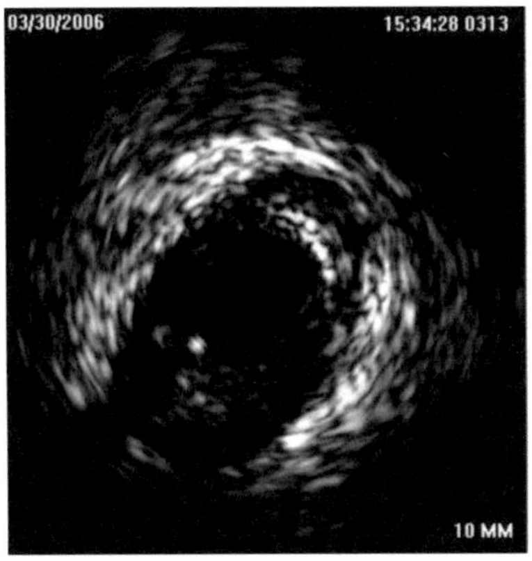

Fig. 13. Large plaque compensated by positive vessel remodeling

6. Drug-eluting stent implantation

Drug eluting stents (DES) significantly reduce the risk of in stent restenosis compared to BMS[76-78]. IVUS guidance seemed to be needless for DES excellent results. However, several issues are still a problem even with the use of DES and some of them, like in stent thrombosis, seem to be more important than in BMS .

In stent restenosis still exists and it´s incidence is 5-10% in selected populations[79-80]. It seems to be more pronounced in paclitaxel eluting stent than sirolimus eluting stents[81]. Minimum stent area that best separates restenosis from no restenosis in DES is between 5.0-6.0 mm^2 [82,83].

The occurrence of in stent thrombosis (IST) in DES is 1-1.5%[84]. The main cause of IST is stent under expansion. DES with further IST development showed significantly lower MSA (4.3-4.6 mm^2). Further risk factor for IST development is residual edge stenosis, defined as a MLA < 4 mm^2 and a plaque burden > 70%[85,74]. These risk factors remain the same like in BMS, where the presence of dissection, thrombus or tissue prolaps into the stent were recognized as further risk factors for IST development[86,87]. The occurrence of IST in BMS is estimated at 0.9%[88].

The risk factors for IST development can be revealed by IVUS control after stent implantation. Roy et al.[89] published study, where IVUS guidance of DES implantation reduced development of IST in 30 days (0.5% in IVUS vs. 1.5% in angio guided group) and 12 month (0.7% in IVUS vs. 2.0% in angio guided group), as well as decreased need for revascularization and MACE in 30 day. Unfortunately, there were no clear criteria for adequate stent deployment in this study. Claessen et al.[90] published a study comparing angio and IVUS guidance in 1504 sirolimus eluting stent implantation in the MATRIX (Comprehensive Assessment of Sirolimus-Eluting Stents in Complex Lesions) registry. They found significantly lower occurrence of myocardial infarction and combined endpoint of myocardial infarction and death in IVUS guided group. Hur et al.[91] published their enormous registry of angio (3744 patients) versus IVUS (4627 patients) guided stent implantation. The main finding of this study is lower mortality in IVUS guided group. This result was seen mainly in DES implantation, because mortality in BMS group was the same. However, the explanation of this interesting finding is not clear, because the occurrence of myocardial infarction, target vessel revascularization and in stent thrombosis was without significance differences between angio and IVUS group. Based on aforesaid trials we can conclude, that IVUS guidance of DES implantation probably improves patient's outcome, but further trials are needed for better understanding of this phenomenon.

Important phenomenon in DES implantation is incomplete stent apposition (ISA), which means, that at least one strut is not adequately apposed to vessel wall. One should distinguish between acute stent malapposition, which is present immediately after stent implantation, late stent malapposition (LSM), which can be persistent , it means that acute malapposition is not healed and late-acquired stent malapposition (LASM), which develops despite normal finding after stent implantation. The mechanism of LASM development is not known, several mechanisms are thought:

- positive vessel remodeling leading to vessel enlargement
- decrease of plaque volume behind the stent caused by antiproliferative effect of DES
- thrombus dissolution after PCI of thrombus containing lesions

The frequency of LSM is not clear, a quite broad range for this phenomenon was published (4-21%)[92,93]. LSM is not found only in DES, but also in BMS, where it's incidence is 4.4-5.4%[94,95]. Empty space behind stent struts can lead to decrease of blood flow in this region and cause development of thrombosis. However, this theoretic concept was not proved in any study following the natural course of patients with LSM. Hong et al.[96,97] did not find any clinical adverse event in patient with LSM during 10 months follow up. On the other hand Cook et al.[98] published correlation between LSM and very late IST. Moreover, Hassan et al.[99] published meta-analysis of 17 randomized trials focusing on LSM in BMS as well as DES. They found four times higher risk of LASM in patients with DES compared to BMS and LSM (acquired or persistent) increased significantly risk for (very) late in stent thrombosis (OR 6,51).

A rare complication (1.25%) of DES implantation is development of coronary aneurysm. The definition of aneurysm is focal enlargement of vessel lumen, which is 50% larger than adjacent reference vessel. Coronary aneurysm is not a benign finding as up to 40% of patients needed revascularization in a study done by Alfonso et al.[100].

7. Ivus guided pci in specific situation

7.1 PCI of bifurcation lesions

PCI in bifurcation is a more challenging procedure with a risk of compromising flow in side branch (SB) and with higher rate of restenosis. The "classical" mechanisms of worsening flow in side branch were thought [101]

- plaque compression in ostial part of SB during dilatation in main vessel (MV). The presence of diffuse ostial plaque (*figure 14*) has higher risk for TIMI 2 flow after stenting than presence of eccentric plaque[102]
- plaque shifting from the MV to SB during dilatation in MV ("snow-plow" phenomenon)
- interposition of stent struts across the ostium of SB

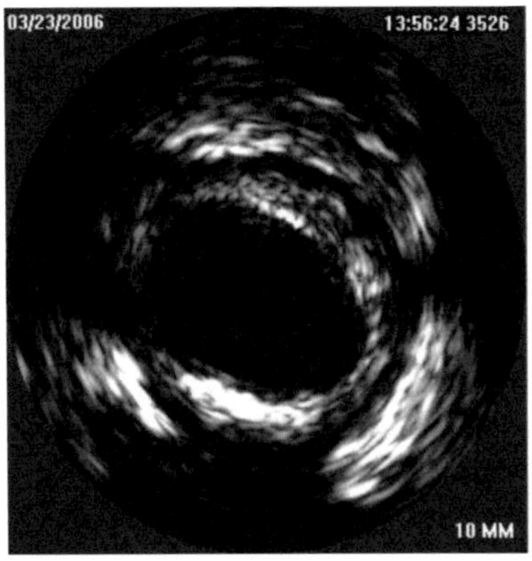

Fig. 14. Bifurcation with diffuse impairment of side branch ostium.

Plaque in bifurcation is mainly localized in counter carina[103]. However, Medina et al.[104] proved the presence of plaque also in carina. They found plaque in 32% of bifurcations and moreover, in 16% of bifurcations the plaque in the carina was larger than in counter carina area. Furthermore, authors showed, that the mechanism of ostial SB damage after stent implantation in the MV was always due to displacement of the carina and no cases of plaque shifting were found. Further interesting finding of this study is that plaque in the carina was greater in the bifurcations that had maximum stenosis located distal to the carina in the MV. Authors explain this finding by hypothesis of different flow velocity patterns in these lesions. Atheroprotective high shear stress can be transformed into an atero-prone low shear stress. Authors describe less damage of SB ostium after stenting of lesions with plaque at the carina. Plaque probably makes carina more resistant and does not allow carina shifting, which is now thought to be a dominant mechanism causing damage to the SB ostium when a stent is implanted into the MV.
Important contribution for planning of PCI in bifurcations is a study done by Costa et al[105]. They found that the part of MV just behind the origin of SB (so called "lower diamond" or "polygon of confluence") is more prone for small minimal stent area after dilatation of SB ostium, which is not reverted even after kissing balloon dilatation. Kang et al.[106] published a study assessing the IVUS predictors for side branch compromise after single-stent crossover technique and found two predictors for post stenting FFR<0.8: MLA 2.4mm^2 and PB > 51% in SB ostium.

Main role of IVUS guidance in bifurcation PCI is precise assessment of atherosclerotic burden of main vessel, carina, ostial part of side branch and the choice of the best strategy based on these findings. IVUS can improve the choice of ideal stent diameter, because bifurcation area is frequently affected by negative remodeling, which is not visible in routine angiography[107].

IVUS should be used of most cases of uncertain atherosclerotic distribution in bifurcation lesions, because in case of favorable finding in SB ostium a planned complex procedure can be converted to a simple one with just stenting of MV.

7.2 PCI of chronic total occlusion

The main disadvantage for IVUS guidance of chronic total occlusion (CTO) interventions is the lateral view of IVUS probe. A prototype of forward-looking IVUS system was developed, but till now it has never been commercialized. IVUS can help during wire introduction to the proximal fibrous cap of CTO in presence of side branch just proximal to occluded segment. IVUS is introduced to this side branch and from this location the wire reaching the origin of total occlusion can be visualized (*figure 15*). IVUS also can help with re-introduction of wire from false lumen to the true lumen, but it is necessary to introduce the IVUS probe to the false lumen after its predilatation with small balloon[108]. This technique unfortunately increases risk of vessel perforation.

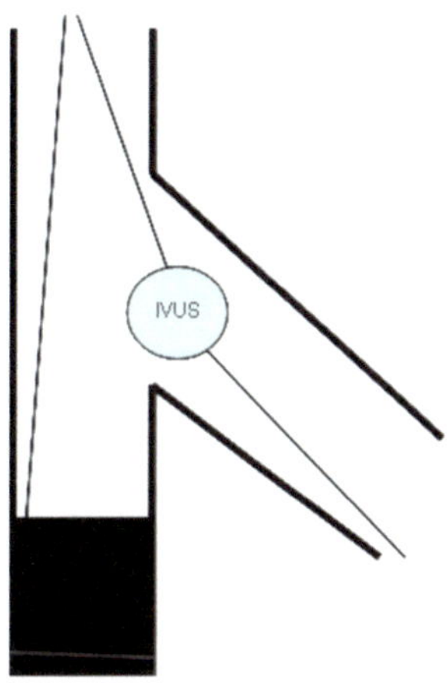

Fig. 15. Schema of IVUS guidance during PCI of chronic total occlusion.

8. Complications

8.1 Dissections

Dissections are tears in the plaque that are parallel to the vessel wall with blood flow in the false lumen and tend to occur at the junction of elements with different compliance (plaque and normal vessel wall, edges of stents) (*figure 16, 17*). Dissections can be described as proximal or distal to the lesion; epicardial or myocardial; and according to length, circumferential arc, depth, lumen compromise, bulkiness and mobility of the flap[5]. The major predictor of an unfavorable prognosis of dissection is a decreased blood flow in affected coronary artery. This situation must be solved immediately. IVUS can also detect dissections, which are not visible on angiography and it is questionable how many of them should be treated. Nishida et al.[109] followed 124 patients with non-flow limiting dissection (65% of them were after stenting). They found that dissection can be let untreated if the residual lumen is more than 6 mm^2 and lumen area is more than 40% of the EEM area. The edge dissections after stenting, which can be visualized only by IVUS and are not apparent during angiography, are not indicated for any intervention, because of good prognosis by spontaneous healing[110].

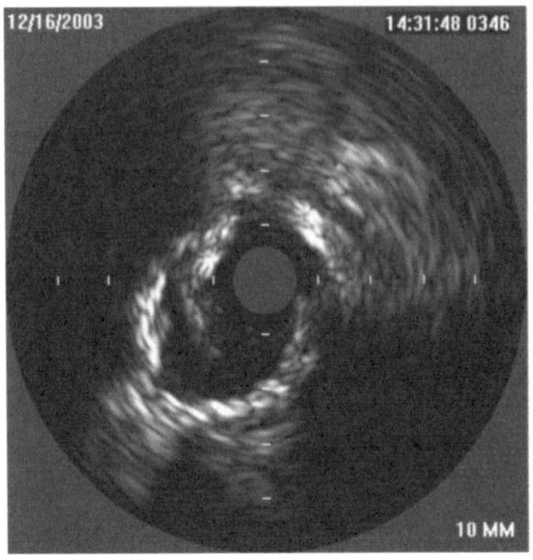

Fig. 16. Dissection with tear reaching to the media.

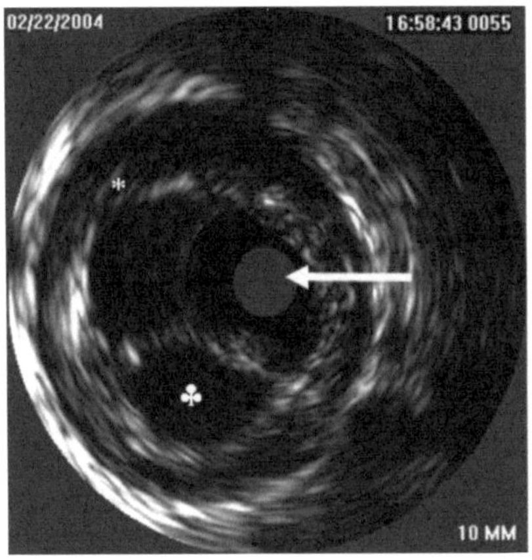

Fig. 17. Complex dissection with IVUS probe in true lumen, one false lumen is located down to true lumen (♣) and another entry to the false lumen is located above the true lumen (*).

8.2 Intramural hematomas

Intramural hematoma is a variant of a dissection. The angiographic appearance ranges from a dissection, thrombus, and abrupt closure to non-significant abnormality. The EEM expands outwards and the intima is pushed inwards and straightens to cause lumen compromise (figure 18). Blood accumulates in the space caused by the split in the media and becomes static and echogenic. The hematoma can propagate antegrade or retrograde, but tends to be stopped by branches or severely diseased parts of the vessel (particularly calcified plaques). In a study, which included more than 1000 patients with IVUS control after PCI, an intramural hematoma was found in 6.7 % with a high rate of clinical events[5, 111].

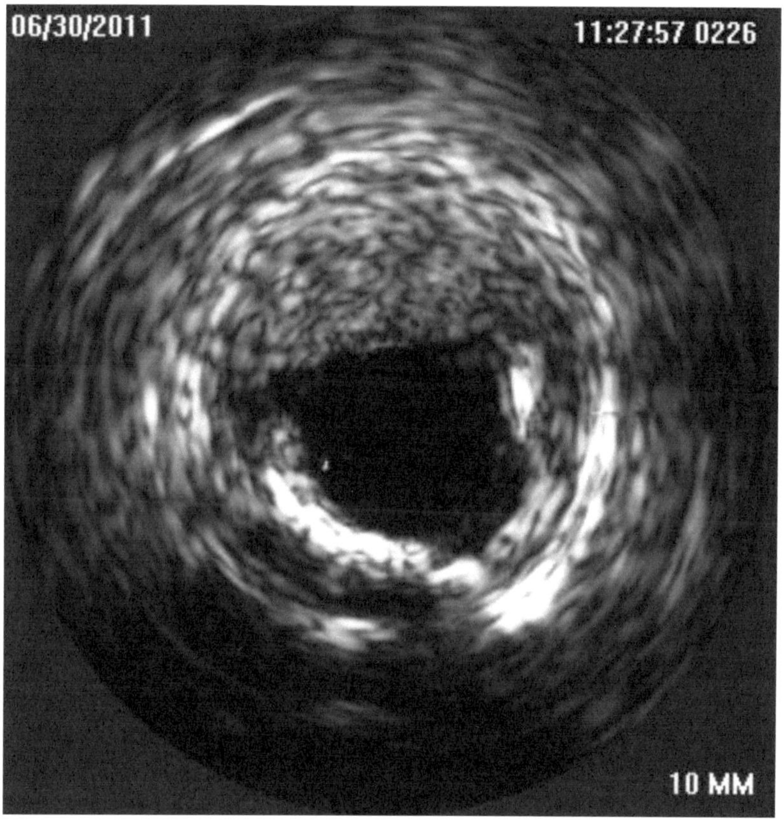

Fig. 18. Intramural haematoma. Bleeding to the media and adventicia is compromising lumen.

8.3 Haziness

IVUS is a very useful tool for diagnosis of underlying processes causing a hazy appearance of lesions after PCI. The most common findings are large residual plaque burden, dissection and plaque protrusion. Rarely stent deformation or intramural hematoma can be found. Intimal wrinkling can occur when a vessel is straightened by a guidewire. It reverses when the wire is removed or when the stiff wire is exchanged for a soft one. A narrowing of the lumen with a straightening of a normal-looking intima, behind which is an echolucent zone can be seen in IVUS picture. Discontinuity of the EEM can be found, which is caused by simultaneously visualized both sides of fold in the artery. Finally, it is important to recognize an angiographic pseudo complication with normal IVUS finding[5].

9. Conclusions

Based on studies focusing on IVUS guidance of stent implantation we can summarize:

1. Based on IVUS criteria we can probably safely defer PCI
2. Satisfactory IVUS finding after balloon dilatation has same results as a stenting with BMS
3. IVUS guidance decreases angiographic restenosis and consequently the revascularization and MACE rate

4. IVUS guidance decreases rate of in stent thrombosis
5. Contraindication for IVUS guidance are small vessels, tortuous vessels and degenerated vein grafts

This summary raises the question why IVUS is not used routinely during all PCI procedures. The answers can be divided into two groups. First there are the lessons we have learned from IVUS and this phenomenon is known as an "IVUS eye". We know that vessels are bigger than they look on angio and we are using bigger stents than before IVUS studies. We know, that without high pressure post dilatation we are not able to achieve sufficient stent diameter despite information derived from manufacturer's compliance charts. These factors dramatically contributed to lowering of in stent restenosis and therefore it is difficult to find statistical significant difference between IVUS and angio guided interventions, like it was described in OPTICUS trial. However, IVUS is still irreplaceable during investigation of unclear finding during angiography (like hazy lesions) or after stenting. IVUS is especially recommended during PCI of left main, the last remaining coronary artery and PCI in patients who are contraindicated for dual antiplatelet therapy for avoiding stent implantation. Furthermore, precise assessment of bifurcation can change the strategy from more complex to simple one in case of low risk profile of ostial part of side branch

The group of arguments against routine use of IVUS during PCI is cost of IVUS catheter, longer procedural time and higher contrast dye consumption. Moreover IVUS guided PCI are more complex and need more skills than angio guided ones. However, in indicated cases IVUS guidance undoubtedly improves short as well as long term of coronary interventions.

10. References

[1] Pijls NH, de Bruyne B, Peels K et al, Measurement of Fractional Flow Reserve to Assess the Functional Severity of Coronary-Artery Stenoses. NEJM 1996; 334: 1703–1708

[2] Topol EJ, Nissen SE.Our preoccupation with coronary luminology. The dissociation between clinical and angiographic findings in ischemic heart disease. *Circulation* 1995;92:2333-2342

[3] Vlodaver Z, Frech R, Van Tassel RA, et al. Correlation of the antemortem coronary angiogram and the postmortem specimen. *Circulation* 1973;47:162-169

[4] Mintz GS, Nissen SE, Anderson WD, Erbel R, Fitzgerald PJ, Pinto FJ, Rosenfiels K, Siegel K, Tuzcu EM, Yock PG. American College of Cardiology Clinical Expert Consensus Document on Standards for Acquisition, Measurement and Reporting of Intravascular Ultrasound Studies (IVUS) A Report of the American College of Cardiology Task Force on Clinical Expert Consensus Documents. *JACC* 2001;37:1478-1492

[5] Mintz GS. Intracoronary ultrasound. Taylor & Francis 2005

[6] Briguori C, Anzuini A, Airoldi F, et al. Intravascular Ultrasound Criteria for the Assessment of the Functional Significance of Intermediate Coronary Artery Stenoses and Comparison with Fractional Flow Reserve. *Am J Cardiol* 2001;87:136-141

[7] Abizaid A, Mintz GS, Pichard A, et al. Clinical, Intravascular Ultrasound, and Quantitative Angiographic Determinants of the Coronary Flow Reserve Before and After Percutaneous Transluminal Coronary Angioplasty. Am J Cardiol 1998;82:423-428

[8] Nishioka T, Amanullah A, Luo H, et al. Clinical Validation of Intravascular Ultrasound Imaging for Assessment of Coronary Stenosis Severity. Comparison With Stress Myocardial Perfusion Imaging. *J Am Coll Cardiol* 1999;33:1870-1878

[9] Takagi A, Tsurumi Y, Suzuki K, et al. Clinical Potential of Intravascular Ultrasound for Physiological Asessment of Coronary Stenosis. *Circulation* 1999;100:250-255
[10] Lee Ch, Tai B, Soon Ch, Low A, Poh K, Yeo T, Lim G, Yip J, Omar A, Teo S, Tan H. New set of intravascular ultrasound-derived anatomic criteria for defining functionally significant stenoses in small coronary arteries (results from intravascular diagnostic evaluation of atherosclerosis in Singapore [IDEAS] Study). *Am J Cardiol* 2010;105:1378-1384
[11] Abizaid A, Mintz GS, Mehran R, et al. Long Term Follow-up After Percutaneous Transluminal Coronary Angioplasty Was Not Performed Based on Intravascular Ultrasound Findings. *Circulation* 1999;100:256-261
[12] Jasti V, Ivan E, Yalamanchili V, et al. Correlation between fractional flow reserve and intravascular ultrasound in patients with an ambiguous left main coronary artery stenosis. *Circulation* 2004;110:2831-2836).
[13] Abizaid A, Mintz GS, A.Abizaid, et at. One-Year Follow-up After Intravascular Ultrasound Assessment of Moderate Left Main Coronary Artery Disease in Patients With Ambiquous Angiograms. *J Am Coll Cardiol* 1999;34:707-715
[14] Kang SJ, Lee JY, Ahn JM, Mintz GS, Kim WJ, Park DW, Yun SCh, Lee SW, Kim YH, Lee ChW, Park SW, Park SJ. Validation of Intravascular Ultrasound–Derived Parameters With Fractional Flow Reserve for Assessment of Coronary Stenosis Severity. *Circulation: Cardiovascular Interventions* 2011; 4: 65-71
[15] Ben-Dor I, Torguson R, Gaglia MA, Gonzales MA, Maluenda G, Bui AB, Xue Z, Satle LF, Suddath WO, Lindsay J, Pichard AD, Waksman R. Correlation between fractional flow reserve and intravascular ultrasound lumen area in intermediate coronary artery stenosis. *Eurointervention* 2011;7:225-233
[16] Ahn JM. Kang SJ, Mintz GS, Oh JH, Kim WJ, Lee JY, Park DW, Lee SW, Kim YH, Lee ChW, Park SW, Moon DH, Park SJ. Validation of minimal lumen area measured by intravascular ultrasound for assessment of functionally significant coronary stenoses. *JACC Cardiovasc Interv* 2011;4:665-671
[17] Stone GW, Maehara A, Lansky A, de Bruyne B, Cristea E, Minth GS, Mehran R, McPherson J, Farhat N, Marso SP, Parise H, Templin B, White R, Zhankg Z,Serruys PW. A prospective natural-history study of coronary atherosclerosis.NEJM 2011;364:226-235
[18] Fearon WF, Bornschein B, Tonino PA, Gothe RM, Bruyne BD, Pijls NH, Siebert U; Fractional Flow Reserve Versus Angiography for Multivessel Evaluation (FAME) Study Investigators. Economic evaluation of fractional flow reserve-guided percutaneous coronary intervention in patients with multivessel disease.*Circulation* 2010;122:2545-50
[19] Nam ChW, Yoon HJ, ChoYK, Park HS, Kim H, Hur SH, Kim YN, Chung IS, Koo BK, Tahk SJ, Fearon WF, Kim KB. Outcomes of percutaneous coronary intervention in intermediate coronary artery disease. Fractional flow reserve-guided versus intravascular ultrasound-guided. JACC Cardiol Intv 2010;3:812-817
[20] Ricciardi M, Meyers S, Choi K, et al. Angiographically silent left main disease detected by intravascular ultrasound: A marker for future adverse cardiac events. *Am Heart J* 2003;146:507-512
[21] Hermiller JB, Buller CE, Tenaglia AN, et al. Unrecognized left main artery disease in patients undergoing interventional procedures. *Am J Cardiol* 1993;71:173-176

[22] Ge J, Liu F, Görge G, et al. Angiographically „silent" plaque in the left main coronary artery detected by intravascular ultrasound. *Coronary Artery disease* 1995;6:805-810
[23] Russo RJ, Wong SC, Marchant D, et al. Intravascular ultrasound-directed clinical decision making in the setting of an inconclusive left main coronary angiogram: final results from the Left Main IVUS Registry. Circulation 2004;108:IV-462
[24] Suter Y, Schoenenberger AW, Toggweiler S, Jamshidi P, Resink T, Erne P. Intravascular ultrasound-based left main coronary artery assessment: comparison between pullback from left anterior descending and circumflex arteries. *J Invasive Cardiol* 2009;21:457-460
[25] Oviedo C, Maehara A, Mintz GS, Tsujita K, Kubo T, Doi H, Castellanos C, Lansky AJ, Mehran R, Dangas G, Leon MB, Stone G, Templin B, Araki H, Ochiai M, Moses JW. Is accurate intravascular ultrasound evaluation of the left circumflex ostium from a left anterior descending to left main pullback possible? *Am J Cardiol* 2010;105:948-95
[26] Park SJ, Kim YH, Park DW, Lee SW, Kim WJ, Suh J, Yun SCh, Lee CHW, Hong MK, Lee JH, Park SW; MAIN-COMPARE Investigators. Impact of intravascular guiaxdance on Long-term mortality in stenting for unprotected left main coronary artery stenosis. *Circ Cardiovasc Interv* 2009;2:167-177
[27] Kotani J, Mintz GS, Rai P, et al. Intravascular ultrasound assessment of angiographic filling defects in native coronary arteries: Do they always contain thrombi ? *JACC* 2004;44:2087-2089
[28] Kobayashi Y, De Gregorio J, Kobayashi N, et al. Stented segments length as an independent predictor of restenosis. *J Am Coll Cardiol* 1999:34:651-659
[29] Grewal J, Ganz P, Selwyn A, et al. Usefulness of intravascular ultrasound in preventing stenting of hazy areas adjacent to coronary stents and its support of support spot-stenting. *Am J Cardiol* 2001;87:1246-1249
[30] Ziada KM, Tuzcu EM, De Franco AC, et al. Intravascular ultrasound assessment of the prevalence and cause of angiographic „haziness" following high-pressure coronary stenting. *Am J Cardiol* 1997;80:116-121
[31] Maehara A, Mintz GS, Ahmed JM, et al. An intravascular ultrasound classification of angiographic coronary artery aneurysms. *Am J Cardiol* 2001;88:365-370
[32] Mizuno K, Kurita A, Imazeki N. Pathological findings after percutaneous transluminal coronary angioplasty. *Br Heart J* 1984;52:588-590
[33] Honey J, Mahon D, Jain A, et al. Morphological effects of coronary balloon angioplasty in vivo assessed by intravascular ultrasound imaging. Circulation 1992;85:1012-1025
[34] Stone G, Hodgson J, Goar F, et al. Improved procedural results of coronary angioplasty with intravascular ultrasound-guided balloon sizing. The CLOUT Pilot Trial. *Circulation* 1997;95:2044-2052
[35] Haase K, Athanasiadis A, Mahrholdt H, et al. Acute and one year follow-up results after vessel size adapted PTCA using intravascular ultrasound. Eur Heart J 1998;19:263-272
[36] Schroeder S, Baumbach A, Haase K, et al. Reduction of restenosis by vessel size adapted percutaneous transluminal coronary angioplasty using intravascular ultrasound. *Am J Cardiol* 1999;83:875-879

[37] Abizaid A, Pichard A, Mintz GS, et al. Acute and long-term results of an intravascular ultrasound-guided percutaneous transluminal coronary angioplasty/provisional stent implantation strategy. Am J Cardiol 1999;84:1298-1303

[38] Schiele F, Meneveau N, Gilard M, et al. Intravascular ultrasound-guided balloon angioplasty compared with stent. Immediate and 6-month results of the multicenter, randomized balloon equivalent to stent study (BEST). *Circulation* 2003;107:545-551

[39] Frey A, Hodgson J, Muller Ch, et al. Ultrasound-guided strategy for provisional stenting with focal balloon combination catheter. Results from the randomized strategy for intracoronary ultrasound-guided PTCA and stenting (SIPS) trial. *Circulation* 2000;102:2497-2502

[40] Gaster A, Skjoldborg S, Larsen J, et al. Continued improvement of clinical outcome and cost effectiveness following intravascular ultrasound guided PCI: insight from a prospective, randomized study. *Heart* 2003;89:1043-1049

[41] Mueller Ch, Hodgson J, Schindler Ch, et al. Cost-effectiveness of intracoronary ultrasound for percutaneous coronary interventions. *Am J Cardiol* 2003;91:143-147

[42] Colombo A, De Gregorio J, Moussa I, et al. Intravascular ultrasound-guided percutaneous transluminal coronary angioplasty with provisional spot stenting for treatment of long coronary lesion. *J Am Coll Cardiol* 2001;38:1427-1433

[43] von Birgelen, Mintz GS, Eggebrecht H, et al. Preintervention arterial remodeling affects vessel stretch and plaque extrusion during coronary stent deployment as demonstrated by three-dimensional intravascular ultrasound. *Am J Cardiol* 2003;92:130-135

[44] Ahmed JM, Mintz GS, Weissman NJ, et al. Mechanism of lumen enlargement during intracoronary stent implantation. An intravascular ultrasound study. *Circulation* 2000;102:7-10

[45] Costa JR, Mintz GS, Carlier SG,Costa RA, Fujii K,Sano K, Kimura M, Lui J, Weisz G, Moussa I, Dangas G, Mehran R, Lansky AJ, Kreps EM, Collins M, Stone GW, Moses JW, MD, Leon MB. Intravascular Ultrasonic Assessment of Stent Diameters Derived from Manufacturer's Compliance Charts. *Am J Cardiol* 2005;96:74 -78

[46] Ponde CK, Aroney CN, McEniery PT, et al. Plaque prolapse between struts of the intracoronary Palmaz-Schatz stent: report of two cases with a novel treatment of this unusual problem. *Cathet Cardiovasc Diagn* 1997;40:353-357

[47] Colombo A, Hall P, Nakamura S, et al. Intracoronary stenting without anticoagulation accomplished with intravascular ultrasound guidance. *Circulation* 1995;91:1676-1688

[48] Gorge G, Haude M, Ge J, et al. Intravascular Ultrasound After low and high inflation pressure coronary artery stent implantation. *J Am Coll Cardiol* 1995;26:725-730

[49] Choi JW, Vardi GM, Meyers SH, et al. Role of intracoronary ultrasound after high-pressure stent implantation. *Am Heart J* 2000;139:643-648

[50] de Jaegere P, Mudra H, Figulla H, et al. Intravascular ultrasound-guided optimized stent deployment. Immediate and 6 months clinical and angiographic results from the Multicenter Ultrasound Stenting in Coronaries Study (MUSIC Study). *Eur Herat J* 1998;19:1214-1223

[51] Blasini R, Neumann FJ, Schmitt C, et al. Restenosis rate after intravascular ultrasound-guided coronary stent implantation. *Cathet Cardiovasc Diagn* 1998;44:380-386

[52] Schiele F, Meneveau N, Vuillemenot A, et al. Impact of intravascular ultrasound guidance in stent deployment on 6 month restenosis rate: a multicenter, randomized study comparing two strategies-with and without intravascular ultrasound guidance. *J Am Coll Cardiol* 1998;32:320-328

[53] Mudra H, di Mario C, de Jaegere P, et al. Randomized comparison of coronary stent implantation under ultrasound or angiographic guidance to reduce stent restenosis (OPTICUS study). Circulation 2001;104:1343-1349

[54] Fitzgerald PJ, Oshima A, Hayase M, et al. Final Results of the Can Routine Ultrasound Influence Stent Expansion (CRUISE) Study. *Circulation* 2000;102:523-530

[55] Russo RJ, Silva PD, Teirstein PS, Attubato MJ, Davidson CJ, De-Franco AC, Fitzgerald PJ, Goldberg SL, Hermiller JB, Leon MB, Ling FS, Lucisano JE, Schatz RA, Wong SC, Weissman NJ, Zientek DM;AVID Investigators. A randomized controlled triual of angiography versus intravascular ultrasound-directed bare-metal coronary stnet placement (the AVID trial). *Circ Cardiovasc Interv* 2009;2:113-123

[56] Oemrawsingh PV, Mintz GS, Schalij M, et al. Intravascular ultrasound guidance improves angiographic and clinical outcome of stent implantation for long coronary artery stenoses. Final results of a Randomized Comparison With Angiographic Guidance (TULIP Study). *Circulation* 2003;107:62-67

[57] Orford J, Denktas A, Williams B, et al. Routine intravascular ultrasound scanning guidance of coronary stenting is not associated with improved clinical outcomes. *Am Heart J* 2004;148:501-6

[58] Gil RJ, Pawlowski T, Dudek D, Horszczaruk G, Zmudka K, Lesiak M, Witkowski A, Ochala A, Kubica J; Investigators of Direct Stenting vs. Optimal Angioplasty trial (DIPOL). Comparison of angiographically guided direct stenting technique with direct stenting and optimal balloon angioplasty guided with intravascular ultrasound: the multicenter, randomized trial results. *Am Heart J* 2007;154:669-675

[59] Gaster AL, Slothuus U, Larsen J, Thayssen P, Hagfelt TH. Cost-effectiveness analysis of intravascular ultrasound guided percutaneous coronary intervention versus conventional percutaneous coronary intervention. *Scand Cardiovasc J* 2001;35:80-85.

[60] Gaster AL, Slothuus Skjoldborg U, Larsen J, Korsholm L, von Birgelen C, Jensen S, Thayssen P, Pedersen KE, Hagfelt TH. Continued improvement of clinical outcome and cost effectiveness following intravascular ultrasound guided PCI: insight from a prospective, randomized study. *Heart* 2003;89:1043-1049

[61] Katritsis D, Ioannidis J Korovessis S, et al. Comparison of myocardial fractional flow reserve and intravascular ultrasound for the assessment of slotted-tube stents. *Cathet Cardiovasc Intervent* 2001;52:322-326

[62] Fearon W, Luna J, Samady H, et al. Fractional flow reserve compared with intravascular ultrasound guidance for optimizing stent deployment. *Circulation* 2001;104:1917-1922

[63] Hanekamp CE, Koolen JJ, Pijls NH, Michels HR, Bonnier HJ. Comparison of quantitative coronary angiography, intravascular ultrasound, and coronary pressure measurement to assess optimum stent deployment. *Circulation* 1999;99:1015-21

[64] Moussa I, Moses J, di Mario C, et al. Does the specific intravascular ultrasound criterion used to optimize stent expansion have an impact on the probability of stent restenosis ? *Am J Cardiol* 1999;83:1012-1017

[65] Hoffmann R, Mintz GS, Mehran R, et al. Intravascular ultrasound predictors of angiographic restenosis in lesions treated with Palmaz-Schatz stents. *J Am Coll Cardiol* 1998;31:43-49

[66] Hong MK, Park SW, Mintz GS, et al. Intravascular ultrasonic predictors of angiographic restenosis after long coronary stenting. *Am J Cardiol* 2000;85:441-445

[67] de Feyter PJ, Kay P, Disco C, et al. Reference chart derived from post-stent-implantation intravascular ultrasound predictors of 6-moth expected restenosis on quantitative coronary angiography. *Circulation* 1999;100:1777-1783

[68] von Birgelen C, Mintz GS, Bose D. et al. Impact of moderate lesion calcium on mechanism of coronary stenting as assessed with three-dimensional intravascular ultrasound in vivo. *Am J Cardiol* 2003;92:5-10

[69] Hong MK, Park SW, Lee CW, et al. Preintervention arterial remodeling as a predictor of intimal hyperplasia after intracoronary stenting: a serial intravascular ultrasound study. *Clin Cardiol* 2002;25:11-15

[70] Endo A, Hirayama H, Yoshida O, et al. Arterial remodeling influences the development of intimal hyperplasia after stent implantation. *JACC* 2001;37:70-75

[71] Shiran A, Weissman NJ, Leiboff B, et al. Effect of preintervention plaque burden on subsequent intimal hyperplasia in stented coronary lesions. *Am J Cardiol* 2000;86:1318-1321, 69/ Alfonso F, Garcia P, Pimental G, et al. Predictors and implications of residual plaque burden after coronary stenting: an intravascular ultrasound study. *Am Heart J* 2003;145:254-261

[72] Shiran A, Mintz GS, Waksman R et al. Early lumen loss after treatment of in-stent restenosis: an intravascular ultrasound study. *Circulation* 1998;98:200-203

[73] Okabe T, Mintz GS, Buch A, et al. Intravascular ultrasound parameters associated with stent thrombosis after drug-eluting stent deployment. Am J Cardiol 2007;4:615-620

[74] Cheneau E, Leborgne L, Mintz GS, et al. Predictors of subacute stent thrombosis. Results of a systematic intravascular ultrasound study. *Circulation* 2003;108:43-47

[75] Parise H, Maehara A, Stone GW, Leon MB, Mintz GS. Meta-analysis of randomized studies comparing intravascular ultrasound versus angiographic guidance of percutaneous coronary intervention in pre-drug-eluting stent era. *Am J Cardiol* 2011;107:374-382

[76] Sousa JE, Costa MA, Abizaid A , et al. Lack of neointimal proliferation after implantation of sirolimus-coated stents in human coronary arteries: a quantitative coronary angiography and three-dimensional intravascular ultrasound study. *Circulation* 2001;103:192-195

[77] Holmes DR Jr, Leon MB, Moses JW, Popma JJ, Analysis of 1-year clinical outcomes in the SIRIUS trial: a randomized trial of a sirolimus-eluting stent versus a standard stent in patients at high risk for coronary restenosis. *Circulation* 2004;109:634-40

[78] Hong MK, Minz GS, Lee ChW, et al. Paclitaxel coating reduces in-stent intimal hyperplasia in human coronary arteries. A serial volumetric intravascular ultrasound analysis from the aSian Paclitaxel-Eluting Stent Clinical Trial (ASPECT). *Circulation* 2003;107:517-520

[79] Moses JW, Leon MB, Popma JJ, Fitzgerald PJ, Holmes DR, O'Shaughnessy C, Caputo RP, Kereiakes DJ, Williams DO, Teirstein PS, Jaeger JL, Kuntz RE. Sirolimus-eluting stents versus standad stents in patients with stenosis in a native coronary artery. *N Engl J Med.* 2003; 349:1315–1323

[80] Stone GW, Ellis SG, Cox DA, Hermiller J, O'Shaughnessy C, Mann JT,Turco M, Caputo R, Bergin P, Greenberg J, Popma JJ, Russel ME. Apolymer-based, paclitaxel-eluting stent in patients with coronary artery disease. *N Engl J Med.* 2004;350:221–230
[81] Cervinka P, Costa MA, Angiolillo DJ, Spacek R, Bystron M, Kvasnak M, Veselka J, Nadna H, Futamatsu K. Head-to-Head Comparison Between Sirolimus-Elutingand Paclitaxel-Eluting Stents in Patients With Complex Coronary Artery Disease: An Intravascular Ultrasound Study. Catheterization and Cardiovascular Interventions 2006;67:846–851
[82] Sonoda S, Morino Y, Jako J, et al. Impact of final stent dimensions on long-term results following sirolimus-eluting stent implantation. Serial intravascular ultrasound analysis from the SIRIUS trial. *J Am Coll Cardiol* 2004;43:1959-1963,
[83] Moses JW, Dangas G, Mehran R, Mintz GS. Drug-eluting stents in real world: how intravascular ultrasound can improve clinical outcome. *Am J Cardiol* 2008;102[suppl]:24J-28J
[84] Jeremias A, Sylvia B, Bridges J, et al. Stent thrombosis after successful sirolimus-eluting stent implantation. *Circulation* 2004;109:1930 –2
[85] Fuji K, Carlier SG, Mintz GS, et al. Stent under expansion and residual reference segment stenos are related to stent thrombosis after sirolimus- eluting stent implantation: an intravascular ultrasound study. *JACC* 2005;45:995-998
[86] Uren NG, Schwarzacher P, Metz JA, et al. Predictors and outcomes of stent thrombosis. An intravascular ultrasound registry. *Eur Heart J* 2002;23:124-132
[87] Cheneau E, Leborgne L, Mintz GS, et al. Predictors of subacute stent thrombosis. Results of a systematic intravascular ultrasound study. *Circulation* 2003;108:43-47
[88] Cutlip DE, Baim DS, Ho KK, Popma JJ, Lansky AJ, Cohen DJ, Carrozza JP Jr, Chauhan MS, Rodriguez O, Kuntz RE. Stent thrombosis in the modern era: a pooled analysis of multicenter coronary stent clinical trials. Circulation 2001;103: 1967–1971.
[89] Roy R, Steinberg DH, Sushinsky SJ, Okabe T, Slottow TP, Kaneshige K, Xue Z, Satler LF, Kent KM, Suddath WO, Pichard AD, Weissman NJ, Lindsay J, Waksman R. The potencial clinical utility of intravascular ultrasound guidance in patients undergoing percutaneous coronary intervention with drug-eluting stents. *European Heart J* 2008;29:1851-1857
[90] Claessen BE, Mehran R, Mintz GS, Weisz G, Leon MB, Dogan O, de Ribamar Costa J, Stone GW, Apostolidou I, Morales A, Chantziara V, Syros G, Sanidas E, Xu K, Tijssen JG, Henriques JP, Piek JJ, Moses JW, Meahara A, Dangas DG. Impact of intravascular ultrasound imaging on early and late clinical outcomes following percutaneous coronary intervention with drug-eluting stents. *JACC Cardiovasc Interv.* 2011;4:974-981
[91] Hur SH, Kang SJ, Kim YH, Ahn JM, Park DW, Lee SW, Yun SC, Lee CW, Park SW, Park SJ. Impact of intravascular ultrasound-guided percutaneous coronary intervention on long-term clinical outcomes in a real world population. *Catheter Cardiovasc Interv* 2011; ahead of print
[92] Degertekin M, Serruys PW, Tanabe K, et al. Long-term follow-up of incomplete stent apposition in patients who received sirolimus-eluting stent for de novo coronary lesions. An intravascular ultrasound analysis. *Circulation* 2003;108:2747-2750
[93] Serruys PW, Degertekin M, Tanabe K, et al. Intravascular ultrasound findings in the multicenter, randomized, double-blind RAVEL (RAndomized study with the

sirolimus-eluting VElocity balloon-expandable stent in the treatment of patients with de novo native coronary artery Lesions) trial. *Circulation.* 2002;106:798–803
[94] Shah VM, Mintz GS, Apple S, et al. Background incidence of late malapposition after bare-metal stent implantation. *Circulation* 2002;106:1753-175
[95] Tanabe K, Serruys P, Degertekin M, et al. Incomplete stent apposition after implantation of paclitaxel-eluting stents or bare metal stents. Insights from the randomized TAXUS II trial. *Circulation* 2005;111:900-90
[96] Hong MK, Mintz GS, Lee ChW, Park DW, Park KM, Lee BK, Kim YH, Song JM, Han KH, Kang DH, Cheong SS, Song JK, Kim JJ, Park SW, Park SJ. Late Stent Malapposition After Drug-Eluting Stent Implantation An Intravascular Ultrasound Analysis With Long-Term Follow-Up. *Circulation* 2006; 113:414-419
[97] Kimura M, Mintz GS, Carlier S, Takebayashi H, Fujii K, Sano K, Yasuda T, Costa RA, Costa JR, Quen J, et al. Outcome after acute incomplete sirolimus-eluting stent apposition as assessed by serial intravascular ultrasound. *Am J Cardiol* 2006;98: 436-442
[98] Cook S, Wenaweser P, Togni M, et al. Incomplete stent apposition and very late stent thrombosis after drug-eluting stent implantation. *Circulation* 2007;115:2426 -36
[99] Hassan AK, Bergheanu SC, Stijnen T, van der Hoeven BL, Snoep JD, Plevier JW, Schalij MJ, Wouter Jukema J.Late stent malapposition risk is higher after drug-eluting stent compared with bare-metal stent implantation and associates with late stent thrombosis. *European Heart Journal* 2010;31:1172-1180
[100] Alfonso F, Pérez-Vizcayno MJ, Ruiz M, Suarez S, Cazares M,, Hernandez R, Escaned J, Bañuelos C, Jiménez-Quevedo P, Macaya C. Coronary Aneurysms After Drug-Eluting Stent Implantation Clinical, Angiographic, and Intravascular Ultrasound Findings. *J Am Coll Cardiol* 2009;53:2053–60
[101] Aliabadi D, Tilli FV, Bowers TR, Benzuly KH, Safian RD, Goldstein JA, et al. Incidence and angiographic predictors of side branch occlusion following high-pressure intracoronary stenting. *Am J Cardiol* 1997;:80:994-997
[102] Furukawa E, Hibi K, Kosuge M, et al. Intravascular Ultrasound Predictors of side branch occlusion in bifurcation lesions after percutaneous coronary intervention. *Circulation Journal* 2005;69:325-330
[103] Stankovic G, Darremont O, Ferenc M, Hildick-Smith D, Louvard Y, Albiero R,e t al. Percutaneous coronary intervention for bifurcation lesions: 2008 consensus document from the fourth meeting of the European Bifurcation Club. *Eurointervention* 2009;5:39-49
[104] Medina A, Martin P, de Lezo JS, Novoa J, Melian F, Hernandez E, de Lezo JS, Pan M, Burgos L, Amador C, Morera O, Garcia A. Ultrasound study of the prevalence of plaque at the carina in lesions that affect the coronary bifurcation: implications for treatment with provisional stent. *Rev Esp Cardiol* 2011;64:43-50
[105] De Lezo JS, Medina A, Martin P, et al. Ultrasound findings during percutaneous treatment of bifurcated coronary lesions. *Rev Esp. Cardiol.* 2008;61:930-935
[106] Kang SJ, Mintz GS, Kim WJ, Lee JY, Park DW, Lee SW, Kim YH, Lee ChW, Park SW, Park SJ. Preintervention angiographic and intravascular ultrasound predictors for side branch compromise after a single-stent crossover technique. *Am J Cardiol* 2011 ahead of prints

[107] Fujii K, Kobayashi Y, Mintz GS, et al. Dominant contribution of negative remodeling to development of significant coronary bifurcation narrowing. *Am J Cardiol* 2003;92: 59-61

[108] Ito S, Suzuki T, Ito T, Katoh O, Ojio S, Sato H, Ehara M, Suzuki T,Kawase Y, Myoishi M, Kurokawa R, Ishihara Y, Suzuki Y, Sato K, Toyama S, Fukutomi T, Itoh M. Novel Technique Using Intravascular Ultrasound-Guided Guidewire Cross in Coronary Intervention for Uncrossable Chronic Total Occlusions. *Circ J* 2004; 68: 1088 -1092

[109] Nishida T, Colombo A, Briguori C, et al. Outcome of nonobstructive residual dissections detected by intravascular ultrasound following percutaneous coronary intervention. *Am J Cardiol* 2002;89:1257-1262

[110] Sheris SJ, Canos MP, Weissman NJ, et al. Natural history of intravascular ultrasound-detected edge dissections from coronary stent deployment. *Am Heart J* 2000;139:59-63

[111] Maehara A, Mintz GS, Bui AB, et al. Incidence, morphology, angiographic findings, and outcomes of intramural hematomas after percutaneous coronary interventions: an intravascular ultrasound study. *Circulation* 2002;105:2037-2042

9

Oral Rapamycin to Reduce Intimal Hyperplasia After Bare Metal Stent Implantation - A Prospective Randomized Intravascular Ultrasound Study

Carmelo Cernigliaro, Mara Sansa,
Federico Nardi and Eugenio Novelli
Department of Cardiology, Clinica San Gaudenzio Novara, Italy

1. Introduction

Coronary artery disease is a major health problem throughout the world. Important advances in diagnosis and treatment of atherosclerotic disorders have been made over the last five decades. Coronary angiography, introduced by Mason Sones in 1958 has been very effective on expanding the diagnosis and treatment of coronary lesions. The introduction of conventional balloon percutaneous transluminal coronary angioplasty (PTCA) by Andreas Grüntzig in 1977, represented an innovative and quite efficient non surgical treatment of angina pectoris and acute myocardial infarction. This procedure was however frequently complicated by an abrupt vessel closure, coronary dissections and a high incidence of restenosis (up to 40 - 50 % of cases) (Grüntzig et al., 1979). In 1986 the first coronary Wallstent was implanted in Toulouse by Jacques Puel and Ulrich Sigwart (Sigwart et al., 1987) and in 1994 Palmaz-Schatz stents were approved by FDA in the United States. Coronary stents improved the immediate and long-term results of coronary angioplasty, reducing immediate complications of the procedure like coronary dissection and abrupt closure and the incidence of restenosis. However, despite technical advances in stent delivery systems and design the rate of restenosis after stent implantation remained 20-30% especially in the high risk patients subsets (Serruys et al., 1994; Fischman et al., 1994). To overcome the problem of restenosis the drug eluting stents Cypher and Taxus were approved in 2003 and 2004 respectively. The initial studies with these stents demonstrated a marked major advance in reducing restenosis (Bailey, 1997; Serruys et al., 2002). Later studies however confirmed that despite these advances, in the real world, stent thrombosis (acute, subacute and late) and instent restenosis still remain a great clinical challenge (Daemen et al., 2007). The process of restenosis is complex. Restenosis may ensue mainly because of: a) patients-related factors (diabetes, restenosis after PTCA, chronic renal insufficiency, high serum PCR etc), b) vessel factors (chronic occlusion, vessel involved e.g. LAD, SVG etc, vessel < 3.0mm diameter, lesion length > 30 mm, bifurcation lesion, ostial lesion), c) procedure factors (post-stent MLD < 3mm, multiple stents, stent underexpansion or malapposition, stent fracture).

2. Cellular mechanism of restenosis

The restenosis process is a combination of inflammatory and reparative reaction at the site of stent implantation that may produce after weeks or months intimal hyperplasia or vascular remodelling.
In the porcine coronary after implantation of a metallic stent, restenotic neointima forms within one month and has a histopathologic appearance similar to human restenosis.
Three distinct stages in the genesis of neointima have been described: thrombosis, cellular recruitment, cellular proliferation.
Thrombosis: the earliest response to arterial injury is the formation of a thrombus, which is pale and platelet-rich microscopically. Erythrocytes and fibrin deposit on platelets and produce a heterogeneous microscopic appearance. By 24 hours the thrombus becomes denser as platelets and erythrocytes lyse and agglutinate. Platelet lysis results in discharge of granules and release of bioactive substances including platelet-derived growth factor (PDFG) (Ross et al., 1986; Williams, 1989).
Cellular recruitment: in this stage the thrombus itself becomes covered by the endothelium. Monocytes and lymphocytes are attracted by the flowing blood to the newly formed endothelial surface and pass through the endothelium into the degenerating fibrin thrombus. The monocytes become macrophages. Both macrophages and lymphocytes release a variety of growth factors and cytokines that are involved in smooth muscle cells migration and proliferation. Macrophages and lymphocytes also elaborate fibrinolytic enzymes. Over time these cells are found at deeper levels within the degenerated thrombus from the luminal (endothelium) direction toward the media of the artery.
Cellular proliferation: in the next stage cells form an intimal cap on the luminal side of the healing mass. The thickness of the cap is proportional to lesion age. Residual thrombus is gradually resorbed and replaced by neointima. An extracellular matrix consisting of collagen and glycosaminoglycans is present presumably secreted by vascular smooth muscle cells.
In early experiments, elimination of smooth muscle cells from media by intraluminal microwave heat energy applied in pig arteries after balloon injury was thought to prevent intimal hyperplasia because no cells would be available to migrate and proliferate. After one month however a large volume of neointima was observed at the burn sites where most of the cells had been killed as if migration of smooth muscle cells into the neointima may still occur from a distant uninjured medial site.
To summarize this interesting information, smooth muscle cells forming neointima do not necessarily originate at the site of medial injury. Endothelized and degenerating thrombus, colonized by monocytes and lymphocytes, provides a matrix where smooth muscle cells migrate and proliferate and synthetize extracellular matrix. The thrombus burden that accumulates at the arterial injury site determines the volume of eventual neointimal volume (Schwartz et al., 1992).

3. Alternative therapies to prevent stent restenosis

These data would favour a systemic approach with drugs that reduce intracoronary inflammation and neointimal proliferation also at sites distant from that injured by stent implantation. Stents that elute loco-regionally drugs such rapamycin or placlitaxel (DES), even if in multiple large randomized studies, demonstrate superiority over conventional bare metal stents (BMS) with regard to clinical endpoints such as target vessel or target lesion revascularization are still subjected to failure and restenosis. Interestingly, limited evidence directly comparing DES implantation to vascular brachytherapy (locally applied beta or gamma radiations) in patients with stent restenosis, has shown no direct benefit of one approach to the other (Torguson et al., 2006).

A systemic approach with oral antiproliferative agents like oral sirolimus or newer inhibitors of cytokines could more effectively reduce vascular smooth cell proliferation, migration and invasion process even at a distant site from the injured media (Kuchulakanti & Waksman, 2004). The oral approach has been so far reported in small size studies. The studies suggest that a course of 30 days of oral therapy is both safe an effective and that efficacy is tied to serum blood levels of the drug (Brara et al., 2003; Cernigliaro et al., 2010; Chaves et al., 2005; Fox et al., 2009; Gallo et al., 1999; Guarda et al., 2004; Hausleiter et al., 2004; Munk et al., 2009; Rodriguez et al., 2003; Rodriguez et al., 2005; Rodriguez et al., 2006; Rodriguez, 2009; Rodriguez et al., 2009; Jennings & Kalus 2010; Stojkovic et al., 2010; Waksman et al., 2004; Waksman et al., 2006).

Future investigation into the efficacy of oral antiproliferative agents also during the periprocedural period of BMS or DES implantation is still needed.

Recent studies have investigated adjunctive therapies that could potentially reduce stent restenosis. Addition of cilostazol to aspirin and a thienopyridine (triple antiplatelet therapy) demonstrated reduction of angiographic restenosis at 6 months follow-up over patients receiving dual antiplatelet therapy regardless of whether a bare metal stents or a drug-eluting stents was implanted (Jennings & Kalus 2010).

Oral inhibitors of up-regulated chemokines for reduction of restenosis rates following implantation of BMS without increase in late thrombosis are being utilized in clinical trials.

Chemokines have a crucial role in the initiation and progression of neointima formation by controlling the vascular remodelling in response to various noxious stimuli. It has been demonstrated that eliminating the MCP-1 gene or blocking MCP-1 signaling decreases neointimal hyperplasia after balloon and stent induced injury in several animal models.

In addition, elevated circulating levels of MCP-1 are observed in patients with restenosis after coronary angioplasty. The induction of MPC-1 correlates with macrophages accumulation and there is strong evidence for an important role of MPC-1 in vascular smooth muscle cells (VSMC) proliferation and migration. One of these oral inhibitors have demonstrated anti-inflammatory activity in a number of experimental diseases, with no induction of systemic immunosuppression and no effect on arachidonic acid metabolism.

In vitro it reduces rat vascular smooth muscular proliferation migration, and invasion processes. In a porcine model of in-stent restenosis the product inhibits in-stent neointimal restenosis. Treatment of rats at a dose of 200mg/Kg/day significantly reduces balloon injury-induced intima formation by 39% at day 14 without affecting re-endothelization and reduces the number of medial and neointimal proliferating cells at day 7 by 54% and 30% respectively. A human Phase II trial of 120 patients receiving BMS is ongoing.

The toxicological profile of the drug is safe and patients with rheumatoid arthritis and lupus nephritis have shown that the product is well tolerated and that urinary MCP-1 and albumin excretion in kidney disease is reduced.

The drug can be taken in combination with all the drugs taken by cardiological patients. It is administered b.i.d for 6 months after stent implantation and can be used in combination with BMS as an alternative to DES (Fox et al., 2009).

Regular high intensity exercise training is associated with a significant reduction of late luminal loss following BMS or DES implantation. Patients enrolled into the high-intesitive training group also demonstrated a significantly lower cardiac event rate. The hypothesis surrounding the potential benefit of a high intensity exercise training is that such activity may be beneficial in minimizing endothelial dysfunction after stent implantation (Munk et al., 2009).

4. Current imaging modalities

Coronary angiography objectively assess the long-term outcome after stent implantation. It provides a silhouette of the intravascular space of coronary arteries. Many important features of the lesion that could influence intimal hyperplasia development after intervention may however not be identifiable with coronary arteriography alone.

Angioscopy is an invasive technique that allows an operator to visualize directly the interior of the vessel that can be seen through the fiberoptic eyepiece, or, using electronic chip camera technology. This allows improved understanding of the pathophysiology of coronary arteries. It identifies the presence of morphological features like thrombus or mural haemorrhage and disrupted atheromas that protrude into lumen. Such disruptions may appear angiographically as luminal haziness.

Grayscale intravascular ultrasonography (IVUS) is an invasive, catheter-based imaging procedure that uses sound waves to see inside the vessels within the body. IVUS is most commonly performed in conjunction with conventional coronary angiography for evaluating vessel pathology, atherosclerotic burden, and lesion severity. As compared with angiography, IVUS can provide more detail of the vessel architecture, including the cross-sectional composition of the lumen and wall and the presence and composition of plaque. Atheroma can be interrogated thouroughly to reveal the nature of the lesion (e.g. soft with high lipid content or fibrotic and calcified). Although IVUS is an invasive imaging modality, reports of major clinical complications are rare despite increasing clinical use. When performed by experienced operators, most major and acute procedural complications associated with IVUS imaging occur during interventional cases. The most frequently encountered complication is coronary spasm, which occurs in approximately 2-3% of patients during interventional and diagnostic procedures and usually responds rapidly to the administration of intracoronary nitroglycerin (Figure 1a, Figure 1b).

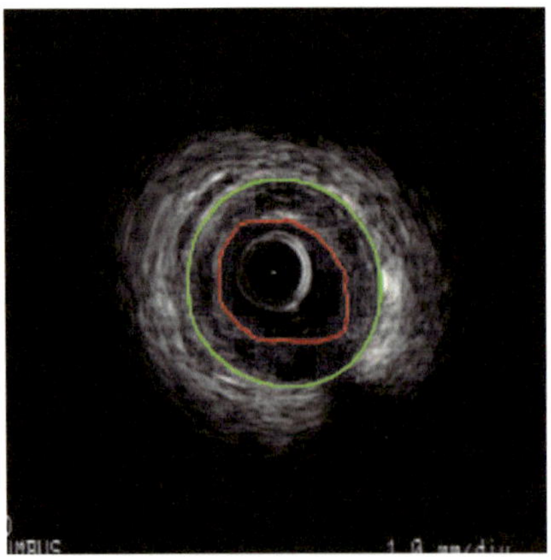

Fig. 1a) Cross sectional IVUS image of a coronary artery with colour coding delineating the lumen (red) the external elastic membrane (green) and the atherosclerotic burden of the media

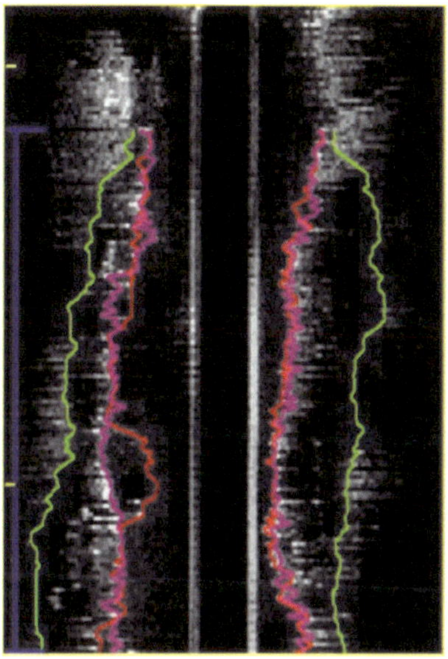

Fig. 1b) Longitudinal display during monitorized pullback of the same artery

Both non invasive and invasive methods have been proposed to aid in visualizing vessel morphology. Noninvasive alternatives to IVUS may include magnetic resonance imaging (MRI), computed tomography (CT) and Doppler ultrasound. Studies support IVUS as the "gold" reference standard when planning, guiding and assessing percutaneous coronary interventions. Multislice CT has moderate to good sensitivities and specificities for the visualization of coronary plaques compared with IVUS as the reference standard. Quantitative 64-channel CT angiography obtained with an effective radiation dose to patients in the range of 3 mSv, can obtain reliable measures in multiple views of reference diameter, minimum lumen diameter, and percent stenosis of coronary arteries before and after intervention (Figure 2a, Figure 2b, Figure 2c, Figure 2d).

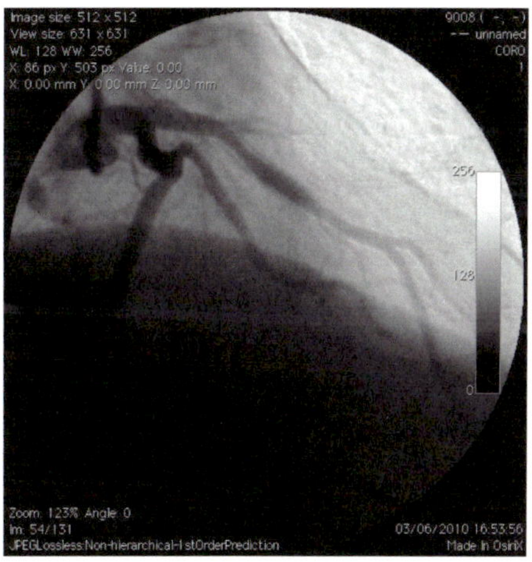

Fig. 2a) Coronary angiography of a Left Anterior Descending Artery with two overlapped DES showing proximal intrastent hyperplasia

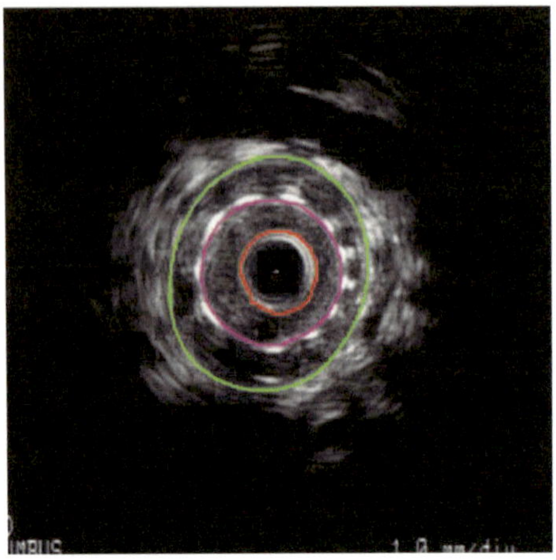

Fig. 2b) Cross sectional IVUS image of the same LAD artery with intrastent intimal hyperplasia

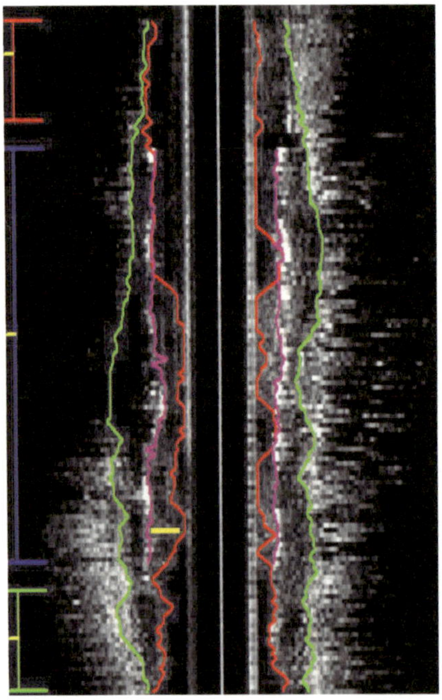

Fig. 2c) Longitudinal IVUS image of the same LAD artery: intimal hyperplasia encroaches the stent (yellow line)

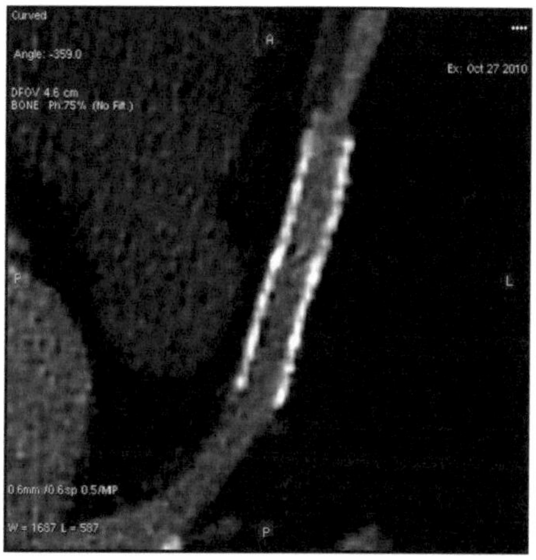

Fig. 2d) 64-CT angiography of the same LAD artery. Intimal hyperplasia encroaches the stent struts as islets of tissue imaged as intraluminal black spots by the struts

Novel invasive imaging technologies include optical coherence tomography (OCT), which measures the intensity of back-reflected light in a similar way to that by which IVUS measures acoustic waves; intracoronary thermography; and spectroscopy (reflected light is collected and launched into a spectrometer.)
Virtual Histology (OCT) analyzes radiofrequency ultrasound signals and provides real-time maps by classifying atherosclerotic plaque into tissue types of fibrous, fibro-fatty, dense calcium, and necrotic-core. VH IVUS is intended to be used in conjunction with imaging catheters during diagnostic ultrasound imaging of the peripheral and coronary vasculature to semi-automatically visualize boundary features and perform spectral analysis of radiofrequency ultrasound signals of vascular features that the user may wish to examine more closely during routine diagnostic ultrasound imaging examinations.

5. Intimal hyperplasia imaging

Coronary arteries architecture consists of an external layer the adventitia, the outer covering of the artery the media, the actual wall of the artery the intima, a layer of endothelial cells that make direct contact with the blood and the lumen. The intima in normal arteries is thin; in diseased arteries is thickened by plaques or other tissue growth often eccentric or asymmetrical. The term intimal hyperplasia applies to any cells that form a multi-layer compartment internally to the elastic membrane of the arterial wall. Standard coronary angiography shows the lumen of the artery and lumen narrowings when present by the injection of contrast dye as well as a dynamic picture of the blood flow. If the intima is thickened by plaques or other tissue growth that are not evenly distributed, coronary angiography will show an eccentric lumen and depending on the angle of the view the artery could show less or more stenosis than it really is. The intima layer is best visualized by the intravascular ultrasound (IVUS) that allows a vision of the coronary artery from the inside-out. The cross-section view obtained by IVUS shows the single circular layers of the artery using shades of gray or colors in real time. In a normal artery the intima will appear thin, in a diseased artery the intima is thickened by plaques as the lumen diameter is reduced. Low-dose quantitative 64-channel CT angiography can be a reasonable alternative to invasive IVUS to evaluate the extent of intimal hyperplasia (Figure 3a, Figure 3b).

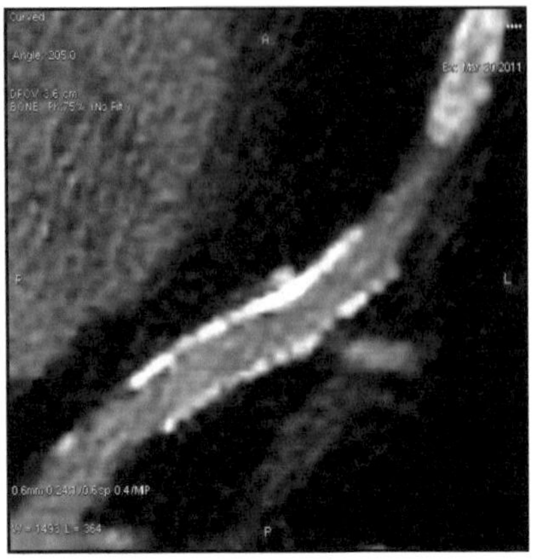

Fig. 3a) 64-CT angiography of a BMS stented Obtuse Margin artery. Intimal hyperplasia is represented as less dense islets of tissue imaged as intraluminal black spots by the struts

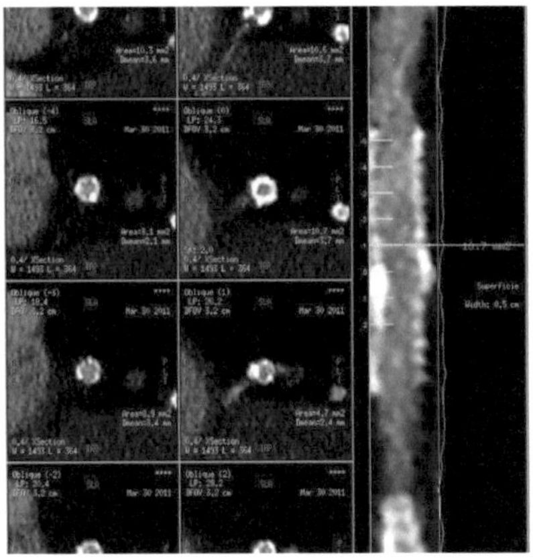

Fig. 3b) 64-CT angiography of the same Obtuse Margin artery in a cross sectional and a longitudinal (right) view

6. The intravascular ultrasound study of oral rapamycin to reduce restenosis after bare metal stent implantation

The aim of our study was to verify if rapamycin, an antiproliferative and antiflammatory drug given orally at a dosage of 2 mg/day for one month was capable to reduce intimal hyperplasia in bare metal stents at 6-month after implantation. Intima hyperplasia in the stented segment of the coronary artery was detected and measured using the intravascular ultrasound technique.

6.1 Methods and results

In this placebo-controlled randomized study, 108 consecutive patients (164 lesions) were enrolled in two groups: oral Rapamycin (54 patients, 83 lesions; 4 mg loading dose on the day of the procedure followed by 2 mg daily for 30 days) and Placebo (54 patients, 81 lesions; 2 mg daily of sodium bicarbonate for 30 days). The angiographic in-segment binary restenosis rate at follow-up angiography was the primary study endpoint. Restenosis was significantly reduced from 36.8% in the Placebo group to 14.3% in the Rapamycin group (p=0.003).

6.2 Intravascular ultrasound analysis

Image acquisition was performed in all cases with a 2.6F 40 MHz Atlantis (Boston Scientific, Natick, Ma) mechanical intravascular ultrasound (IVUS) catheter, interfaced to an Insight III ultrasound consolle (Cardio Vascular Imaging Systems, Boston Scientific, Natick, Ma). The guidewire was threaded through a short monorail close to the probe. The imaging catheter was then advanced beyond the stented segment, as far as possible, after intracoronary injection of 200µg nitroglycerin and after administration of heparin 5000 IU. Motorized transducer pullbacks were performed at a speed of 0.5 mm/sec and recorded on S-VHS videotapes for off-line quantitative analysis.

Videotaped recordings of IVUS pullbacks were digitalized by using Echo-CMS (Medis, The Netherlands), a Windows-based 3D image acquisition software. The IVUS pullback and frame-grabbing rates were constant, and each segment obtained thus represented a 200µm-thick slice. We used QCU-CMS (Medis, The Netherlands), a contour detection program for automated 2D and 3D IVUS analysis of the digitalized segment. Two-dimensional parameters were measured in all slices of the stented segment, and proximal and distal reference segments, according to the ACC Consensus Document for Intravascular Ultrasound. Volume data was then calculated as $V = \sum_{i=1}^{n} A_i \times H$, in which V = volume (lumen, stent or vessel), A = area in each slice, H = slice thickness, and n = number of analyzed slices.

All IVUS analyses were performed by an independent core lab (Mediolanum Cardio Research, Milan, Italy) blinded to the patients' treatment.

6.3 Study endpoints and definitions

Intravascular ultrasound end-points were the volume of neointimal hyperplasia, minimum residual stent area and percentage in-stent volume obstruction, obtained after IVUS analysis by dividing IH volume by stent volume.

The primary end-point was the rate of binary restenosis (percentage diameter stenosis >50%) at 6-month angiographic follow-up.

Additional end-points were the 18-month rates of target vessel failure: death, myocardial infarction (new onset of Q waves on a 12-lead ECG, or CK enzyme elevation > 2 upper limit of normality, with CK-MB fraction >5%), and repeat target vessel revascularization, including coronary artery bypass graft surgery and percutaneous coronary intervention. Intravascular ultrasound end-points were the volume of neointimal hyperplasia, minimum residual stent area, and percentage in-stent volume obstruction, obtained after IVUS analysis by dividing IH volume by stent volume (Figure 4a and Figure 4b).

6.4 Statistical analysis

All analyses were performed on an intention-to-treat basis. Kolmogorov-Smirnov test was used to assess variables normality. Normally distributed variables were compared by Student's T-test, whereas the Mann-Whitney U-test was utilized for not normally distributed variables.

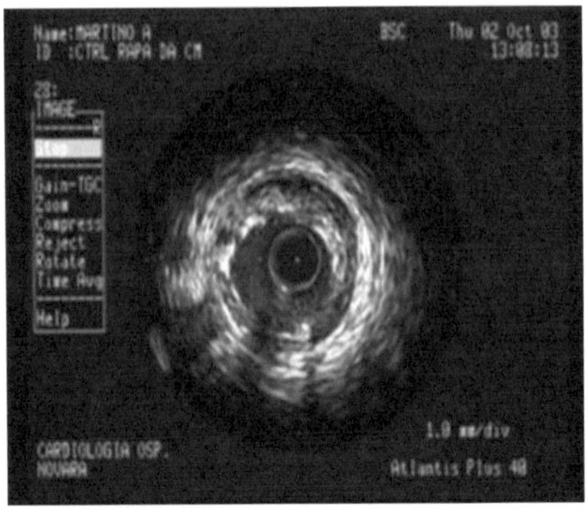

Fig. 4a) Cross sectional IVUS image of a coronary artery of a patient 6 month after BMS implantation and rapamicyn medication: no visible intimal hyperplasia across the stent struts

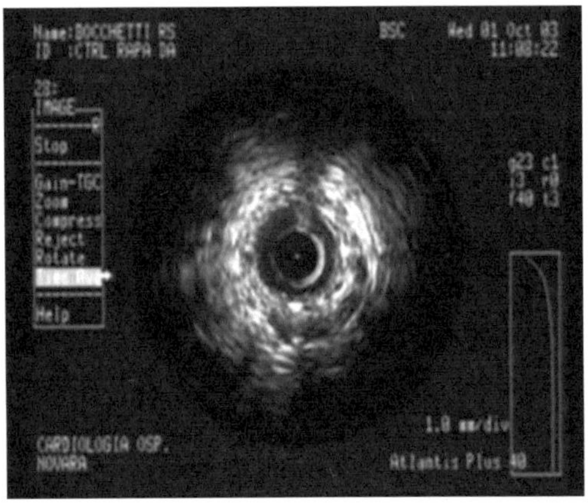

Fig. 4b) Cross sectional IVUS image of a coronary artery of a patient 6 month after BMS implantation and placebo medication: abundant intimal hyperplasia encroaches the stent struts

Discrete baseline characteristics were compared with the use of the chi-square test, Yates corrected when necessary. Statistical significance was accepted for a value of $p<0.05$. Data analysis were performed by SPSS statistical software (version 12.0; SPSS Inc, Chicago, IL).

6.5 Results

Intravascular ultrasound analysis was performed in a total of 93 lesions, 48 in the Rapamycin group and 45 lesions in the Placebo group. The two groups were similar with regard to all baseline clinical and angiographic characteristics. IVUS was attempted but not performed due to inability to advance the catheter across the restenotic lesion in 6 cases (11.1%) in the Rapamycin group and 4 cases (8.2%) in the Placebo group (p=ns). The results for the IVUS analysis at 6-month follow-up are summarized in Table 1.

Serum Rapamycin dosage was performed in a total of 53 patients. Serum Rapamycin levels > 5 ng/ml have been reported to be associated to a lower rate of restenosis. In our series, binary in-stent restenosis was significantly higher in patients with rapamycin blood concentration < 5 ng/ml than in patients with > 5 ng/ml rapamycin (33.3% vs. 7.7%, p=0.044).

	Rapamycin (n=48 lesions)	Placebo (n=45 lesions)	*p*
Mean Vessel CSA (mm^2)	18.70 ± 5.71	16.18 ± 4.32	0.043
Mean Stent CSA (mm^2)	8.93 ± 3.13	7.27 ± 2.35	0.007
Minimum Stent CSA (mm^2)	7.59 ± 2.94	6.20 ± 1.94	0.033
Stent Length (mm)	15.2 ± 7.58	14.5 ± 5.38	ns
Stent Volume (mm^3)	139.2 ± 83.1	111.1 ± 62.9	ns
Minimum Lumen CSA (mm^2)	4.76 ± 2.84	3.68 ± 1.79	0.031
Intimal Hyperplasia Volume (mm^3)	28.04 ± 24.9	33.46 ± 32.4	ns
% Volume Obstruction	18.06 ± 10.7	27.06 ± 15.7	0.008

CSA: cross-sectional area.

Table 1. Results for the IVUS analysis at 6-month follow-up.

There were no serious adverse events during the 18-month period of follow-up. Significant changes in the serum creatinine, cholesterol, triglyceride as well as red and white blood cell counts, fibrinogen, ESR, hepatic enzymes at 15, 30 days and 6 month were not observed. Two patients, one in the Rapamycin group and one in the placebo group, respectively 2 weeks and 3 weeks after treatment, stopped the medication because of severe heartburn.

6.6 Discussion

Purpose of our study was to evaluate the anti-restenotic properties of orally administered Rapamycin after bare metal stent placement, assessed by quantitative angiography and intravascular ultrasound analysis performed at 6 month follow-up angiography, and by assessing the clinical event rates at 5-year follow-up. This study demonstrates that oral administration of Rapamycin at the doses tested results in statistically significant inhibition of neo-intimal hyperplasia, with a reduction in binary restenosis from 36.8% to 14.3% at 6-month follow-up. Percentage volume obstruction at follow-up IVUS was reduced from 27% in the Placebo Group to 18% in the Rapamycin Group. This was associated with a reduction in target vessel failure at 18-month clinical follow-up respectively from 38.8% to 24.1%.
Rapamycin is a macrolide analogue that binds to and inhibits mTOR (mammalian Target of Rapamycin), which is a kinase ultimately involved in the phosphorilation of the 40S ribosomal subunit. By inhibiting mTOR, Rapamycin halts cell proliferation by blocking the cell cycle in the G1/S phase. Experimental studies have shown that Rapamycin inhibits vascular smooth muscle cell proliferation, migration, and differentiation, thus leading to an inhibition of intrastent neointimal hyperplasia proliferation, and consequently a reduced restenosis rate.

6.7 Conclusion

Our study shows that oral adminstration of Rapamycin at the doses tested results in an inhibition of neointimal hyperplasia at 6-month angiographic and IVUS follow-up, after coronary stent placement for de novo native coronary artery lesions. This leads to a reduction in angiographic restenosis, and clinical events, mainly target lesion revascularization, which persists at 5-year follow-up. The degree of inhibition of NIH achieved by orally administered Rapamycin appears inferior to that achieved by locally delivered Rapamycin from drug-eluting stents. An optimization of the dosage regimen is still necessary. However, oral administration of Rapamycin associated to bare metal stent implantation could be a competitive strategy even in the drug-eluting stent era. Randomized clinical trials comparing these strategies are warranted. Another possible direction is combination therapy between orally administered Rapamycin and drug-eluting stents in patient or lesion subsets at particularly high risk of restenosis.

7. References

Bailey S.R. (1997) Local drug delivery: current applications. *Prog Cardiovasc Dis*, Vol.40, pp. 183–204.

Brara P.S., Moussavian M., Grise M.A., Fernandez M., Schatz R.A. & Brara P.S. (2003) Pilot trial of oral rapamycin for recalcitrant restenosis. *Circulation*, Vol.107, pp. 1722-4.

Brito F.S., Rosa W.C., Arruda J.A., Tedesco H., Pestana J.O. & Lima V.C. (2005) Efficacy and safety of oral sirolimus to inhibit in-stent intimal hyperplasia. *Catheter Cardiovasc Interv*, Vol.64, pp. 413-8.

Cernigliaro C., Sansa M., Vitrella G., Verde A., Bongo A.S., Giuliani L. and Novelli E. (2010) Preventing restenosis after implantation of bare stents with oral rapamycin: a randomized angiographic and intravascular ultrasound study with a 5-year clinical follow-up. *Cardiology*, Vol.115, pp. 77-86.

Chaves A.J., Sousa A.G., Mattos L.A., Abizaid A., Feres F., Staico R., Centemero M., Tanajura L.F., Abizaid A.C., Rodrigues A., Paes A., Mintz G.S. & Sousa J.E. (2005) Pilot study with an intensified oral sirolimus regimen for the prevention of in-stent restenosis in de novo lesions: a serial intravascular ultrasound study. *Catheter Cardiovasc Interv*, Vol.66, pp. 535-40.

Daemen J., Wenaweser P., Tsuchida K., Abrecht L., Vaina S., Morger C., Kukreja N., Jüni P., Sianos G., Hellige G., van Domburg R.T., Hess O.M., Boersma E., Meier B., Windecker S. & Serruys P.W. (2007) Early and late coronary stent thrombosis of sirolimus-eluting and paclitaxel-eluting stents in routine clinical practice: data from a large two institutional cohort study. *Lancet*, Vol.369, pp. 667-78.

Fischman D.L., Leon M.B., Baim D.S., Schatz R.A., Savage M.P., Penn I., Detre K., Veltri L., Ricci D., Nobuyoshi M., et al. (1994) A randomised comparison of coronary stent placement and balloon angioplasty in the treatment of coronary artery disease. *N Engl J Med*, Vol.331, pp. 496–501.

Fox D.J., Reckless J., Lingard H., Warren S. & Grainger D.J. (2009) Highly potent, orally available anti-inflammatory broad-spectrum chemokine inhibitors. *J Med Chem*, Vol.52, pp. 3591-5.

Gallo R., Padurean A., Jayaraman T., Marx S., Roque M., Adelman S., Chesebro J., Fallon J., Fuster V., Marks A. & Badimon J.J. (1999) Inhibition of intimal thickening after balloon angioplasty in porcine coronary arteries by targeting regulators of the cell cycle. *Circulation*, Vol.99, pp. 2164-70.

Grüntzig A.R., Senning A. & Siegenthaler WE. (1979) Non-operative dilatation of coronary artery stenosis: percutaneous transluminal coronary angioplasty. *N Engl J Med,* Vol.301, pp. 61–68.

Guarda E., Marchant E., Fajuri A., Martínez A., Morán S., Mendez M., Uriarte P., Valenzuela E., Lazen R. (2004) Oral rapamycin to prevent human coronary stent restenosis: a pilot study. *Am Heart J,* Vol.148:e9.

Hausleiter J., Kastrati A., Mehilli J., Vogeser M., Zohlnhöfer D., Schühlen H., Goos C., Pache J., Dotzer F., Pogatsa-Murray G., Dirschinger J., Heemann U. & Schömig A.; OSIRIS Investigators. (2004) Randomized, double-blind, placebo-controlled trial of oral sirolimus for restenosis prevention in patients with in-stent restenosis: the Oral Sirolimus to Inhibit Recurrent In-stent Stenosis (OSIRIS) trial. *Circulation,* Vol.110, pp. 790-5.

Jennings D.L. & Kalus J.S. (2010) Addition of cilostazol to aspirin and a thienopyridine for prevention of restenosis after coronary artery stenting: a meta-analysis. *J Clin Pharmacol,* Vol.50, pp. 415-21.

Kuchulakanti P. & Waksman R. (2004) Therapeutic potential of oral antiproliferative agents in the prevention of coronary restenosis. *Drugs,* Vol.64, pp. 2379-88.

Munk P.S., Staal E.M., Butt N., Isaksen K. & Larsen A.I. (2009) High-intensity interval training may reduce in-stent restenosis following percutaneous coronary intervention with stent implantation A randomized controlled trial evaluating the relationship to endothelial function and inflammation. *Am Heart J,* Vol.158, pp. 734-41.

Rodriguez A.E., Alemparte M.R., Vigo C.F., Pereira C.F., Llaurado C., Russo M., Virmani R. & Ambrose J.A. (2003) Pilot study of oral rapamycin to prevent restenosis in patients undergoing coronary stent therapy: Argentina Single-Center Study (ORAR Trial). *J Invasive Cardiol,* Vol.15, pp. 581-4.

Rodríguez A.E., Rodríguez Alemparte M., Vigo C.F., Fernández Pereira C., Llauradó C., Vetcher D., Pocovi A. & Ambrose J. (2005) Role of oral rapamycin to prevent restenosis in patients with de novo lesions undergoing coronary stenting: results of the Argentina single centre study (ORAR trial). *Heart,* Vol.91, pp. 1433-7.

Rodriguez A.E., Granada J.F., Rodriguez-Alemparte M., Vigo C.F., Delgado J., Fernandez-Pereira C., Pocovi A., Rodriguez-Granillo A.M., Schulz D., Raizner A.E., Palacios I., O'Neill W., Kaluza G.L. & Stone G.; ORAR II Investigators. (2006) Oral rapamycin after coronary bare metal stent implantation to prevent restenosis: the Prospective, Randomized Oral Rapamycin in Argentina (ORAR II) Study. *J Am Coll Cardiol,* Vol.47, pp. 1522-9.

Rodriguez A.E. (2009) Emerging drugs for coronary restenosis: the role of systemic oral agents the in stent era. *Expert Opin Emerg Drugs,* Vol.14, pp. 561-76.

Rodriguez A.E., Maree A., Tarragona S., Fernandez-Pereira C., Santaera O., Granillo A.M., Rodriguez-Granillo G.A., Russo-Felssen M., Kukreja N., Antoniucci D., Palacios I.F. & Serruys P.W.; ORAR III Investigators. (2009) Percutaneous coronary intervention with oral sirolimus and bare metal stents has comparable safety and efficacy to treatment with drug eluting stents, but with significant cost saving: long-term follow-up results from the randomised, controlled ORAR III (Oral Rapamycin in ARgentina) study. *EuroIntervention,* Vol.5, pp. 255-264.

Ross R., Raines E.W. & Bowen-Pope D.F. (1986) The biology of platelet-derived growth factor. *Cell,* Vol.46, pp. 155-69.

Serruys P.W., Jaegere P., Kiemeneij F., Macaya C, Rutsch W, Heyndrickx G, Emanuelsson H, Marco J, Legrand V, Materne Pet al. (1994) A comparison of balloon expandable stent implantation with balloon angioplasty in patients with coronary artery disease. *N Engl J Med*, Vol.331, pp. 489–495.

Serruys P.W., Degertekin M., Tanabe K., Abizaid A., Sousa J.E., Colombo A., Guagliumi G., Wijns W., Lindeboom W.K., Ligthart J., de Feyter P.J. & Morice M.C.; RAVEL Study Group. (2002) Intravascular ultrasound findings in the multicenter, randomized, double-blind RAVEL (RAndomized study with the sirolimus-eluting VElocity balloon-expandable stent in the treatment of patients with de novo native coronary artery Lesions) trial. *Circulation*, Vol.106, pp. 798-803.

Sigwart U., Puel J., Mirkovitch V., Joffre F. & Kappenberger L. (1987) Intravascular stents to prevent occlusion and restenosis after transluminal angioplasty. *N Engl J Med*, Vol.316, pp. 701–706.

Stojkovic S., Ostojic M., Nedeljkovic M., Stankovic G., Beleslin B., Vukcevic V., Orlic D., Arandjelovic A., Kostic J., Dikic M. & Tomasevic M. (2010) Systemic rapamycin without loading dose for restenosis prevention after coronary bare metal stent implantation. *Catheter Cardiovasc Interv*, Vol.75, pp. 317-25.

Schwartz R.S., Huber K.C., Murphy J.G., Edwards W.D., Camrud A.R., Vlietstra R.E. & Holmes D.R. (1992) Restenosis and the proportional neointimal response to coronary artery injury: results in a porcine model. *J Am Coll Cardiol*, Vol.19, pp. 267-74.

Torguson R., Sabate M., Deible R., Smith K., Chu W.W., Kent K.M., Pichard A.D., Suddath W.O., Satler L.F. & Waksman R. (2006) Intravascular brachytherapy versus drug-eluting stents for the treatment of patients with drug-eluting stent restenosis. *Am J Cardiol*, Vol.98, pp. 1340-4.

Waksman R., Ajani A.E., Pichard A.D., Torguson R., Pinnow E., Canos D., Satler L.F., Kent K.M., Kuchulakanti P., Pappas C., Gambone L., Weissman N., Abbott M.C. & Lindsay J. (2004) Oral rapamycin to inhibit restenosis after stenting of de novo coronary lesions: the Oral Rapamune to Inhibit Restenosis (ORBIT) study. *J Am Coll Cardiol*, Vol.44, pp. 1386-92.

Waksman R., Pakala R., Baffour R., Hellinga D., Seabron R., Kolodgie F. & Virmani R. (2006) Optimal dosing and duration of oral everolimus to inhibit in-stent neointimal growth in rabbit iliac arteries. *Cardiovasc Revasc Med*, Vol.7, pp. 179-84.

Williams L.T. (1989) Signal transduction by the platelet-derived growth factor receptor. *Science*, Vol. 243, pp. 1564-70.

10

Effects of Thiazolidinediones on In-Stent Restenosis: A Review of IVUS Studies

Takanori Yasu[1], Hiroto Ueba[2],
Takuji Katayama[2] and Masanobu Kawakami[2]
[1]*University of the Ryukyus, Graduate School of Medicine,*
[2]*Saitama Medical Center, Jichi Medical University,*
Japan

1. Introduction

Patients with metabolic syndrome or type 2 diabetes are at high risk of in-stent-restenosis, although drug-eluting stents reduce the in-stent restenosis rate and target lesion revascularization rate to less than half compared with bare metal stents.(Mintz GS, et al. J Am Coll Cardiol 2006) Most clinical trials of systemic pharmacotherapies with ACE inhibitors, statins and antiplatelet agents to reduce restenosis have yielded disappointing results. Proliferation of vascular smooth muscle cells is the predominant mechanism of neointimal hyperplasia leading to restenosis. Insulin resistance is a major factor in metabolic syndrome and type 2 diabetes, and has been demonstrated to represent an independent risk factor for in-stent-restenosis.(Piatti P, et al. Circulation 2003) Thiazolidinediones are insulin-sensitizing agents, and reportedly inhibit proliferation of vascular smooth muscle cells in vitro and in animal studies. Recent studies, including our own, (Katayama et al. Am Heart J 2007; Takagi et al. J Am Coll Cardiol Intv 2009) have highlighted the beneficial effects of thiazolidinediones in reducing neointimal growth after stent implantation. We review herein IVUS studies regarding the effects of thiazolidinedione therapy on in-stent restenosis after coronary stent implantation.

2. Effects of thiazolidinedione beyond anti-diabetic actions

Thiazolidinediones activate peroxisome proliferator-activated receptor (PPAR)-γ in adipose tissue, improving insulin sensitivity and glucose control in patients with type 2 diabetes mellitus and metabolic syndrome. The first thiazolidinedione described, troglitazone, was removed from the market because of hepatotoxic effects. Two glitazones, pioglitazone (Actos; Takeda/Lilly,) and rosiglitazone (Avandia; GlaxoSmithKline) are now commercially available for treatment of diabetes mellitus. Glitazones have been shown to improve specific lipid abnormalities associated with insulin resistance. Treatment with glitazones elevates serum levels of high-density lipoprotein (HDL) cholesterol, decreases triglyceride levels, and changes the size of low-density lipoprotein (LDL) cholesterol from small particles to large ones, less atherogenic particles. (Hanefeld M, et al. Diabetes Care 2004) Beyond the anti-diabetic activity, thiazolidinediones inhibit inflammatory activity, and migration and proliferation of vascular smooth muscle cells by decreasing matrix metalloproteinase production and inducing cell cycle arrest or apoptosis and atherosclerotic effects in vascular cells in vitro and in diseased animal models. (Marx N, et al. Circ Res 2004)

2.1 Effects of thiazolidinedione on atherosclerosis and cardiovascular events

In the PROactive study, a double-blinded, placebo-controlled investigation, pioglitazone significantly reduced the composite of all-cause mortality, non-fatal myocardial infarction, and stroke in patients with type 2 diabetes, who have a high risk of macrovascular events. (Dormandy JA, et al. Lancet 2005) Nissen et al. conducted a double-blinded, randomized, multicenter trial in 543 patients with coronary disease and type 2 diabetes to compare the effects of an insulin sensitizer, pioglitazone, with an insulin secretagogue, glimepiride, on the progression of coronary atherosclerosis in patients with type 2 diabetes. (Nissen SE, et al. JAMA 2008) Treatment with pioglitazone resulted in a significantly lower rate of progression of coronary atherosclerosis as assessed by intravascular ultrasound (IVUS) compared with glimepiride in patients with type 2 diabetes and coronary artery disease. A meta-analysis showed that pioglitazone did not increase the risk of myocardial infarction or cardiovascular mortality. (Lincoff, et al. JAMA 2007)

In contrast, controversy persists regarding the effects of rosiglitazone therapy on myocardial infarction and cardiovascular mortality. A meta-analysis of 4 randomized controlled trials (N=14 291, including 6421 receiving rosiglitazone and 7870 receiving control therapy, with a follow-up duration of 1-4 years) showed that rosiglitazone use for ≥12 months is associated with a 42% increased risk of acute myocardial infarction and a doubling in the risk of heart failure among patients with impaired glucose tolerance or type 2 diabetes. (Singh S, et al. JAMA 2007) The most recent systematic review by Nissen and Wollski reported that rosiglitazone therapy significantly increased the risk of myocardial infarction (odds ratio (OR), 1.28; 95% confidence interval (CI), 1.02-1.63; P=.04), but not cardiovascular mortality (OR, 1.03; 95% CI, 0.78-1.36; P=.86). (Nissen SE, et al. Arch Intern Med 2010)

Both thiazolidinediones have been shown to increase the risk of heart failure compared with treatment with placebo or other antidiabetes medications. In order to compare the risk of serious cardiovascular harm by rosiglitazone and by pioglitazone, Graham DJ et al. conducted a nationwide, observational, retrospective, inception cohort of 227, 571 Medicare beneficiaries aged 65 years or older who initiated treatment with rosiglitazone or pioglitazone. The adjusted hazard ratio for rosiglitazone compared with pioglitazone was 1.06 (95% confidence interval [CI], 0.96-1.18) for AMI; 1.27 (95% CI, 1.12-1.45) for stroke; 1.25 (95% CI, 1.16-1.34) for heart failure; 1.14 (95% CI, 1.05-1.24) for death; and 1.18 (95% CI, 1.12-1.23) for the composite of AMI, stroke, heart failure, or death. Compared with prescription of pioglitazone, prescription of rosiglitazone was associated with an increased risk of stroke, heart failure, and all-cause mortality and an increased risk of the composite of AMI, stroke, heart failure, or all-cause mortality in patients 65 years or older. (Graham DJ et al. JAMA. 2010)

2.2 Effects of pioglitazone on in-stent restenosis in metabolic syndrome

We first demonstrated that treatment with pioglitazone reduces intimal index as assessed by IVUS as a parameter of neointimal hyperplasia after bare metal stent implantation in patients with non-diabetic metabolic syndrome using an open-labeled randomized controlled study. (Katayama, et al. Am Heart J 2007) Before coronary stenting, 32 patients were randomly assigned to two treatment groups: the pioglitazone group; and the control group. All patients were successfully treated using IVUS-guided coronary stenting. After coronary stenting, patients in the pioglitazone group were treated with 30 mg/day of pioglitazone in addition to standard medications for 6 months, whereas patients in the control group were treated using only standard medications. After intracoronary administration of isosorbide dinitrate, a 40-MHz IVUS catheter was advanced to the distal side beyond the target lesion, and IVUS images were recorded using automatic pullback (0.5 mm/s). The lesion was defined as the site with smallest lumen, and the reference points were defined as the sites with the largest lumen within 10 mm proximal and distal to the lesion. Bare metal stents were implanted based on IVUS measurements. In accordance with the American College of Cardiology Task Force on Clinical Expert Consensus Documents on IVUS, (Mintz S, et al. J Am Coll Cardiol 2001) quantitative IVUS measurements were performed by a single observer who was blinded to the treatment assignments of patients. (Figure 1)

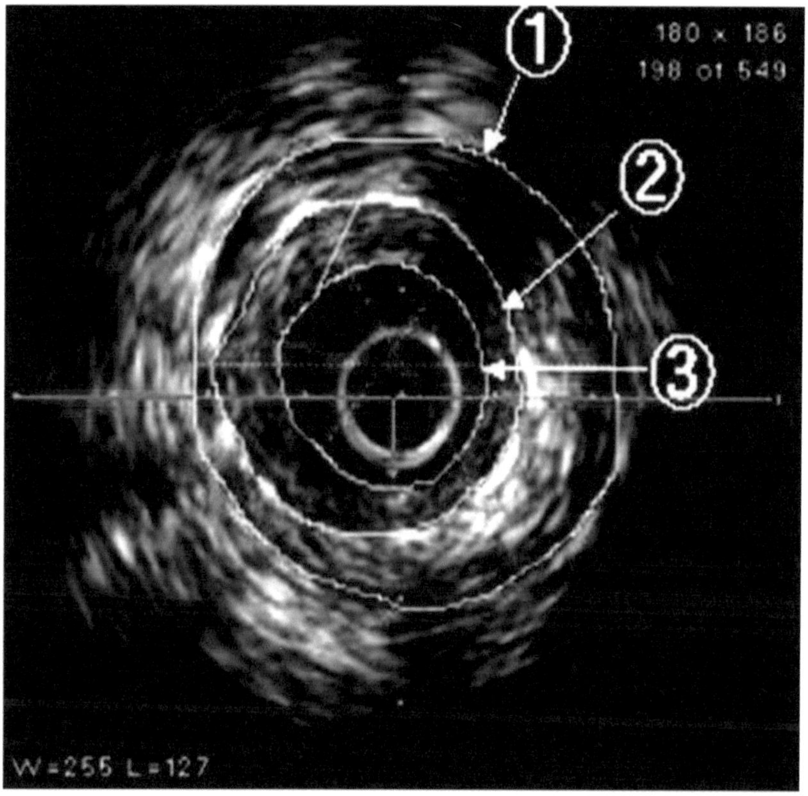

Fig. 1. The following parameters of IVUS were measured at 0.5-mm intervals through the stent site immediately and 6 months after stent implantation. 1) External elastic membrane cross-sectional lumen areas (mm^2); 2) Stent cross-sectional lumen areas (mm^2); 3) Lumen cross-sectional lumen areas (mm^2). Intimal area was calculated as the stent cross-sectional lumen area minus the lumen cross-sectional lumen areas, and the intimal index was defined as the intimal area divided by the stent cross-sectional lumen areas.

Two-dimensional tomographic images from IVUS allowed direct visualization of the 360° characterization of the coronary arterial lumen and neointimal hyperplasia at stent sites. IVUS is a safe, accurate and reproducible method and has thus been recognized as the reference method for quantification of restenosis in trials of anti-restenosis therapeutic interventions. Conversely, angiographic studies of progression/regression are limited because angiography shows the opacified silhouette of only the lumen. Furthermore, the variability of vascular remodeling prevents reliable assessment of plaque dimensions on the basis of lumen narrowing.

The primary end point of this study was the reduction of neointimal hyperplasia as evaluated by intimal index, a prespecified parameter for evaluating neointimal hyperplasia by IVUS. (Katayama, et al. Am Heart J 2007) Intimal index rather than intimal area is considered as a more reliable parameter for the assessment of neointimal hyperplasia. (Mintz GS, et al. J Am Coll Cardiol 2006) Secondary end points were intimal area, late loss of minimal lumen diameter, percentage diameter stenosis, binary restenosis rate, and target vessel revascularization.

Mean intimal index and maximal intimal index by IVUS were significantly reduced in the pioglitazone group compared with controls (Figure 2, panel a). Mean intimal area and maximal intimal area also tended to be reduced in the pioglitazone group compared with controls, but this difference was not significant (Figure 2, panel b). Late loss of minimal lumen diameter and percentage diameter stenosis by quantitative coronary angiography were significantly decreased in the pioglitazone group compared with controls (Figure 2, panels c, d).

The binary restenosis rate was 0% in the pioglitazone group, compared to 31% in controls (P=.043). Three patients in the control group underwent target vessel revascularization, whereas no patients in the pioglitazone group required such interventions. No significant differences in fasting plasma glucose levels, 2-h plasma glucose levels, or hemoglobin (Hb)A1c levels at baseline or follow-up were seen between the 2 groups. On the other hand, fasting insulin levels at baseline were significantly higher in the pioglitazone group compared with controls, and 2-h insulin levels at follow-up were lower in the pioglitazone group than in controls (67.1 ± 28.8 μU/mL vs. 151.9 ± 185.7 μU/mL; P=.027). Visceral fat areas as measured by abdominal computed tomography were significantly decreased at follow-up in the pioglitazone group compared with controls, although no significant differences in plasma lipid profiles (including total cholesterol, LDL, HDL and triglyceride levels) between groups. Pioglitazone treatment improved insulin resistance and decreased visceral fat accumulation, which is closely associated with insulin resistance, without significant changes in glucose or HbA1c levels, or lipid profiles. Our results indicate that reductions in neointimal hyperplasia by pioglitazone in non-diabetic patients with metabolic syndrome are likely attributable to improvements in insulin resistance. Our findings are consistent with previous reports of randomized controlled trials and meta-analyses in patients with impaired glucose tolerance or type 2 diabetes. However, no RCTs have demonstrated that rosiglitazone significantly reduces the risk of repeat target vessel revascularization following implantation of bare metal stents. A meta-analysis by Nishio et al. showed that rosiglitazone does not reduce the risk of repeat target vessel revascularization following PCI (Nishio et al. Cardiovasc Revasc Med 2010). The reasons behind these differing results for prevention of in-stent-restenosis by two thiazolidinediones remain unclear.

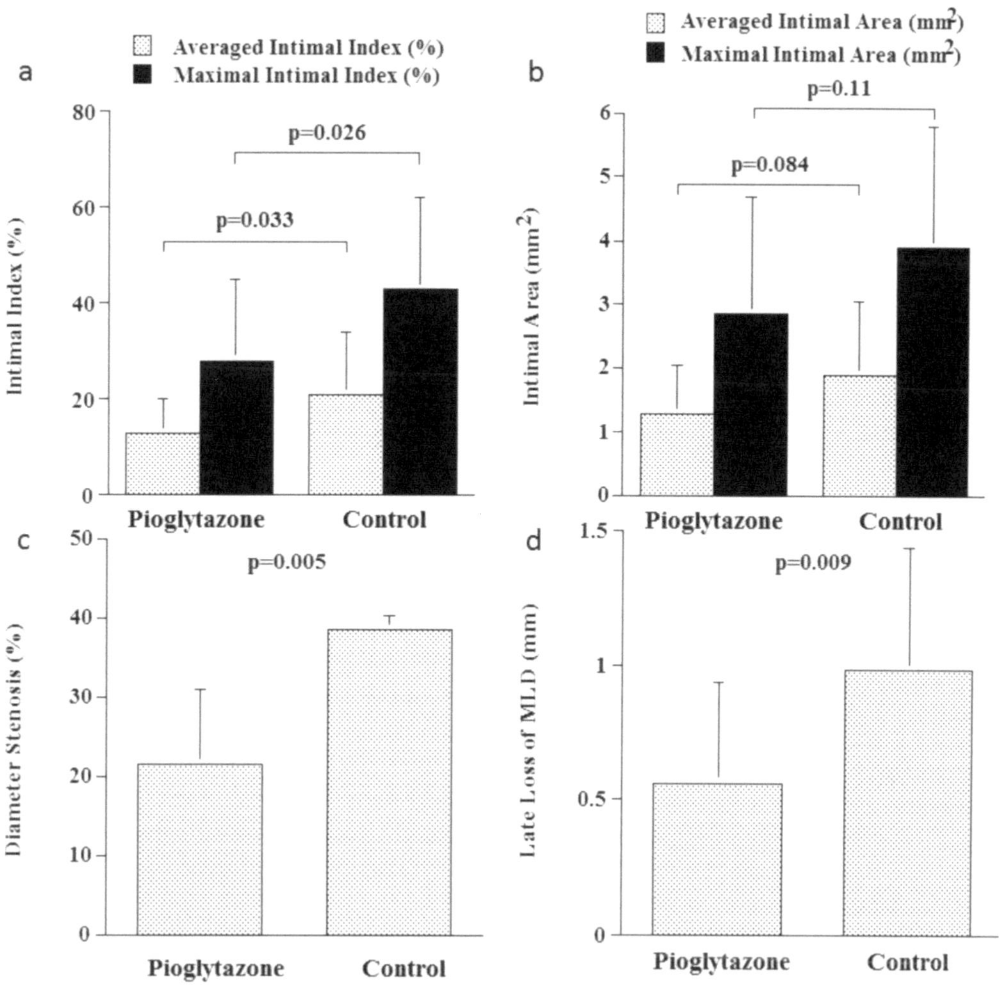

Fig. 2. Intimal index (a) and intimal area (b) as measured by IVUS and late loss (c) and diameter stenosis (d) as assessed by coronary angiography at 6-month follow-up. Mean intimal index and maximal intimal index (a) were significantly reduced in the patient group treated using pioglitazone (n=14) compared with controls (n=14). A non-significant reduction in intimal area was seen in the pioglitazone group compared with controls (b). Late loss of minimum lumen diameter and percentage diameter stenosis as assessed by quantitative coronary arteriography at 6-month follow-up. Late loss of minimum lumen diameter (c) and percentage diameter stenosis (d) were significantly decreased in the pioglitazone group compared with controls.

3. Conclusion

Thiazolidinediones, agonists of peroxisome proliferator-activated receptor (PPAR)-γ, improve insulin sensitivity in patients with type II diabetes mellitus and metabolic syndrome. Beyond the anti-diabetic actions, thiazolidinediones exert anti-inflammatory and anti-atherosclerotic effects in vascular cells in vitro and in diseased animal models. Pioglitazone shows reductions in neointimal hyperplasia leading to in-stent-restenosis after implantation of bare metal stents in patients with type 2 diabetes and metabolic syndrome by IVUS, without unfavorable effects such as increases in myocardial infarction or cardiovascular death. Rosiglitazone shows not only no significant reduction of in-stent-restenosis, but also a strong possibility of increased risk of myocardial infarction and cardiovascular death.

Two-dimensional tomographic imaging by IVUS allows direct visualization of the 360° characterization of coronary arterial lumen and neointimal hyperplasia at the stent sites. IVUS is a safe, accurate and reproducible method and has thus been recognized as the reference method for quantification of restenosis in trials of anti-restenosis therapeutic interventions.

4. References

Mintz GS, Weissman NJ. (2006) Intravascular ultrasound in the drug eluting stent era. *J Am Coll Cardiol* 48:421 -429.

Piatti P, Di Mario C, Monti LD, Fragasso G, Sgura F, Caumo A, Setola E, Lucotti P, Galluccio E, Ronchi C, Origgi A, Zavaroni I, Margonato A, Colombo A. (2003) Association of insulin resistance, hyperleptinemia, and impaired nitric oxide release with in-stent restenosis in patients undergoing coronary stenting. *Circulation* 108:2074 - 2081.

Katayama T, Ueba H, Tsuboi K, Kubo N, Yasu T, Kuroki M, Saito M, Momomura S, Kawakami M. (2007) Reduction of neointimal hyperplasia after coronary stenting by pioglitazone in nondiabetic patients with metabolic syndrome, *Am Heart J* 153: 762.e1-762.e7.

Takagi T, Okura H, Kobayashi Y, Kataoka T, Taguchi H, Toda I, Tamita K, Yamamuro A, Sakanoue Y, Ito A, Yanagi S, Shimeno K, Waseda K, Yamasaki M, Fitzgerald PJ, Ikeno F, Honda Y, Yoshiyama M, Yoshikawa J; POPPS Investigators (2009) prospective, multicenter, randomized trial to assess efficacy of pioglitazone on in-stent neointimal suppression in type 2 diabetes: POPPS (Prevention of In-stent Neointimal Proliferation by Pioglitazone Study) *J Am Coll Cardiol Intv* 2:524–531.

Hanefeld M, Brunetti P, Schernthaner GH, Matthews DR, Charbonnel BH, the QUARTET study group: (2004) One-year glycemic control with a sulfonylurea plus pioglitazone versus a sulfonylurea plus metformin in patients with type 2 diabetes. *Diabetes Care* 27:141–147.

Marx N, Duez H, Fruchart JC, Staels B. (2004) Peroxisome proliferator-activated receptors and atherogenesis: regulators of gene expression in vascular cells. *Circ Res.* 94:1168–1178.

Mintz GS, Nissen SE, Anderson WD, Bailey SR, Erbel R, Fitzgerald PJ, Pinto FJ, Rosenfield K, Siegel RJ, Tuzcu EM, Yock PG.(2001) American College of Cardiology Clinical Expert Consensus Document on Standards for Acquisition, Measurement and Reporting of Intravascular Ultrasound Studies (IVUS). A report of the American College of Cardiology Task Force on Clinical Expert Consensus Documents. *J Am Coll Cardiol* 37:1478-1492.

Marx N, Wohrle J, Nusser T, Walcher D, Rinker A, Hombach V, Koenig W, Hoher M, (2005) Pioglitazone reduces neointima volume after coronary stent implantation: a randomized, placebo-controlled, double-blind trial in nondiabetic patients, *Circulation* 112: 2792–2798.

Dormandy JA, Charbonnel B, Eckland DJ, Erdmann E, Massi-Benedetti M, Moules IK, Skene AM, Tan MH, Lefèbvre PJ, Murray GD, Standl E, Wilcox RG, Wilhelmsen L, Betteridge J, Birkeland K, Golay A, Heine RJ, Korányi L, Laakso M, Mokán M, Norkus A, Pirags V, Podar T, Scheen A, Scherbaum W, Schernthaner G, Schmitz O, Skrha J, Smith U, Taton J; PROactive investigators. (2005) Secondary prevention of macrovascular events in patients with type 2 diabetes in the PROactive Study (PROspective pioglitAzone Clinical Trial In macroVascular Events): a randomised controlled trial. *Lancet* 366: 1279–1289.

Nissen SE, Nicholls SJ, Wolski K, Nesto R, Kupfer S, Perez A, Jure H, De Larochellière R, Staniloae CS, Mavromatis K, Saw J, Hu B, Lincoff AM, Tuzcu EM; PERISCOPE Investigators. (2008) Comparison of pioglitazone vs glimepiride on progression of coronary atherosclerosis in patients with type 2 diabetes: the PERISCOPE randomized controlled trial, *JAMA*; 299:1561–1573.

Lincoff AM, Wolski K, Nicholls SJ, Nissen SE. Pioglitazone and risk of cardiovascular events in patients with type 2 diabetes mellitus: a meta-analysis of randomized trials. *JAMA* 2007;298:1180–1188.

Singh S, Loke YK, Furberg CD.(2007) Long-term risk of cardiovascular events with rosiglitazone: a meta-analysis. *JAMA*.298:1189-1195.

Nissen SE, Wolski K. (2010) Rosiglitazone revisited: An updated meta-analysis of risk for myocardial infarction and cardiovascular mortality. *Arch Intern Med.* 170:1191-1201.

Graham DJ, Ouellet-Hellstrom R, MaCurdy TE, Ali F, Sholley C, Worrall C, Kelman JA. (2010) Risk of acute myocardial infarction, stroke, heart failure, and death in elderly medicare patients treated with rosiglitazone or pioglitazone. *JAMA*.304:411-418.

Riche DM, Valderrama R, Henyan NN. (2007) Thiazolidinediones and risk of repeat target vessel revascularization following percutaneous coronary intervention: a meta-analysis. *Diabetes Care.* 30:384-388.

Nishio K, Kobayashi Y. (2010) Different effects of thiazolidinediones on target vessel revascularization with bare metal stents: a meta-analysis. *Cardiovasc Revasc Med.* 11:227-231.

Part 3

Technical Developments

11

Arterial Plaque Characterization Using IVUS Radio-Frequency Time Echoes

Rafik Borji and Matthew A. Franchek
University of Houston, Department of Mechanical Engineering
USA

1. Introduction

The reported yearly worldwide death tolls and especially in the US about cardio-vascular disease is the leading factor that motivated scientists to invest time and money in order to find innovative ways that enable accurate and early detection of such diseases (American Heart Association [AHA], 2006; AHA, 2008). Since CVD occurs within the human body, imaging modalities were invented to present a picture of the artery as close as possible to its real status. These imaging methods accompanied with continuous developments have helped tremendously in the improvement of proactive health care and early interventions before aggravations. Intravascular Ultrasound (IVUS) is one of the cost effective modalities that have been extensively used for diagnostics purposes (Gaster et al., 2003; Mueller et al., 2003). Although IVUS has the advantage of differentiating between all the artery cross-section components in terms of geometry (Nissen & Yock, 2001), the composition and mechanical properties of each component is still a subject of discussion and research. In fact, an objective classification of plaques based on both mechanical and acoustic properties is not reached yet. For instance, echogenicity of luminal tissue in most cases is the same for a plaque composed of high lipid depositions (Stary, 1992; Stary et al., 1994; Stary et al., 1995). Thus ultrasound wave propagation and transmission should be studied fundamentally in the human tissues and specifically through the artery cross-sections. The only way these ultrasonic waves could be studied meticulously is by solving the propagation governing equations, i.e., through the wave equation. Finding the analytical solution of these waves contributes definitely in understanding the propagation fashion and behavior inside the medium. Finding analytical solution of the wave equation is highly dependent on the medium. In the case of artery cross-section in a human body, there exist numerous geometric irregularities. These irregular shaped components of the artery make the wave equation unsolvable analytically. Consequently numerical methods are employed to find discrete solutions of the ultrasound waves.
The inability of discriminating most plaque types from the grayscale images has fostered researchers to think about the content and information that the IVUS backscattered radio-frequency (RF) ultrasound waves could offer. Studies have shown that RF signals possess valuable information in terms of plaque composition (Normal, fatty, fibro-fatty, fibrous, fibrous with calcification). It has been noticed that there is a difference between these RF echoes coming from various plaque types (Urbani et al., 1993).

Integrated backscatter IVUS (IB IVUS) was introduced and calculated based on these RF signals. Despite the accurate differentiation between all plaque types (calcification, mixed lesion, fibrous tissue, lipid core and thrombus) using IB IVUS, the angle dependency between ROI's and catheter axis makes this classification unstable and sensitive (Urbani et al., 1993; Picano et al., 1983; Sarnelli et al.,1986; Landini et al., 1986; Barzilai et al., 1987; De Kroon et al., 1991; Picano et al., 1994). Moreover the high resolution dictated for plaque detection necessitates high frequency ultrasound signals which affect the penetration depth of these transmitted ultrasonic pulses.

In addition to the use of IB as a determinant parameter by which plaques were classified, new research directions has been inspired from the elastic property that could characterize each plaque type. This gave rise to what is called **intravascular elastography** (also known as **IVUS elastography**) (Cespedes et al., 1991). In fact, investigators have taken advantage of the possibility of recording the RF echoes to use them for displacements or strain determination (Ryan & Foster, 1997; De Korte et al., 1998; Schaar et al., 2003; Saijo et al., 2004; Shapo et al., 1996). Despite the striking difference of the strain values for various plaques, most of the studies were performed in vitro where the temperature is different from in vivo case. Additionally excised arteries were used after freezing and thawing which influences the values of elastic modulus. Elastography has also been criticized for its inability of discriminating between normal artery and Fibrous caps (De Korte et al., 2000).

The use of the RF echoes content has also been used further. A method called **virtual histology** (also called **VH IVUS**) based on these IVUS-RF-ultrasonic waves has been developed. This tissue characterization technique is based on the frequency spectrum analysis (Koenig & Klauss, 2007; Nair et al., 2002). Several limitations accompanied the development of VH IVUS. In fact, virtual histology gives an axial resolution which is too low to detect fibrous cap thickness. In addition the detection between soft plaque material and thrombus is not possible.

Despite this simplicity of image construction from IVUS and the development of some signal processing procedures to overcome the lack of plaque characterization, there are significant challenges which limited the accuracy and clarity of the images produced via IVUS. These challenges are always present in the imaging process. For example, the omnipresence of noise related to the acquisition of the ultrasound waves (due to electronic devices) plays an important role on hiding useful information during the detection process. Moreover uncertainties due to sound speed variation, eccentricity of the transducer as well as scattering (related to small particles such as cells, and irregular surfaces) are important factors which contribute to the limitations of the developed IVUS techniques for the identification of vulnerable plaques. This certainly influences the issues of resolution and inability to adequately discriminate between fibrous and lipid-rich plaques.

The nature of this imaging modality (irregularities in the geometry of the tissues and movement of the catheter tips) and the sensitivity of the recorded RF echoes have motivated other research groups to work on modeling the ultrasound wave propagation in biological tissues and specifically IVUS.

Since the IVUS imaging method is based on ultrasound wave propagation, the only way to sketch a model for this propagation will be dictated from the constitutive laws that govern these waves. To know the complete behavior of the waves towards each tissue component, a solution should be found in time and space for these signals.

Nonlinear propagation mathematical models have been introduced. The most widely used model for modeling finite amplitude sound beam propagation is the so-called Khokhlov, Zabolotskaya and Kuznetsov (KZK) equation (Kuznestov, 1971). Numerous methods to solve this non-linear model have been proposed (Lee & Hamilton, 1995; Tavakkoli et al., 1998). One of the difficulties for these numerical models was the computational aspect. Huge memory and supercomputing machines have to be allocated for the implementation of such nonlinear models. Even using advanced equipments in terms of performance, the computation process of these models can take several hours and even days. This is far from simulating a real time propagation of the ultrasonic waves.
Given the complexity in solving these nonlinear models, other groups of researchers have resorted to the adoption of simple linear wave equation models (Kendall & Weimin, 2001). In fact ultrasound that is propagating in biological tissues generates small fluctuations. The propagation of these fluctuations is governed by what is called the wave equation. The closed form solution of the wave equation here above is unavailable. Thus two main numerical methods were proposed; which are the finite differences and the finite element methods (Guenther & John, 1996; Kendall & Weimin, 2001). The complexity of the models presented problems in terms of real time simulation and computational burden.
A reduced order model called Transmission Line matrix (TLM) method is developed in this chapter to simulate the ultrasound wave propagation. The foundation of the computational method (Transmission Line Matrix Method) that is used to model IVUS in a simple regular medium (rectangular shape) is first developed. A new TLM model in polar coordinates (circular shape to model the artery cross-section) is then outlined. The TLM model will subsequently be modified to model IVUS. The system identification methodology used to construct a parametric model that characterizes a plaque for specific mechanical and acoustic properties is demonstrated in the last part of the chapter.

2. TLM model

Transmission Line Matrix concept was based on transmission lines (Fig. 1).

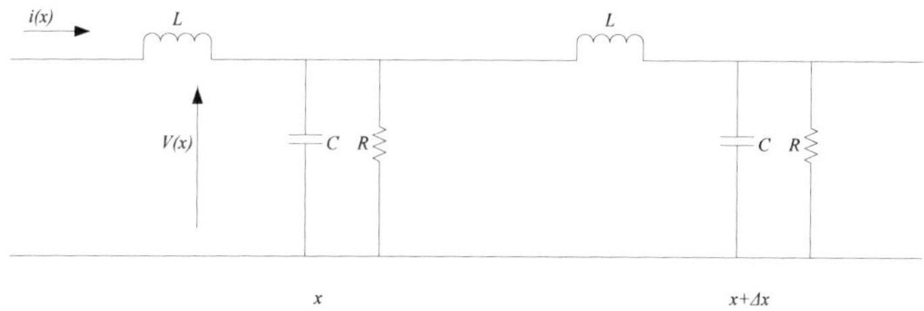

Fig. 1. A simple transmission line circuit between points x and x+Δx

The idea of using electrical circuits for TLM came from the analogy that was established between the current or voltage propagating in this line from one point to another and the electromagnetic field (EMF) governing equations (Christos, 1995). Besides this analogy, TLM was based on the Huygens principle where each point of a wave front is regarded as a secondary wave source point and the surface tangent to the secondary wave fronts is used to determine the future position of wave front (Fig. 2).

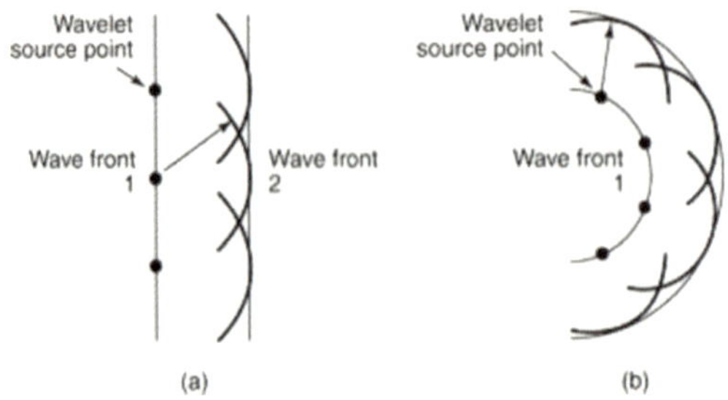

Fig. 2. Schematics of the Huygens principle for wave propagation (CliffsNotes. Wave Optics, 2010)

TLM models this physics principle by discretizing the medium into a mesh grid and replacing the wave amplitudes by voltages and currents traveling from one node to another (Fig. 3).

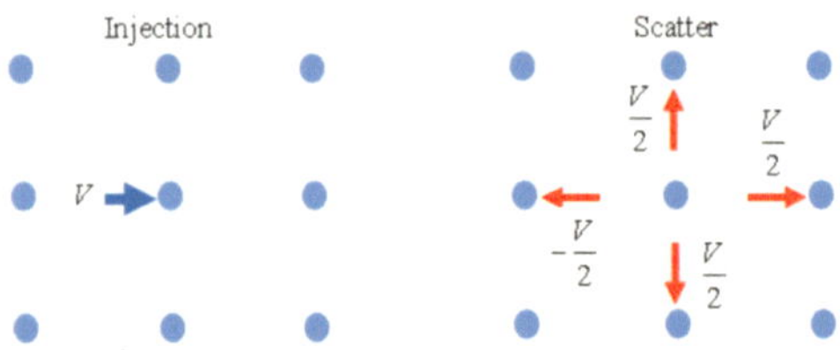

Fig. 3. Propagation in TLM model

2.1 Rectangular TLM

The 2-D TLM method has been widely developed and studied in the literature because of its importance in terms of treating wave propagation in the two dimensional space (Christos, 1995; De Cogan et al., 2006). As mentioned previously the use of TLM method for wave propagation purposes was first inspired from the analogy that was found between the electric circuit variables and the EMF problem. A two dimensional element of a medium of dimensions u and v , is represented by a node intersected by two transmission lines in the x and y directions (Fig. 4).

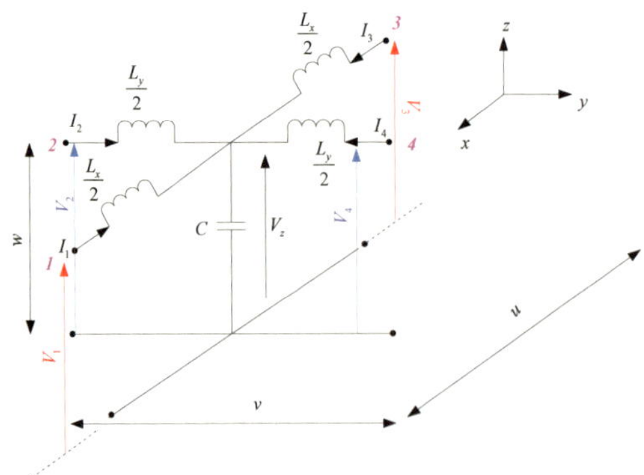

Fig. 4. Shunt TLM node

If C is the total capacitance of this element and L_x, L_y are the total inductances for the two lines in x and y directions respectively, then the voltage/current differential equations are

$$\begin{cases} \dfrac{\partial V_z}{\partial x} = -\dfrac{L_x}{u}\dfrac{\partial I_x}{\partial t} \\ \dfrac{\partial V_z}{\partial y} = -\dfrac{L_y}{v}\dfrac{\partial I_y}{\partial t} \\ -u\dfrac{\partial I_x}{\partial x} - v\dfrac{\partial I_y}{\partial y} = C\dfrac{\partial V_z}{\partial t} \end{cases}, \quad (1)$$

where I_x and I_y are the current traveling in the lines in x and y directions respectively and V_z is the total voltage in the element. Recall that the governing equations for EMF and Sound wave problems in the 2-D configuration are the following.

$$\begin{cases} \dfrac{\partial E_z}{\partial x} = \mu\dfrac{\partial H_y}{\partial t} \\ \dfrac{\partial E_z}{\partial y} = -\mu\dfrac{\partial H_x}{\partial t} \\ \dfrac{\partial H_y}{\partial x} - \dfrac{\partial Hx}{\partial y} = \varepsilon\dfrac{\partial E_z}{\partial t} \end{cases}. \quad (2)$$

$$\begin{cases} \dfrac{\partial P}{\partial x} = -\rho\dfrac{\partial U_x}{\partial t} \\ \dfrac{\partial P}{\partial y} = -\rho\dfrac{\partial U_y}{\partial t} \\ -\dfrac{\partial U_x}{\partial x} - \dfrac{\partial U_y}{\partial y} = \sigma\dfrac{\partial P}{\partial t} \end{cases}. \quad (3)$$

Where E and H are the Electric and magnetic fields, μ and ε are the permeability and permittivity of the space. P is the pressure, U_x and U_y are the pressure velocity components in x and y directions, ρ is the density of the medium and σ is the compressibility of the medium.

The system of equations in (1) is transformed to equation (4)

$$\begin{cases} \dfrac{\partial\left(\dfrac{V_z}{w}\right)}{\partial x} = \dfrac{L_x v}{uw}\dfrac{\partial\left(-\dfrac{I_x}{v}\right)}{\partial t} \\ \dfrac{\partial\left(\dfrac{V_z}{w}\right)}{\partial y} = -\dfrac{L_y u}{vw}\dfrac{\partial\left(\dfrac{I_y}{u}\right)}{\partial t} \\ \dfrac{\partial\left(-\dfrac{I_x}{v}\right)}{\partial x} - \dfrac{\partial\left(\dfrac{I_y}{u}\right)}{\partial y} = \dfrac{Cw}{uv}\dfrac{\partial\left(\dfrac{V_z}{w}\right)}{\partial t} \end{cases}. \quad (4)$$

Here w is an arbitrary distance inserted to retain the correct dimensionality when dividing I_x and I_y by v and u respectively (Al-Mukhtar & Sitch, 1981). Comparing equations (2), (3) and (4), the analogy between EMF, sound propagation and electric circuits is established in Table 1. From this analogy the electric and magnetic fields of the EMF problem could be solved through the TLM method by considering them as the transmission line voltage and currents respectively. The same thing applies for the sound wave problem (wave equation), where the amplitudes are calculated via the voltages traveling in the TLM model.

EMF parameters	Sound wave parameters	Electric Circuit Parameters for the Transmission Line (TL)
E_z	P	V_z/w
$-H_y$	U_x	I_x/v
H_x	U_y	I_y/u
μ	ρ	$L_y u/vw$ or $L_x v/uw$
ε	σ	Cw/uv

Table 1. Analogy between EMF, Sound wave and TL parameters

In a regular mesh, each node is characterized by equally spaced nodes related to each other by four lines (in the x and y directions) as illustrated in Fig. 4. This shunt node in a Cartesian regular mesh is presented by four transmission line segments each of characteristic impedance $Z_i, i=1,2,3,4$. These four lines have the same length (i.e. same impedance). The scattering is calculated based on the incident $\left({}_kV_i^I\right)$ and reflected $\left({}_kV_i^R\right)$ pulses to the node and the relationship between them. This relationship between $\left({}_kV_i^I\right)$ and $\left({}_kV_i^R\right)$ is derived using a general approach based on replacing each of the line segment by its Thevenin equivalent (U.A. Bakshi & V.U. Bakshi, 2009). For each segment, this consists of a voltage $2{}_kV_i^I$ in series with the impedance Z_i (Fig. 5).

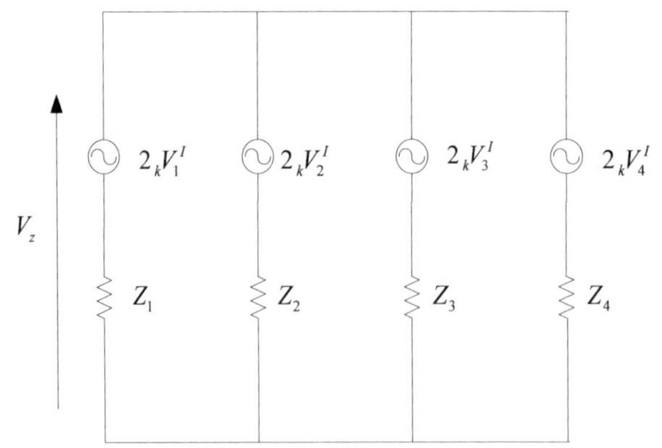

Fig. 5. Thevenin equivalent circuit for the 4 lines intersecting the shunt node of the mesh

The scattering matrix for the shunt node

$$\begin{bmatrix} {}_kV_1^R \\ {}_kV_2^R \\ {}_kV_3^R \\ {}_kV_4^R \end{bmatrix} = 0.5 \begin{bmatrix} -1 & 1 & 1 & 1 \\ 1 & -1 & 1 & 1 \\ 1 & 1 & -1 & 1 \\ 1 & 1 & 1 & -1 \end{bmatrix} \begin{bmatrix} {}_kV_1^I \\ {}_kV_2^I \\ {}_kV_3^I \\ {}_kV_4^I \end{bmatrix}. \quad (5)$$

There are applications, such as arteries, when the medium geometry is complex (curved or circular shapes), where the use of the regular TLM method is not appropriate to solve numerically the sound wave equation. This restriction on the shape and size of the mesh affects the capability of the conventional regular TLM method. Moreover the employment of the conventional TLM where the shape is irregular necessitates the use of finer meshes to represent these irregularities accurately. This represents a burden in terms of memory use and run time for numerical computations. Hence a new TLM mesh and model will be developed for the whole artery cross-section in the next section.

2.2 Cylindrical TLM

A two dimensional element of a medium having differing dimensions u and v, is represented by a node intersected by two transmission lines in x and y directions (Fig. 6).

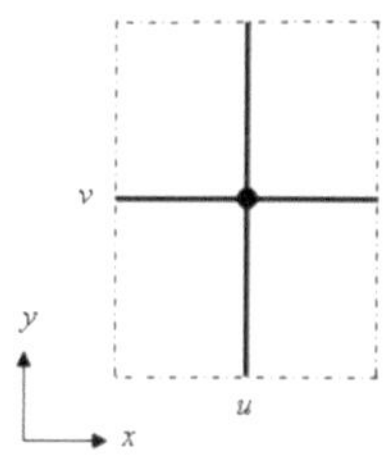

Fig. 6. Irregularly spaced element

From Table 1, the following relationships are obtained

$$\begin{cases} C = \sigma \dfrac{uv}{w} \\ L_x = \rho \dfrac{uw}{v} \\ L_y = \rho \dfrac{vw}{u} \end{cases}. \quad (6)$$

Time synchronism is conserved in the TLM (Christos, 1995). In fact, the transmitted pulse from one node must reach its surrounding nodes at the same time regardless the lines lengths linking these nodes in all direction (x and y directions in the 2-D case). This means that the velocity of propagation of the voltage is dependent on the lines lengths. Since the velocity is function of the total inductance and capacitance of the line ($V = \frac{1}{\sqrt{LC}}$), the inductance term is fixed and capacitance is calculated for each direction by taking into account the relationship between inductance, capacitance and velocity.

Given the inductances in both directions, the capacitances per unit length in these lines are obtained.

$$\begin{cases} C_x = \dfrac{\sigma_0 v}{u^2 h \rho_r w} \\ C_y = \dfrac{\sigma_0 u}{v^2 h \rho_r w} \end{cases} . \tag{7}$$

Due to the irregular mesh grid, the total capacitances found in x and y directions, C_x and C_y are sometimes less than the total capacitance of the element C. A residual capacitance C_s is defined and modeled by an open-circuit stub at each node of the mesh (Fig. 7).

$$C_s = \sigma \frac{uv}{w} - \frac{\sigma_0 \left(u^2 + v^2\right)}{uvh\rho_r w} \tag{8}$$

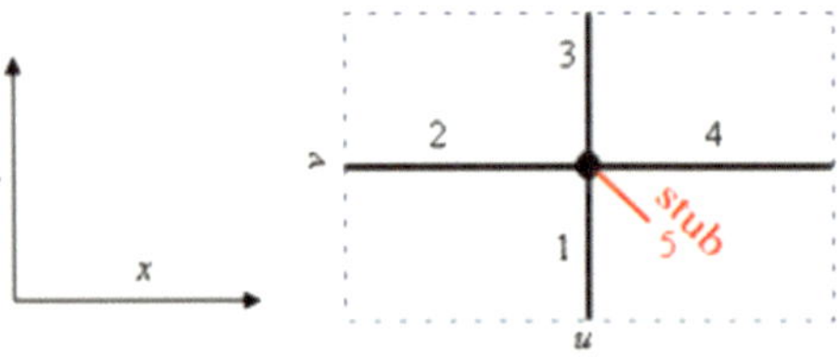

Fig. 7. Stub represented by a new line at each node

The artery cross-section is presented by a disk. The coordinates system is characterized by the angle θ and the radial position r (polar coordinates). In the TLM method, the discretization process of the medium will lead to an irregular gridding (Fig. 8).

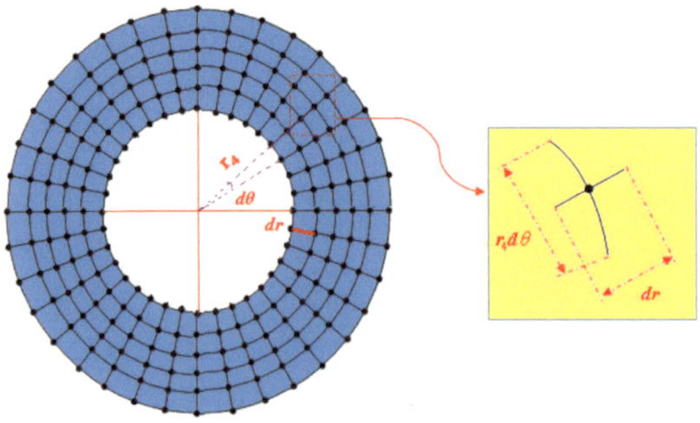

Fig. 8. Irregular structure of a circular element of the cylindrical TLM model

In general for an arbitrary node that has a radial position r the element is characterized by the following lines lengths

$$\begin{cases} u_r = dr \\ u_\theta = rd\theta \end{cases} \tag{9}$$

Obviously the nodes in this case are not equally spaced. Therefore the TLM model corresponds exactly to the same formulation. Consequently a stub line must be added to compensate for the residual capacitance caused by the length difference of the radial and angular lines of each element in the mesh. The element is characterized by radial and angular impedances and a stub admittance Z_r, Z_θ and Z_5.

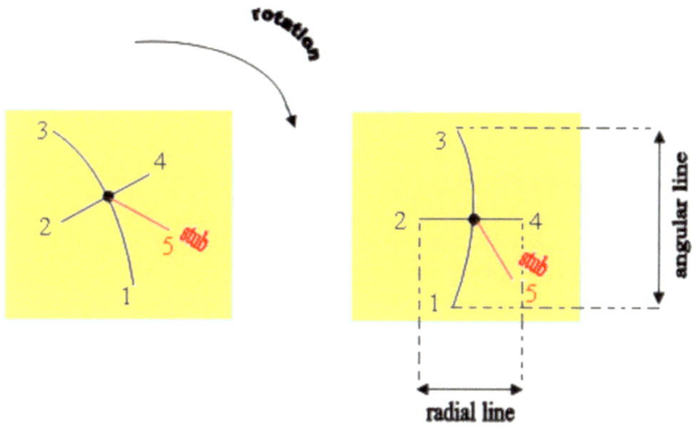

Fig. 9. Added stub line to a circular element

In Fig. 9, the radial line $[2,4]$, the angular line $[1,3]$ and the stub line are characterized respectively by Z_r, Z_θ and Z_5. The radial, angular impedances and the stub admittance can be derived by replacing u by dr and v by $rd\theta$.

$$\begin{cases} Z_r = \dfrac{wdr\rho_r}{rd\theta} Z_{ref} \\ Z_\theta = \dfrac{wrd\theta\rho_r}{dr} Z_{ref} \\ Z_5 = \dfrac{2\left[\sigma(dr)^2(rd\theta)^2 h\rho_r - \sigma_0\left((dr)^2+(rd\theta)^2\right)\right]}{(dr)(rd\theta)w\sigma_0\rho_r} \end{cases} , \qquad (10)$$

where $\rho_r = \dfrac{\rho}{\rho_0}$ is the ratio of a line inductance with respect to the smallest line inductance and $Z_{ref} = \sqrt{\dfrac{h\rho_0}{\sigma_0}}$ is the characteristic impedance of the smallest line in the mesh grid of the artery cross-section. ρ_0 and $\dfrac{\sigma_0}{h}$ are the inductance and capacitance of the reference line (i.e. smallest line).

For both Cartesian and cylindrical geometry, each TLM element is thus characterized by a circuit structure of five transmission lines (Fig. 10).

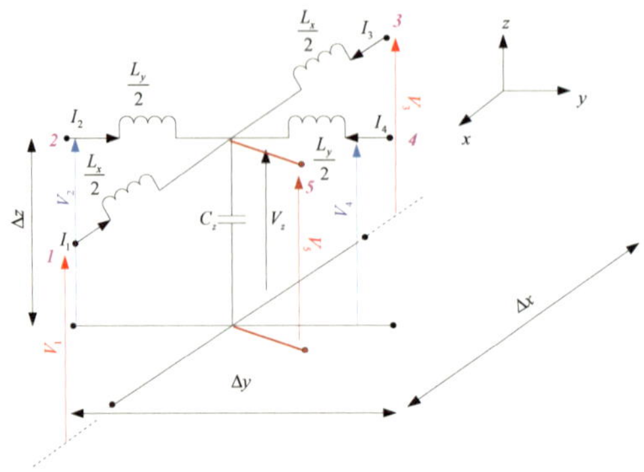

Fig. 10. Shunt node for irregular TLM

The equivalent Thevenin circuit is composed of five Thevenin sources in series with five equivalent impedances corresponding to the five lines (Fig. 11).

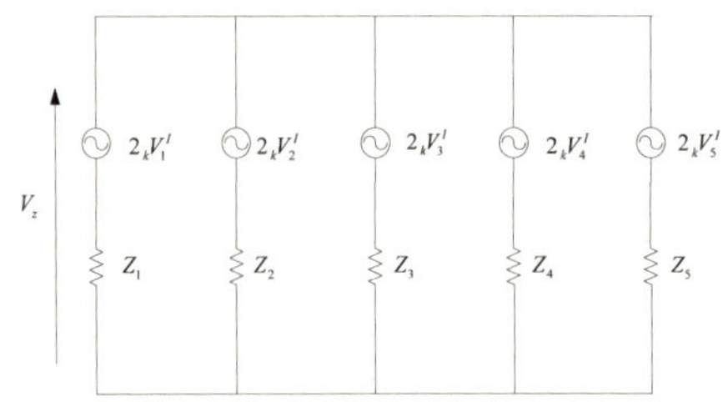

Fig. 11. Thevenin equivalent circuit for the 5 lines intersecting an arbitrary node of the irregular mesh

The scattering matrix equation in this case is

$$\begin{bmatrix} {}_kV_1^R \\ {}_kV_2^R \\ {}_kV_3^R \\ {}_kV_4^R \\ {}_kV_5^R \end{bmatrix} = \frac{1}{D}\begin{bmatrix} 2Z_1 - D & 2Z_2 & 2Z_3 & 2Z_4 & 2Z_5 \\ 2Z_1 & 2Z_2 - D & 2Z_3 & 2Z_4 & 2Z_5 \\ 2Z_1 & 2Z_2 & 2Z_3 - D & 2Z_4 & 2Z_5 \\ 2Z_1 & 2Z_2 & 2Z_3 & 2Z_4 - D & 2Z_5 \\ 2Z_1 & 2Z_2 & 2Z_3 & 2Z_4 & 2Z_5 - D \end{bmatrix}\begin{bmatrix} {}_kV_1^I \\ {}_kV_2^I \\ {}_kV_3^I \\ {}_kV_4^I \\ {}_kV_5^I \end{bmatrix}. \tag{11}$$

${}_kV_i^R$ and ${}_kV_i^I$ are the reflected and incident voltages to an arbitrary node of the line i at time k and $D = \sum_{i=1}^{5} Z_i$ is the sum of the impedances of the four lines and the stub admittance.

3. TLM IVUS model

Ultrasound waves have the same properties as sound waves. They obey the same wave propagation law. In this section a physics-based numerical model is developed using TLM method to mimic the ultrasound wave propagation inside the arterial wall. Both rectangular and cylindrical TLM models will be employed to model IVUS. The first TLM model is used by considering a small portion of the artery cross-section that has a rectangular shape (Fig. 14). However the second TLM model (cylindrical) takes into account the whole artery cross-section geometry. These codes were developed in Matlab. In order to construct the TLM models many basic parameters should be provided. The size of the medium, the gridding rate, the boundary termination, the wave source location and the traveling process are the most important data to be known in the modeling process.

The medium is automatically generated from the developed TLM codes once the dimensions are specified. Given the inner and outer radii of the artery cross-section, an automated mesh is generated. Since TLM model is based on the nodes and lines of the discretized medium, the number of nodes in both directions as well as the lines lengths are function of the indicated gridding rates. In the cylindrical TLM model, the choice of the gridding rate is essential for capturing the propagation of the ultrasound wave. The wave should reach the outer edge of the artery cross-section. In fact for an arbitrary mesh the propagation trend of the ultrasound wave is more pronounced in the angular direction of the circular medium. The choice of the mesh grid must be generated in a way that guarantees a conic wave propagation of the TLM method. This means that the propagation should occur in a conic way in the radial direction. The propagation as developed previously in the TLM model depends on the scattering matrix which is function of the lines impedances. These impedances are function of the gridding rates in both radial and angular directions. Thus a specific mesh grid should be developed to ensure this numerical stability. The propagation of the sound wave is expected to be like the one illustrated by Fig. 12.

Investigations have shown that the angular deviation of the propagation occurs when the radial position is characterized by $\frac{Z_r}{Z_\theta} = 0.633$. Since $\frac{Z_r}{Z_\theta} = \frac{(dr)^2}{(Rd\theta)^2}$, after this radial position, the ratio between the gridding rates has this condition $\frac{dr}{Rd\theta} < 0.8$. The mesh grid is designed such that $\frac{dr}{Rd\theta} \geq 0.8$. By imposing this numerical condition on the mesh grid, the propagation occurs in a conic fashion as illustrated in Fig. 12.

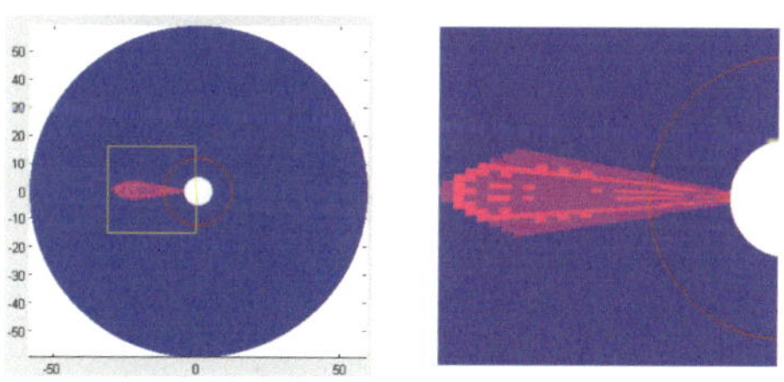

Fig. 12. Conic propagation of the sent wave through the circular medium

As the TLM is a numerical method, the medium should be of a finite size. This is known as **medium termination**. This is presented by a wall that is characterized by the same acoustic impedance of the terminated medium. For example if the external medium that comes after the artery is air, then the wall that models the termination of air is characterized by the acoustic impedance of the air. For all the developed simulations the surrounding media impedances will be taken in such a way the boundary reflection effect is attenuated so that these reflected components do not influence the wave propagation inside the artery cross-section.

The design of **the wave source** has been widely studied for the IVUS. In the TLM model, flexibility is given in the code to design any kind of source waves. Since Matlab is the platform where the code was developed, SIMULINK toolbox is used for the source wave specifications. This toolbox offers a variety of signals some of them are illustrated in Fig. 13. In addition to the wide range of source waves, this model gives the possibility of specifying any location in the mesh to be the source point where the ultrasonic wave starts to propagate. For instance the source could be in one node of the edges of the medium, inside the medium or in different nodes at the same time.

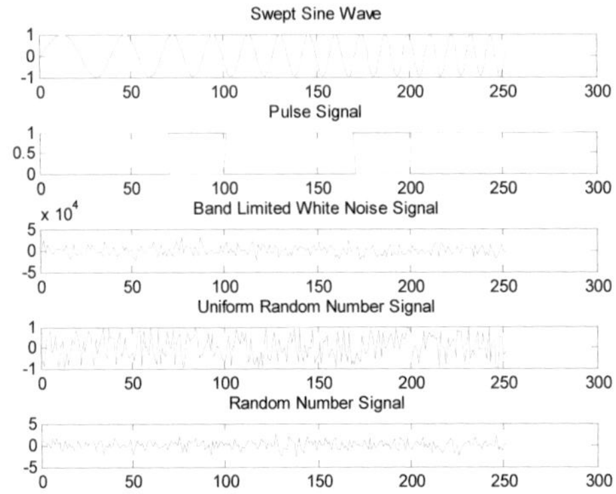

Fig. 13. Examples of different source waves designed by Simulink

The propagation process is based in the Huygens principle where for a given node in the mesh, the reflected amplitudes going out at time k will serve as the incident waves to the surrounding nodes at time $k + 1$. For the rectangular and cylindrical TLM models, it is given by equations (12) and (13).

$$\begin{cases} {}_kV_1^R(x_0,y_0) = {}_{k+1}V_3^I(x_0,y_0-\Delta y) \\ {}_kV_2^R(x_0,y_0) = {}_{k+1}V_4^I(x_0-\Delta x,y_0) \\ {}_kV_3^R(x_0,y_0) = {}_{k+1}V_1^I(x_0,y_0+\Delta y) \\ {}_kV_4^R(x_0,y_0) = {}_{k+1}V_2^I(x_0+\Delta x,y_0) \end{cases} \tag{12}$$

$$\begin{cases} {}_{k+1}V_1^I(r_0,\theta_0+d\theta) = {}_kV_3^R(r_0,\theta_0) \\ {}_{k+1}V_2^I(r_0+dr,\theta_0) = {}_kV_4^R(r_0,\theta_0) \\ {}_{k+1}V_3^I(r_0,\theta_0-d\theta) = {}_kV_1^R(r_0,\theta_0)\,. \\ {}_{k+1}V_4^I(r_0-dr,\theta_0) = {}_kV_2^R(r_0,\theta_0) \\ {}_{k+1}V_5^I(r_0,\theta_0) = {}_kV_5^R(r_0,\theta_0) \end{cases} \tag{13}$$

The IVUS TLM models can represent both healthy and abnormal artery cross-sections. In the healthy case the TLM model is described by a medium that has constant acoustic impedance ($Z = \rho c$, ρ is the medium density and c is the acoustic speed in the medium). However the abnormal artery is modeled by an inclusion that is inserted in the healthy medium. This inclusion is characterized ban acoustic impedance that is different from the one of the healthy medium. Illustrated in Fig. 14 is the case where artery contains a plaque (Yellow colored region).

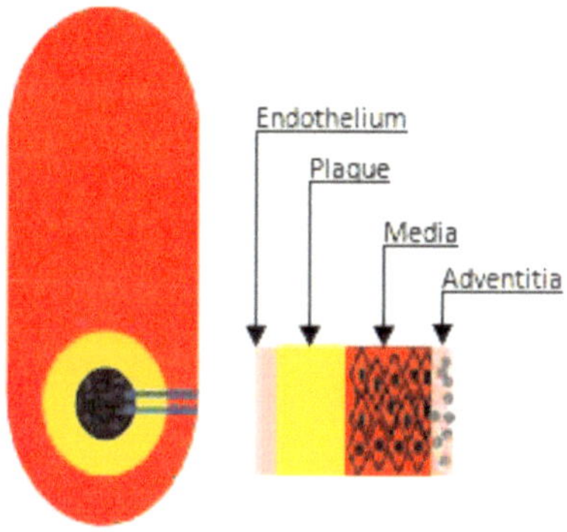

Fig. 14. Plaque in the artery

The TLM model will consider the plaque as a rectangular object that is inserted inside the artery portion presented by the rectangular medium. The plaque (inclusion) that is formed inside the artery is characterized by different acoustic properties. In fact the ultrasound speed and density are not the same as of the normal tissue (i.e. different acoustic impedances). This will produce a boundary between the healthy portion of the artery and the abnormality edge. This boundary characterizes a change in impedances. A reflection/transmission phenomenon takes place due to this change along the four edges of the plaque. Considering $Z_{Plaque} = c_{Plaque}\rho_{PLaque}$ and $Z_{Artery} = c_{artery}\rho_{Artery}$ to be the acoustic impedances of the plaque and artery, then the reflection and transmission coefficients are

$$R = \frac{Z_{Plaque} - Z_{Artery}}{Z_{Plaque} + Z_{Artery}}$$
$$T = 1 - \frac{Z_{Plaque} - Z_{Artery}}{Z_{Plaque} + Z_{Artery}} . \quad (14)$$

The transmission and reflection that occur on both sides of the boundary are function of these coefficients. Depending on the acoustic characteristics of the plaque the propagation of the wave will show different behavior. As an example to illustrate the effect of the plaque, three different acoustic impedances are taken. A swept sine wave is designed to be the source signal at the node (1st horizontal, 45th vertical). The medium is composed of 751 by 76 nodes and the plaque is located between the 20th and 30th node in the horizontal direction and the 25th and 65th node in the vertical direction (Fig. 15).

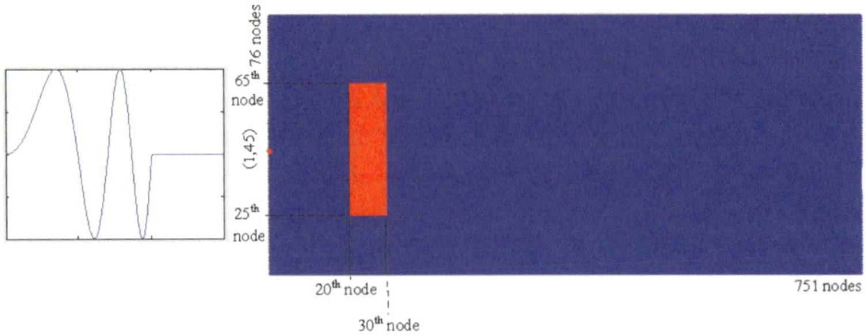

Fig. 15. Plaque example generated by the developed 2-D rectangular TLM model

Fig. 16 is an illustration of the plaque influence on the determination of the wave shape using regular TLM model. This model could be extended to study numerous cases where all combinations of abnormalities can be constructed.

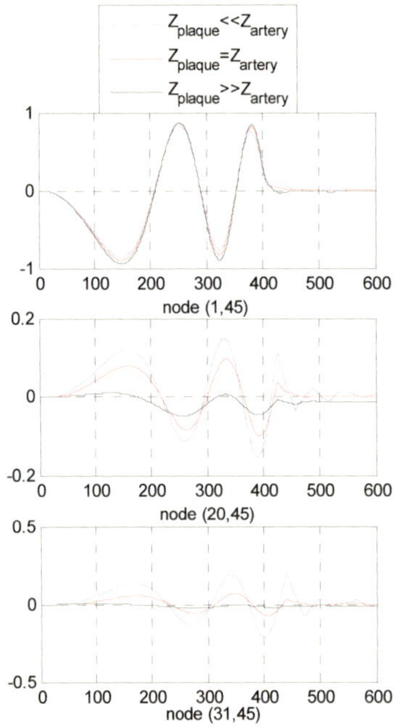

Fig. 16. Comparison of the time signals using the rectangular TLM model ($Z_{Hardinclusion} = 7.4Z_{Healthyartery}$ and $Z_{Softinclusion} = 0.074Z_{Healthyartery}$)

Also using the cylindrical TLM model, an inclusion was inserted in the circular medium between the 70th and 130th angular nodes and 20th and 30th radial nodes. A sine wave is injected from the inner radius (node (1st radial direction, 100th angular direction)) and the wave propagation is recorded. It can be shown from Fig. 17, the effect of the acoustic properties of the inclusions that form inside the artery. These models will be employed in the next section to analyze these recorded signals and build a lumped parameter model of the different tissues types based on their size and acoustic properties.

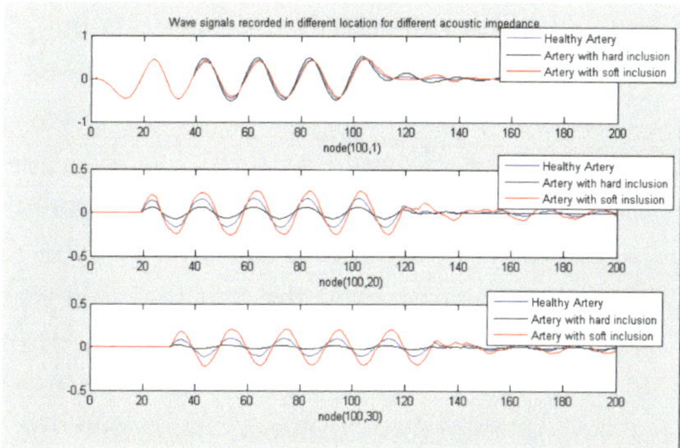

Fig. 17. Time signals record of the wave propagation at different locations having different inclusion ($Z_{Hardinclsuion} = 7.4Z_{\text{healthy artery}}$ and $Z_{Softinclsuion} = 0.074Z_{\text{healthy artery}}$)

4. Plaque characterization

This section departs from the traditional approaches appearing in the literature by considering the inclusion within a medium to be a dynamic system. A system identification approach will be adopted to characterize the dynamics of the plaque (Soderstrom & Stoica, 2001). Thus, the TLM models developed in the previous sections are used as a mean of acquiring the time signals transmitted and reflected in a region of interest within the medium (plaque or inclusion location). These signals will be considered as inputs and outputs to the dynamic system where digital signal processing techniques are employed to identify a parametric model for these plaques.

4.1 Persistency of excitation of the input signal

Any input signal used in the context of system identification must meet certain condition. In particular, the input signal should be **persistently exciting** (Ljung, 1999). The frequency domain condition enforcing a persistency of excitation is:

A signal $u(t)$ characterized by its spectrum $\Phi_u(\omega)$ is said to be persistently exciting if

$$\Phi_u(\omega) > 0 \qquad \textit{for almost all } \omega$$

Thus the spectrum may be zero on a set of number of points (almost all definition).

One classical frequency-rich signal is the swept sine signal which is also known as the "chirp signal". The chirp signal is a single sine wave with a frequency that is changing continuously as a function of time. The general mathematical presentation of the swept sine wave is

$$u(k) = A\sin\left(2\pi\beta(k) * \frac{(k-1)}{f_s} + \varphi\right) + B$$

$$\beta(k) = f_{\min} + \frac{(f_{\max} - f_{\min})}{2t_{target}}\left(\frac{k-1}{f_s}\right) \quad \text{where } f_s \geq 2f_{\max}$$

Where A is the wave amplitude, B is the signal bias term, φ is the phase angle of the wave and $\beta(k)$ is the time varying frequency of the swept sine in Hertz. The frequency f_s is the sampling frequency. The frequency $\beta(k)$ in this case is a linearly varying frequency over the interval $[f_{\min}, f_{\max}]$. The target time, denoted as t_{target}, is the time for which the upper bound of the frequency range is achieved. During the system identification process of the plaque and healthy tissue characterization, a swept sine will be designed as the source signal (the choice of the swept sign came from the fact that this wave was the only signal that was consistent in terms of constancy of the model structure). From literature, the frequency range used in the signal processing for the soft tissue is in the range of $\left[10^5, 10^7\right] Hz$. The swept sine is therefore designed such that the frequency covers this range. This signal will be combined with a zero-element vector. As illustrated in Fig. 18, a swept sine is designed to be the source signal of the simulation part for the TLM models. The sampling time of this signal is equal to 10^{-9} sec.

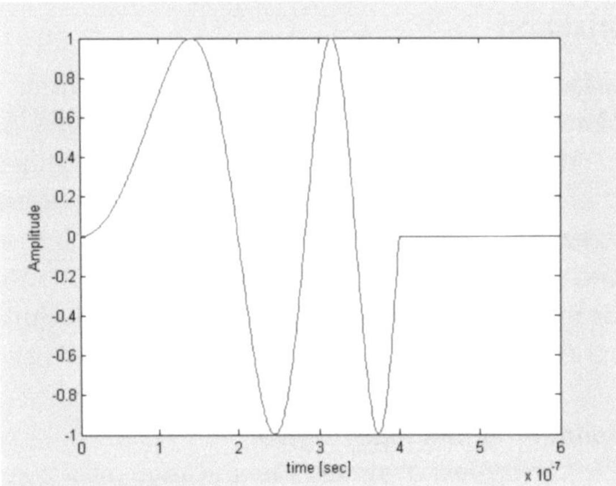

Fig. 18. Constructed swept sine pulse

4.2 System identification method

This process is composed of two stages. In the first stage, the identification technique that is used for modeling purposes is the so-called *Orthogonal Least Squares* (OLS) method (Korenberg et al., 1988; Chen et al., 1989). This method is a discrete time domain based approach where the time signals are used for model determination. In fact, the transient time domain information generated from the TLM artery models and their delayed components will be used as possible input regressors. This method will determine the most significant regressors from a broad range of possible candidates to identify the best parametric model. The general model structure can be linear or nonlinear. However for this work, it is anticipated that only a linear model will be needed.

A discrete time model generally resembles a polynomial structure. Considering a general case, a discrete system model with unknown coefficients (model parameters to be estimate) can be transformed into the linear-in-the-parameters representation by means of the expansion

$$z(k) = \sum_{i=1}^{M} p_i(k)\theta_i + \xi(k), \quad k = 1,\ldots,N, \tag{15}$$

where $z(k)$ is the output, $p_i(k)$ are the monomials of the different inputs up to certain degree M, θ_i are the unknown parameters of the model to be estimated, $\xi(k)$ is the modeling error and N is the data length. Equation ,(15) can be transformed to the matrix form

$$Z = P\Theta + \Xi . \tag{16}$$

Given this formulation, a linear least squares problem emerges. The proposed OLS method systematically searches the entire regressor space (monomials) as precised in equation (16) to find the best error reduction set, transforms these optimal regressors into orthogonal components, and then perform final regressor identification based on the new orthogonal system. These estimates will be mapped back to the original parameter estimates with their relative regressors given in equations ,(15) and .(16). This is called Parameter Estimation (PE). Structure Selection (SS) algorithm is then applied where it is anticipated that a linear model will emerge. This procedure takes the estimated parameters and statistically prioritizes these regressors into the most significant regressor, second most significant regressor and so on until accuracy of the model output is realized.
The second stage is characterized by the estimation of the model coefficients. A second system identification technique called *recursive least squares* (RLS) is used (Ljung, 1999). This method departs from a system of linear equations in the matrix form

$$Y = P\Theta , \tag{17}$$

where $\Theta \in \Re^{M\times 1}$ is the unknown parameters of the model to be determined, $Y \in \Re^{N\times 1}$ is the output vector $P \in \Re^{N\times M}$ is the information matrix which is function of the input and output vectors.
The utility of this method is to calculate the inverse of the information matrix. Based on an algorithm that is composed of three equations, the inverse matrix is simply calculated by means of additions and multiplications. Finally once the inverse of the information matrix is found, the model coefficient vector Θ can be calculated from equation (17).

4.3 Tissue characterization using regular and cylindrical irregular TLM models

A set of inputs were designed. This set was composed of a swept sine, a Schroeder wave, a pulse and a band limited white noise. Swept sine and Schroeder wave signals were the more appropriate candidates since they are characterized by their frequency-rich content and their persistent excitation property. During the model structure identification all the considered inputs except the swept sine gave different model structure of the plaque while its properties were changed. That is why, the swept sine signal was considered to be the best input that captures the dynamics of the studied plaques. The OLS algorithm is applied to the input/output sets of data and a discrete parametric model is established for the plaque. The following simple first order linear model is generated for the different plaques

$$y(k) = a_1 y(k-1) + b_0 u(k) , \tag{18}$$

where $y(k)$ is the model output of the plaque and $u(k)$ is the input to the plaque. In order to investigate the effect of plaque acoustic properties variation on the model, a first order continuous model is derived from the input/output data sets

$$\tau\dot{y}(t) + y(t) = du(t)\,. \tag{19}$$

d is the DC gain and τ the time constant.
The DC gain and the time constant are determined using different approximations of the first derivative of the output, $\dot{y}(t)$. These approximations calculations were performed to test the robustness of the model coefficients when recovering continuous model from discrete model. Multiple first time derivate approximations were performed to recover the continuous model calculations (Centered first order derivative approximation, Forward second order derivative approximation, Backward second order derivative approximation and Centered fourth order derivative approximation). The model coefficients were calculated and compared using these approximations and the error variation was negligible.
The characterization of the plaque will be linked to the model coefficients and mainly the DC gain. The DC gain is expected to decrease if the impedance is increasing. This is explained by the fact that if the acoustic impedance is going up then the density of the plaque is increasing, meaning that this portion of tissue is getting harder and denser mechanically. A denser material has a repulsive effect and the transmitted signal into it is minor. This means that the denser the material is the more resistive effect it shows. Therefore if the impedance goes up then the DC gain is expected to decrease.
In the TLM model, the plaque acoustic impedance is increased gradually and the input/output data sets to this plaque are recorded. The model coefficients (DC gain and pole location) are calculated.
Table 2 illustrates the results of the first order model of the plaque that is obtained from the rectangular TLM model. This model is characterized by a medium that is composed of 90 by 300 nodes in the horizontal and vertical directions respectively and a plaque that is located between the 10th and 30th horizontal nodes and 25th and 65th vertical nodes. The designed swept sine signal is composed of 600 data points with a sampling time that is equal to 10^{-9} sec and a frequency range of $\left[10^4, 10^7\right] Hz$. This input was injected at the 1st horizontal and 45th vertical node. The 45th vertical direction coincides with the middle line crossing the plaque. The input (10th radial position) and output (31st radial position) signals to the plaque were recorded.

Acoustic Impedance $[Kgm^{-2}s^{-1}]$	DC gain d	Time constant τ
$Z_{healthyTissue}$=1559216	0.5634	22.15
Z=1.2x$Z_{healthyTissue}$	0.5171	21.95
Z=1.4x$Z_{healthyTissue}$	0.4778	21.81
Z=1.6x$Z_{healthyTissue}$	0.4442	21.71
Z=1.8x$Z_{healthyTissue}$	0.4149	21.64
Z=2x$Z_{healthyTissue}$	0.3893	21.61

Table 2. Time constant and DC gain variation as function of the acoustic impedance of the plaque (rectangular TLM model)

Table 2 confirms that the DC gain is indeed decreasing when the acoustic impedance of the plaque in increased. Moreover, the time constant τ (indicator of the time response of the system) is decreasing likewise the DC gain when the acoustic impedance is increased. This is explained physically by the fact that the increase of the hardness of the tissue (the plaque) will affect the speed of the system response. The coefficients percentage variations are summarized in Table 3.

Acoustic Impedance $[Kgm^{-2}s^{-1}]$	Acoustic impedance change [%]	DC gain d	DC gain change [%]	Time Constant τ	Time Constant change [%]
$Z=1.2xZ_{healthyTissue}$	20	0.5171	-8.22	21.95	-0.90
$Z=1.4xZ_{healthyTissue}$	40	0.4778	-15.19	21.81	-1.50
$Z=1.6xZ_{healthyTissue}$	60	0.4442	-21.16	21.71	-1.99
$Z=1.8xZ_{healthyTissue}$	80	0.4149	-26.36	21.64	-2.30
$Z=2xZ_{healthyTissue}$	100	0.3893	-30.90	21.61	-2.44

Table 3. DC gain and Time constant variation in percentage (rectangular TLM model)

Using the cylindrical irregular TLM model, the same plaque size and location as of the regular TLM model is considered. The plaque is located between the 10th and 30th radial nodes and 25th and 65th angular nodes. The same designed swept sine signal is injected at the 1st radial and 45th angular node. The 45th angular direction coincides with the middle line crossing the plaque. The input (10th radial position) and output (31st radial position) signals to the plaque are recorded. To study the plaque type effect on the model coefficients, the variation of the DC gain and pole location is studied as function of the plaque density variation. Therefore the speed is set constant and the density of the plaque is varying with respect the healthy tissue density. The same approximations are used to determine the coefficients of the continuous model. As in the case of the regular TLM model section, it is expected that both the DC gain and the time constant to decrease when the acoustic impedance of the plaque is increased and this is what is presented in Table 4.

Acoustic Impedance $[Kgm^{-2}s^{-1}]$	DC gain d	Time Constant τ
$Z_{healthyTissue}=1559216$	0.5275	26.42
$Z=1.2xZ_{healthyTissue}$	0.5224	25.04
$Z=1.4xZ_{healthyTissue}$	0.5090	23.28
$Z=1.6xZ_{healthyTissue}$	0.4910	21.34
$Z=1.8xZ_{healthyTissue}$	0.4699	19.30
$Z=2xZ_{healthyTissue}$	0.4472	17.28

Table 4. DC gain and Time constant variation as function of the acoustic impedance of the plaque (cylindrical irregular TLM model)

It can be seen from both models that a plaque could be characterized by a first order system. In fact the coefficients variation of this model is inversely proportional to the acoustic impedance variation. The coefficients variations are summarized in Table 5.

Acoustic Impedance $[Kgm^{-2}s^{-1}]$	Acoustic impedance change [%]	DC gain d	DC gain change [%]	Time Constant τ	Time Constant change [%]
$Z=1.2xZ_{healthyTissue}$	20	0.5224	-0.97	25.04	-5.22
$Z=1.4xZ_{healthyTissue}$	40	0.5090	-3.51	23.28	-11.88
$Z=1.6xZ_{healthyTissue}$	60	0.4910	-6.92	21.34	-19.23
$Z=1.8xZ_{healthyTissue}$	80	0.4699	-10.92	19.30	-26.95
$Z=2xZ_{healthyTissue}$	100	0.4472	-15.22	17.28	-34.60

Table 5. DC gain and Time constant variation in percentage (cylindrical irregular TLM model)

Considering the model structure found during the tissue characterization, the plaque can be viewed as *a first order low pass filter*. This first order filter illustrated in Fig. 19 is characterized by a DC gain and a time constant that decrease when the resistance R_1 is increasing.

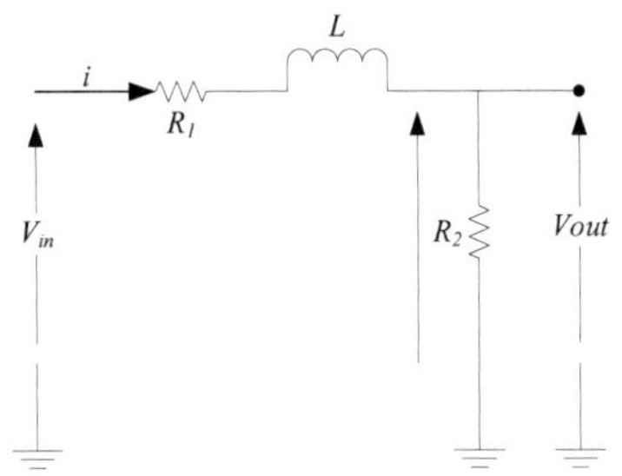

Fig. 19. RL low pass filter

The transfer function of this filter is the following

$$TF = \frac{\frac{R_2}{R_1+R_2}}{1+\frac{L}{R_1+R_2}s}. \tag{16}$$

The resistance R_1 and R_2 can be linked to the acoustic impedance of the medium. From the transfer function above, if R_1 and R_2 increases the DC gain and the time constant decrease.

5. Conclusions

In this paper, ultrasound wave propagation through biological tissues and specifically through arterial wall was studied. This modeling work was twofold. First it departed from a simple regularly-shaped medium (rectangular geometry) where a transmission line matrix (TLM) model was employed to capture the ultrasound wave propagation. In a second step an irregular TLM model was constructed based on a circular-shaped medium (disk) to simulate IVUS. Both of these models were based on the discretization of the medium where the Huygens principle was applied in the propagation process from one node to another. Moreover the propagating ultrasound waves were recorded in a digitized format in any location at any time specified during the numerical simulation.

Advanced system identification techniques were, then, introduced and applied to characterize tissues. This approach used specific simulated waves in terms of locations to serve as the input/output data sets for the dynamic identification of these regions of interest. This characterization was based upon the construction of parametric models in the form of transfer function where its coefficients are directly related to each plaque type. A first order structure was, thus, found for all plaque types with different DC gain and time constant values depending on the properties of these inclusions.

Finally, a quantitative study was performed to link the variation of these two parameters with respect to acoustic properties. It has been shown consequently that these plaque characteristics were identified quantitatively based on the ultrasound waves using the system identification approach.

6. References

American Heart Association, AHA. (2008). Statistical Update, 2010, Available from: <http://www.americanheart.org/downloadable/heart/1200594755071International%20Cardiovascular%20Disease%20%20Tables.pdf>

American Heart Association, AHA. (2003). Cardiovascular Disease Statistics, 2010, Available from: < http://www.americanheart.org/presenter.jhtml?identifier=4478>

Gaster, A.L.; Skjoldborg, U.S.; Larsen, J.; Lorsholm, L.; Von Birgelen, C.; Jensen, S.;Thayssen, P.; Pederson, K. E. & Haghfelt, T.H. (2003). Continued improvement of clinical outcome and cost effectiveness following intravascular ultrasound guided PCI: insights from a prospective, randomised study. *Heart*, Vol. 89, No. 9, (September 2003), pp. (1043-1049), ISSN 1468-201X

Mueller, C. ;Hodgson, J.Mc. B.;Schindler, C.;Perruchoud, A. P.; Roskamm, H. & Buettner, H. J. (2003). Cost-Effectiveness of Intracoronary Ultrasound for Percutaneous Coronary Interventions. *American Journal of Cardiology*, Vol. 91, No. 2, (January 2003), pp. (143-147), ISSN 0002-9149

Nissen, S.E. & Yock, P. (2001). Intravascular Ultrasound : Novel Pathophysiological Insights and Current Clinical Applications. *Circulation*, Vol. 103, No. 4, (January 2001), pp. (604-616), ISSN 0009-7322

Stary, H. C. (1992). Composition and classification of human atherosclerotic lesions. *Virchows Archiv*, Vol. 421, No. 4, (June 1992), pp. (277-290), ISSN 0945-6317

Stary, H. C.; Chandler, A. B.; Glagov, S.; Guyton, J.R.; Insull, W.Jr.; Rosenfeld, M.E.; Schaffer, S.A.; Schwartz, C.J.; Wagner, W.D. & Wissler, R.W. (1994). A definition of initial, fatty streak, and intermediate lesions of atherosclerosis. A report from the Committee on Vascular Lesions of the Council on Arteriosclerosis, American Heart Association. *Circulation*, Vol. 89, No. 5, (May 1994), pp. (2462-2478), ISSN 0009-7322

Stary, H.C.; Chandler, A.B.; Dinsmore, R.E.; Fuster, V.; Glagov, S.; Insull, W.Jr.; Rosenfeld, M.E.; Schawrtz, C.J.; Wagner, W.D. & Wissler, R.W. (1995). A Definition of Advanced Types of Atherosclerotic Lesions and a Histological Classification of Atherosclerosis : A Report From the Committee on Vascular Lesions of the Council on Arteriosclerosis, American Heart Association. *Circulation*, Vol. 92, No. 5, (September 1995), pp. (1355-1374), ISSN 0009-7322

Urbani, M.P.; Picano, E.; Parenti, G.; Mazzarisi, A.; Fiori, L.; Paterni, M.; Pelosi, G. & Landini, L. (1993). In vivo radiofrequency-based ultrasonic tissue characterization of the atherosclerotic plaque. *Stroke*, Vol. 24, No. 10, (October 1993), pp. (1507-1512), ISSN 00392499

Picano, E.; Landini, L.; Distante, A.; Sarnelli, R.; Benassi, L. & Abbate, A. (1983). Different degrees of atherosclerosis detected by backscattered ultrasound: an in vitro study on fixed human aortic walls. *Journal of Clinical Ultrasound*, Vol. 11, No. 7, (September 1983), pp. (375-379), ISSN 0091-2751

Sarnelli, R.; Landini, L. & Squartini F. (1986). Atherosclerosis detection by ultrasounds. A comparative histologic study on aortic specimens. *Applied Pathology*, Vol. 4, No. 4, (1986), pp. (270-275), ISSN 0252-1172

Landini, L.; Sarnelli, R.; Picano, E. & Salvadori M. (1986). Evaluation of frequency dependence of backscatter coefficient in normal and atherosclerotic aortic walls. *Ultrasound in medicine & biology*, Vol. 12 No. 5, (May 1986), pp. (397-401), ISSN 0301-5629

Barzilai, B.; Saffitz, J.E.;Miller, J.G. & Sobel, B.E. (1991). Quantitative ultrasonic characterization of the nature of atherosclerotic plaques in human aorta. *Circulation Research*, Vol. 60, No. 3, (March 1991), pp. (459-463), ISSN 0009-7330

De Kroon, M.G.M.; Van der Wal, L.F.; Gussenhoven, W.J. & Bom, N. (1991). Angle-dependent backscatter from the arterial wall. *Ultrasound in medicine & biology*, Vol. 17, No. 2, (February 1991), pp. (121-126), ISSN 0301-5629

Picano, E.; Landini, L.; Urbani, M.P.; Mazzarisi, A.; Paterni , M. & Mazzone, A.M. (1994). Ultrasound tissue characterization techniques in evaluating plaque structure. *American Journal of Cardiac Imaging*, Vol. 8, No. 2, (April 1994), pp. (123-128), ISSN 0887-7971

Cespedes, E. I.; Ponnekanti, H.; Yazdi, Y. & Li, X. (1991). Elastography: a quantitative method for imaging the elasticity of biological tissues. *Ultrasonic Imaging*, Vol. 13, No. 2, (April 1991), pp. (111-134), ISSN 0161-7346

Ryan, L.K. & Foster, F.S. (1997). Ultrasonic measurement of differential displacement and strain in vascular model. *Ultrasonic Imaging*, Vol. 19, No. 1, (January 1997), pp. (19-38), ISSN 0161-7346

De Korte, C.L.; Cespedes, E.I.; Van der steen, A.F.; Pasterkamp, G. & Bom, N. (1998). Intravascular ultrasound elastrography: assessment and imaging of elastic properties of diseased arteries and vulnerable plaque. *European Journal of Ultrasound*, Vol. 7, No. 3, (August 1998), pp. (219-224), ISSN 0929-8266

Achaar, J. A.; De Korte, C.L.; Mastik, F.; Strijder, C.; Pasterkamp, G.; Boersma, E.; Seerruys, P.W. & Van Der Steen, A.F. (2003). Characterizing Vulnerable Plaque Features With Intravascular Elastography. *Circulation*, Vol. 108, No. 21, (November 2003), pp. (2636-2641), ISSN 0009-7322

Saijo, Y.; Tanaka, A.; Owada, N.; Akino, Y. & Nitta, S. (2004). Tissue velocity imaging of coronary artery by rotating-type intravascular ultrasound. *Ultrasonics*, Vol. 42, No. 1-9, (April 2004), pp. (753-757), ISSN 0041-624X

Shapo, B.M.; Crowe, J.R.; Erkamp, R.; Emelianov, S.Y.; Eberle, M.J. & O'donnell, M. (1996). Strain imaging of coronary arteries with intraluminal ultrasound: experiments on an inhomogeneous phantom. *Ultrasonic Imaging*, Vol. 18, No. 3, (July 1996), pp. (173-191), ISSN 0161-7346

De Korte, C. L.; Pasterkamp, G.; Van Der Steen, A.F.W.; Woutman, H.A. & Bom, N. (2000). Characterization of Plaque Components With Intravascular Ultrasound Elastography in Human Femoral and Coronary Arteries In Vitro. *Circulation*, Vol. 102, No. 6, (August 2000), pp. (617-623), ISSN 0009-7330

Koenig, A. & Klauss, V. (2007). Virtual Histology. *Heart*, Vol. 93 No. 8, (May 2007), pp. (977-982), ISSN 1468-201X

Nair, A.; Kuban, B.D.; Tuzcu, E.M.; Schoenhagen, P.; Nissen, S.E. & Vince, D.G. (2002). Coronary Plaque Classification With Intravascular Ultrasound Radiofrequency Data Analysis. *Circulation*, Vol. 106, No. 18, (May 2002), pp. (2200-2206), ISSN 0009-7330

Kuznestov, V.P. (1971). Equations of nonlinear acoustics. *Soviet Physics - Acoustics*, Vol. 16, (1971), pp. (467-470), ISSN 0038-562X

Lee, Y.S. & Hamilton, M.F. (1995). Time-domain modeling of pulsed finite-amplitude sound beams. *Journal of the Acoustical Society of America*, Vol. 97, No. 2, (February 1995), pp. (906-917), ISSN 0001-4966

Tavakkoli, J.; Cathignol, D. & Souchon, R. (1998). Modeling of pulsed finite-amplitude focused sound beams in time domain. *Journal of the Acoustical Society of America*, Vol. 104, No. 4, (October 1998), pp. (2061-2072), ISSN 0001-4966

Kendall, A. & Weimin, H. (June 2007). *Theoretical Numerical Analysis- A functional analysis framework*, (Second edition), Springer, ISBN 0387258876, New York, USA

Guenther, R.B. & John, W.L. (1996). *Partial differential equations of mathematical physics and integral equation*. Dover publications, ISBN 9780486688893, New York, USA

CliffsNotes.com. *Wave Optics*. 12 Apr 2011 <http://www.cliffsnotes.com/study_guide/topicArticleId-10453,articleId-10442.html>

Christos, C. (1995). *The Transmission-Line Modeling Method TLM*, John Wiley & Sons, ISBN 0780310179, New York, USA

De Cong, D.; O'Connor, W.J. &Pulko, S. (2006). *Transmission Line Matrix in Computational Mechanics*, Taylor & Francis, ISBN 0415327172, Boca Raton, Florida, USA

Al-Mukhtar, D.A. & Sitch, J.E. (1981). Transmission-line matrix method with irregularly graded space. *IEEE Proc*, Vol. 128, No. 6, (December 1981), pp. (299-305), ISSN 0143-7097

Bakshi, U.A. & Bakshi, V.U. (2009). *Basic Electrical Engineering*, Technical Publications Pune, ISBN 8184312571, India

Soderstrom, T. & Stoica, P. (2001). *System Identification*, Prentice Hall, ISBN 0138812365, New York, USA

Ljung, L. (1999). *System identification: theory for the user*, (Second edition), Prentice Hall, ISBN 0136566952, New York, USA

Korenberg, M.; Billings, S.A.; Liu, Y.P. & McIlroy, P.J. (1988). Orthogonal parameter estimation algorithm for non-linear stochastic systems. *International Journal of Control*, Vol. 48, No. 1, (January 1988), pp. (193-210), ISSN 0020-7179

Chen, S.; Billings, S.A. & Luo, W. (1989). Orthogonal least squares methods and their application to non-linear system identification. *International Journal of Control*, Vol. 50, No. 5, (November 1989), pp. (1873 - 1896), ISSN 0020-7179

12

The Benefits of IVUS Dynamics for Retrieving Stable Models of Arteries

Aura Hernàndez-Sabaté and Debora Gil
Computer Science Dept. and Computer Vision Center, Universitat Autònoma de Barcelona
Bellaterra, Spain

1. Introduction

Artery diseases are mainly caused by the accumulation of plaque (made up of a combination of blood, cholesterol, fat and cells) inside arterial walls (Fuster, 1994). Such plaque accumulation narrows the artery blood flow (stenosis) and makes arteries inflaming and being less flexible (atherosclerosis). Artery blood flow reduction is measured by the percentage of obstruction in vessel sections and is a usual measurement previous to decide which is the best treatment (either surgical or pharmacological) for an atherosclerotic lesion. Depending on the histological composition of the plaque, its (bio-mechanical) physical behavior will be different, making it more or less unstable (vulnerable plaques) and, thus, resulting in a different risk for the patient (Kakadiaris et al., 2006). Early detection of plaque composition is a main step for planning the most suitable treatment (angioplasty, stent apposition, ...) and might prevent further thrombosis potentially leading to a fatal heart attack. Tissue bio-mechanical properties play an important role in the diagnosis and treatment of cardiovascular diseases. The main mechanical properties currently under study are radial strain, which is related to plaque type and vulnerability (Céspedes et al., 2000), and shear stress, which influences the probability of plaque accumulation (Wentzel et al., 2001). Both measures can be computed by means of the study of vessel tissue deformation along the cardiac cycle.

IntraVascular UltraSound (IVUS) is the best choice to study, both, vessel morphology and its bio-mechanical properties. On one hand, inspection of a single IVUS image gives information about the percentage of stenosis. Manual stenosis measurements require a manual tracing of vessel borders (the internal layer, intima, and the most external one, adventitia). This is a very time-consuming task and might suffer from inter-observer variations. On the other hand, inspection of longitudinal views provides information about artery bio-mechanical properties. The assessment of bio-mechanical properties requires exploring the evolution of vessel walls and structures along the sequence. Dynamics due to heart pumping (among others) introduces a misalignment of sequence frames, preventing any feasible volumetric measurement or 3D reconstruction. In particular heart dynamics produce two types of motion: longitudinal motion along the catheter pullback and in-plane motion of each single cross section. Longitudinal dynamics produces a sequence block with spatially shuffled frames, which hinders any analysis along the sequence. Heart pumping also introduces a periodic rotation and translation in IVUS cross-sections, which hinders proper evaluation of tissue bio-mechanical properties. Both 3D reconstructions and bio-mechanical properties

assessment require a compensation of artery dynamics, either by sampling the sequence synchronized with a cardiac phase or by in-plane sequence stabilization.
Since the early years of IVUS imaging, many algorithms for a reliable intima detection (Bouma et al., 1997; Brathwaite et al., 1996; Brathwaite & McPherson, 1998; Brusseau et al., 2004; Dijkstra et al., 2001; Gil et al., 2000; Hansen et al., 2002; Luo et al., 2003; Mendizabal-Ruiz et al., 2008; Sonka et al., 1996; von Birgelen et al., 1996; 1997) and plaque characterization (de Korte et al., 2000; Escalera et al., 2008; Granada et al., 2007; Nair et al., 2002; Okubo et al., 2008) have been proposed. Most of them are based on the appearance of structures in images. Adventitia modeling has been a delicate issue hardly addressed e.g. (Dijkstra et al., 1999; Gil et al., 2006; Haas et al., 2000; Klingensmith et al., 2000; Olszewski et al., 2004; Plissiti et al., 2004; Pujol & Radeva, 2005; Sonka et al., 1995; Takagi et al., 2000), though it is crucial for stenosis measurement. This is due to its weak appearance in IVUS images, which makes appearance-based techniques fail to produce optimal results and forces ad-hoc elaborated strategies. Also, image-based cardiac phase retrieval strategies are based on image appearance and extract cardiac phase by exploring its temporal changes across the sequence (Barajas et al., 2007; Matsumoto et al., 2008; Nadkarni et al., 2005; Sean M. O'Malley, 2006; Zhu et al., 2003). Speckle, texture and morphology introduce non-cardiac irregular variations in appearance patterns that must be carefully filtered.
So far, dynamics has only been considered as an artifact which is, at most, corrected (Hernàndez-Sabaté et al., 2009; Rosales et al., 2004). We claim that rigid motion estimation is a useful tool for exploring, both, vessel structures and cardiac dynamics. The main concern of this chapter is to show the benefits of cardiac dynamics for adventitia segmentation and image-based cardiac phase retrieval.
The general scheme for adventitia segmentation can be split in three main steps sketched in figure 1.

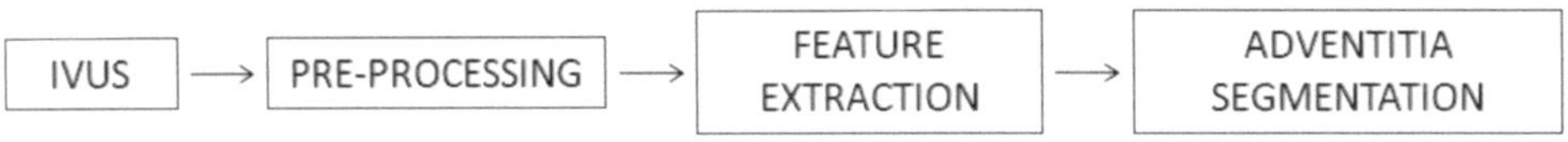

Fig. 1. Pipeline for Adventitia Segmentation

The poor image quality as well as large variety of IVUS artifacts (calcium, side-branches, shadows, catheter guide and blood back scatter) force an elaborated pre-processing step for enhancing adventitia appearance. In order to ensure a good compromise between preservation of the adventitia weak appearance and speckle smoothing, a filtering carefully driven for each image is compulsory (Gil et al., 2006; Unal et al., 2006). This makes the pre-processing stage to be one of the most computationally expensive tasks of the whole scheme. We claim that IVUS (in-plane) rigid motion can significantly improve the smoothing step, since vessel structures follow a periodic motion (induced by heart beat) clearly different from the chaotic random behavior of textured and blood areas. We propose using the mean of stabilized sequence blocks in order to enhance vessel structures while blurring texture and speckle.
Concerning image-based ECG-gating, existing strategies (Barajas et al., 2007; Matsumoto et al., 2008; Nadkarni et al., 2005; Sean M. O'Malley, 2006; Zhu et al., 2003) follow the scheme sketched in figure 2.
First, a signal reflecting cardiac motion is computed from IVUS sequences. Second, the signal is filtered (in the frequency domain) in order to remove non-cardiac phenomena and artifacts. Finally, a suitable sampling of the filtered signal retrieve cardiac phase. All authors agree in

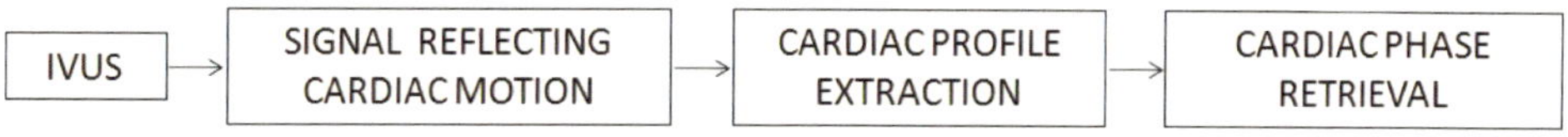

Fig. 2. Pipeline for Image-based Cardiac Phase Retrieval

using a band-pass filter in the second step and the extrema of filtered signals for sampling at end-systole and diastole. The main differences among existing algorithms and thus, the clue for an accurate cardiac phase retrieval, lie in the signal computed from the sequence. Given that in-plane and out-of-plane cardiac motion are coupled, we propose using the periodic component of in-plane motion as the signal reflecting cardiac motion.

In this chapter we propose an integrative framework for retrieving vessel morphology and cardiac phase from IVUS rigid dynamics. Vessel structures extracted from IVUS sequences and stabilized by correcting cardiac dynamics produce stable models of arteries containing deformation along all cardiac cycle and, thus, useful for exploring biomechanics. The collection of vessel structures at frames synchronized at the same fraction of the cardiac cycle provide static models for computing 3D measurements. The pipeline of our integrative framework is sketched in figure 3 where the three clinical tools presented in the chapter are highlighted in orange.

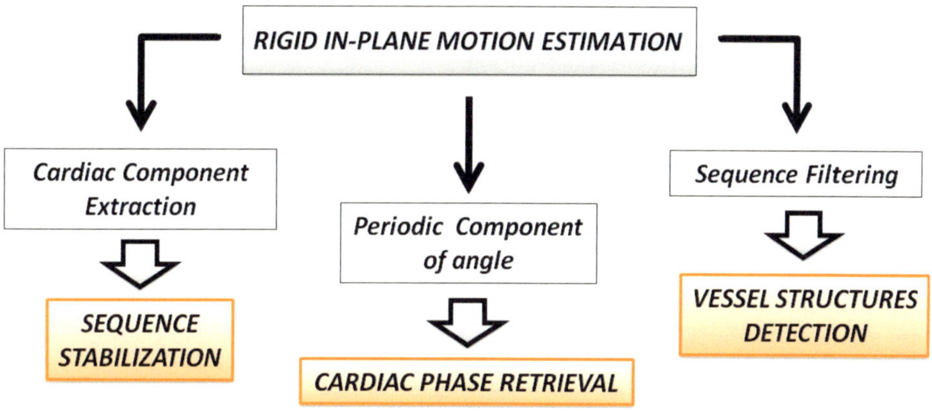

Fig. 3. Pipeline for the Integrative Framework

The remainder of the chapter is structured as follows. In section 2 we sketch the method used to compute rigid in-plane motion (Hernàndez-Sabaté et al., 2009). Section 3 is devoted to detail the three steps which constitute the integrative framework we propose. In section 4 we explain the validation protocol while results are given in section 5. Finally, discussions about the advantages and limitations of using rigid in-plane dynamics compared to appearance methods will be given in the last section of the chapter.

2. Rigid in-plane motion estimation

Different factors such as heart pumping, blood pressure or artery geometric properties mainly contribute to the dynamics of coronary arteries (Holzapfel et al., 2002; Mazumdar, 1992; Nadkarni et al., 2003). The first order approximation to vessel in-plane dynamics is given by a linear transformation combining translation, rotation and scaling (Waks et al., 1996). Dilation is inherent to the elasticity of the vessel itself and it does not preserve the metric. The rigid part of this approximation can be modeled as a rigid body motion and is given by a rotation followed by a translation. Figure 4 shows the physics-based model of the rigid motion of an artery. The computation of the translation and rotation angle is as follows (Hernàndez-Sabaté et al., 2009).

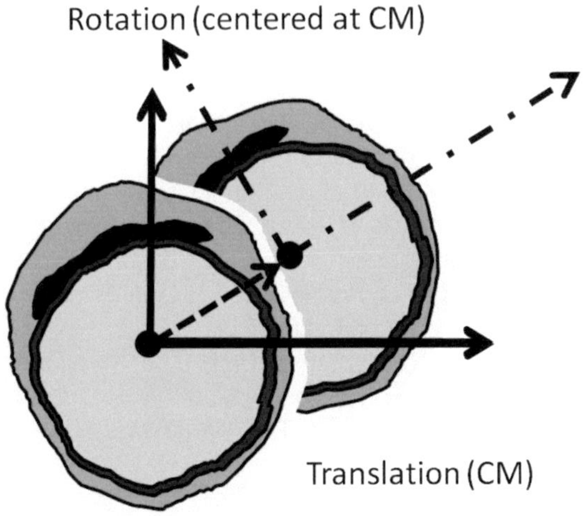

Fig. 4. Physics-based model: rigid solid motion

2.1 Translation

In body dynamics, the point describing the object response to external forces and torques is determined by means of its center of gravity or mass (Goldstein et al., 2002). The difference between its position and the origin of coordinates is identified to the object translation. We note it as VCM which is computed from IVUS frames as follows.

Since grey level reflects tissue mass density due to IVUS images reconstruction, the center of mass given by the image intensity, namely ICM, corresponds to the physical center of gravity of the vessel. However, some acquisition devices allow interactive tuning of the image brightness in order to enhance tissue and vessel structures appearance (Mintz & Nissen, 2001). Given that such intensity gain is radial (Caballero et al., 2006), tissue close to the catheter might look brighter and, for vessels not centered at the catheter, intensity gainings might deviate the position of ICM from the true center of mass. Vessel geometric center, namely GCM, coincides with the vessel center of gravity only in the case of uniform tissue density. However, it serves to compensate the deviation of ICM for non centered vessels. We define the center of mass of the vessel, VCM, by a combination of ICM and GCM achieving a good compromise between vessels whose intensity gain has been tuned and vessels with uniform tissue density.

The center of mass of the image intensities is given by:

$$ICM = \left(\frac{\sum_{i=1}^{n} i \sum_{j=1}^{m} I(i,j)}{\sum_{i=1}^{n} \sum_{j=1}^{m} I(i,j)}, \frac{\sum_{j=1}^{m} j \sum_{i=1}^{n} I(i,j)}{\sum_{i=1}^{n} \sum_{j=1}^{m} I(i,j)} \right)$$

The geometric center of mass of a set of N points roughly lying on the adventitia (the most stable structure along the sequence) (x_k, y_k) is computed as follows:

$$GCM = \frac{1}{N} \left(\sum_{k=1}^{N} x_k, \sum_{k=1}^{N} y_k \right)$$

Finally, the following formula weights both centers of mass, taking into account the deviation of the vessel from the center of the image (Hernàndez-Sabaté et al., 2009):

$$VCM = DR \cdot ICM + (1 - DR) \cdot GCM \tag{1}$$

where DR is the vessel-catheter deviation rate (i.e. the deviation of the vessel from the center of the image). If we consider the maximum, R_{max}, and minimum, R_{min}, distances of the set $(x_k, y_k)_k$ to the image center, DR is defined as:

$$DR = \frac{min_k(\sqrt{x_k^2 + y_k^2})}{max_k(\sqrt{x_k^2 + y_k^2})} = \frac{R_{min}}{R_{max}}$$

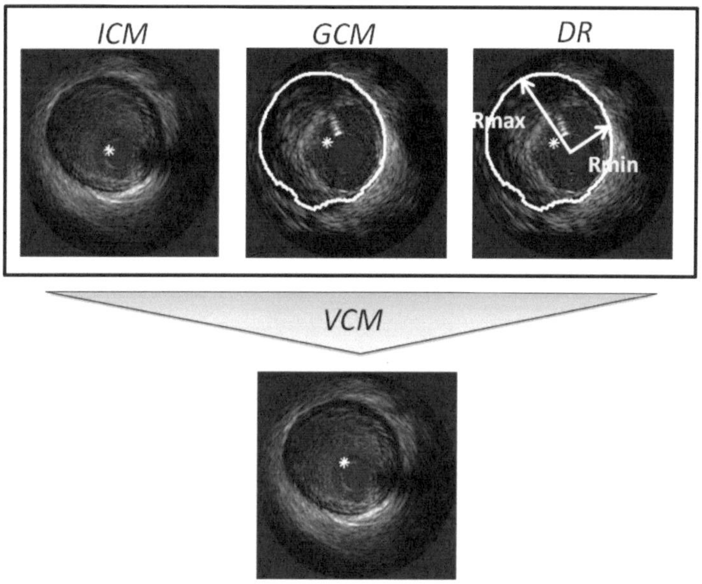

Fig. 5. Computation of the Vessel Center of Mass

We note that in case the artery is centered at the catheter, DR measures its eccentricity. Figure 5 shows the computation of the Vessel Center of Mass from computation of the Image and Geometric Centers of Mass given by formula (1).

2.2 Rotation

Once vessel translation has been compensated, two global motions still remain: rotation and radial scaling. In the polar domain with origin VCM, they convert into a horizontal translation (corresponding to rotation) and a vertical scaling (corresponding to radial scaling). In the case of human coronary arteries, scaling is very close to 1 (Ramírez, 2005), so $\lambda = 1 + \varepsilon$ becomes a perturbation of identity given by ε (Hernàndez-Sabaté, 2009). The horizontal translation is estimated by means of the computation of the phase of the ratio of Fourier transforms of every two consecutive frames (Hernàndez-Sabaté et al., 2009).
That is, if I_1, I_2 are two functions (images) that differ in a pure translation:

$$I_2(i, j) = I_1(i - t_1, j - t_2)$$

the first order approximation to I_2 can be computed by applying the Fourier transform (Oppenheim & Willsky, 1997) and using phase correlation (Kuglin & Hines, 1975). Let $\widehat{I}_1$, $\widehat{I}_2$ be the Fourier transforms of I_1 and I_2, respectively, then they are related via:

$$\widehat{I}_2(\omega) = \widehat{I}_1(\omega)e^{-i\langle \omega,t\rangle}$$

for $\vec{\omega} = (\omega_1, \omega_2)$ the Fourier frequency, $\vec{t} = (t_1, t_2)$ and $\langle \vec{\omega}, \vec{t}\rangle = \omega_1 t_1 + \omega_2 t_2$ the Euclidean scalar product.

If we consider the phase, $\rho(\omega)$, of the ratio between the two Fourier transforms (Alliney, 1993), then we have that:

$$\rho(\omega) = \rho\left(\frac{\widehat{I}_2(\omega)}{\widehat{I}_1(\omega)}\right) = \rho\left(e^{-i\langle \omega,t\rangle}\right) = \langle \omega, t\rangle \ = \omega_1 t_1 + \omega_2 t_2$$

so that the points $(\omega_1, \omega_2, \rho(\omega))$ lie on a plane, Π, with the slopes given by the translation components:

$$\Pi : \rho(\omega) = t_1\omega_1 + t_2\omega_2$$

In practice, noise and texture introduce a scatter in the set $(\omega_1, \omega_2, \rho(\omega))$, especially for

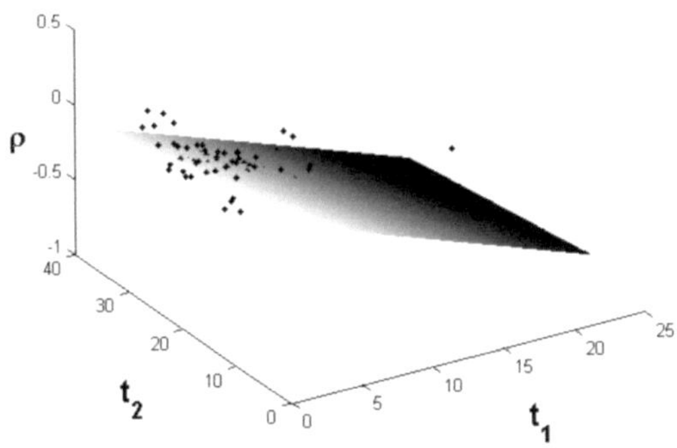

Fig. 6. Regression plane approximating Fourier phase correlation between two shifted images.

those frequencies with smaller amplitudes. We reduce noise-scatter by only considering those frequencies common to both images with an associated amplitude larger than a given percentile. Such frequencies with the phase ρ yield a point cloud, like the one shown in figure 6, which regression plane provides a least-square estimator of the plane Π. The first slope of that regression plane, t_1, estimates the angle of rotation between two consecutive frames.

3. Stable models of arteries

Tissue bio-mechanical properties (like strain and stress) are playing an increasing role in diagnosis and long-term treatment of intravascular coronary diseases. Their assessment strongly relies on estimation of vessel wall deformation along the cardiac cycle. On one hand, image misalignment introduced by vessel-catheter motion is a major artifact for a proper tracking of tissue deformation. On the other hand, longitudinal motion artifacts in IVUS sequences hinders a properly 3D reconstruction and vessel measurements. Furthermore, vessel plaque assessment by analysis of IntraVascular UltraSound sequences is a useful tool for cardiac disease diagnosis and intervention. Manual detection of luminal (inner) and medial-adventitial (external) vessel borders is the main activity of physicians in the process of lumen narrowing (plaque) quantification. Difficult definition of vessel border descriptors, as well as, shades, artifacts, and blurred signal response due to ultrasound physical properties trouble automated adventitia segmentation.

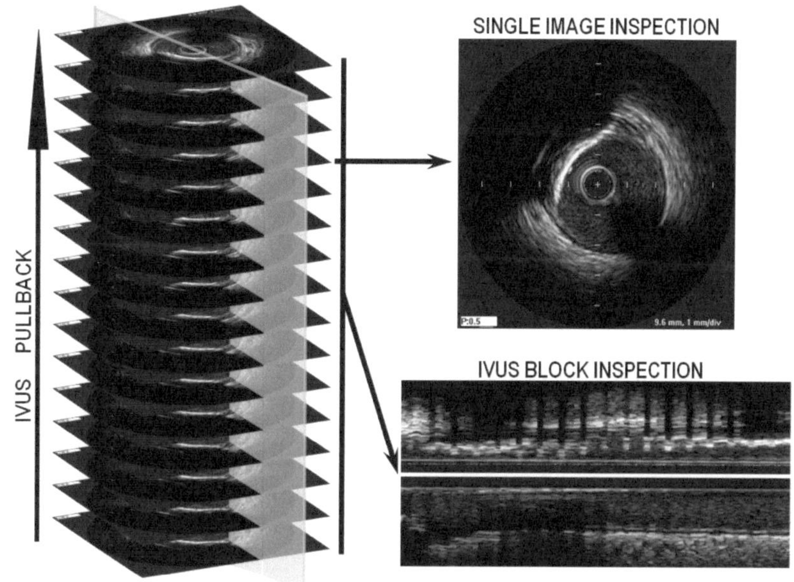

Fig. 7. Images extracted from an IVUS pullback. The left image is a block of 16 IVUS consecutive frames from a constant pullback. The right top image is a single cross-section of the vessel. The right bottom image is a longitudinal view obtained by intersecting 401 frames with the grey plane at the same angle.

Figure 7 shows a block of IVUS images obtained from a pullback (on the left) and the two kind of images derived from them (on the right). Each sequence frame (on the top right) shows a cross-section of the vessel under study with a complete detail of its morphology. The frames on the left can be intersected by a longitudinal plane including the catheter trajectory (grey plane on fig.7, left graphic), defined by a fixed angle on cross sections. The image obtained in this way is called longitudinal cut of the artery (bottom-right image). The image misalignment can be appreciated in the echo-shadowing calcified plaque of the upper profile of the longitudinal cut.

A framework integrating the solution for the three limitations of IVUS (image misalignment, longitudinal motion and adventitia segmentation) should be of utmost importance for clinical practice. In the above section, we have presented a method for assessing IVUS rigid in-plane motion. This estimation allows us to compute the following three steps for achieving an integrative framework of stable models of arteries useful for clinical practice. On one hand, translation and rotation estimation serves to stabilize the sequence by removing cardiac dynamics. On the other side, we present the potential of rigid motion estimation for approaching cardiac phase retrieval from coronary IVUS sequences without ECG signal for correction of longitudinal motion artifacts. Finally, we show the benefits of using stabilized sequences for improving the computational time of automatic adventitia segmentation algorithms.

3.1 Sequence stabilization

The rigid motion that cardiac vessels undergo is a complex dynamical process which results from the combination of several contributions. In general, it presents a geometric component related to the artery 3D shape and a dynamic one induced by breathing and cardiac movements (Rosales et al., 2004). Depending on the particular problem to approach, each of the terms should have a specific treatment. Exploring artery geometry might be derived by analyzing the geometric component (Rotger et al., 2006), whereas extraction of cardiac dynamics concerns the cardiac dynamical contribution (Zhu et al., 2003). In the case of vessel biomechanics analysis, the goal is to produce a static model allowing a better tissue tracking along the segment. Firstly, the reader should note that, without further analysis, the geometric component does not reach a reliable 3D representation of the vessel geometry, which might lead to wrong static models. Secondly, even if one could infer the true 3D geometry from it, by compensating vessel tortuosity there is no guarantee of a better alignment of vessel plaque. This suggests only correcting the dynamical terms of the translation and rotation for stabilizing the sequence.
For that, the signal obtained is decoupled in the Fourier domain into geometric, breathing and cardiac component and the last component serves to stabilize the images along the sequence (Hernàndez-Sabaté, 2009). The translation and rotation parameters are functions of the time s. If the geometric term of a motion parameter is denoted by the subindex $_g$, the cardiac term, induced by heart beating, is denoted by the subindex $_c$ and breathing contributions are denoted by the subindex $_b$, the angle and translation decompose into:

$$\begin{aligned} t(s) &= t_g(s) + t_b(s) + t_c(s) \\ \theta(s) &= \theta_g(s) + \theta_b(s) + \theta_c(s) \end{aligned} \tag{2}$$

Focusing on the Fourier series of these components, breathing and cardiac terms are periodic and, thus, have a discrete Fourier spectrum, whereas geometry has a broad-band (non-discrete) spectrum (Oppenheim & Willsky, 1997). As usual, Fourier transforms are indicated by a hat ($\hat{}$) over functions. Principal harmonics have been learned by supervised classification of the spectrum of a training set of 30 patients without apparent lesions used in a study for assessment of myocardial perfusion in contrast angiography (Gil et al., 2008). Confidence intervals of the 95% yield the expected ranges for the principal frequency of each of the periodic components. For breathing it is $(10, 45)$ repetitions per minute (rpm), while for cardiac motion it is $(45, 200)$ rpm. Thus, cardiac motion principal harmonic, ω_c, is defined as the first local maximum in $I_{\omega_c} = (45, 200)$ rpm and the term is approximated by the first 10 harmonics, $(k\omega_c)_{k=1:10}$. For the sake of an efficient algorithm, ω_c is approximated by the global maximum of Fourier transform amplitude for frequencies in the range $I\omega_c$. It follows that the cardiac motion term of a sequence lasting N_{Sec} seconds is given by:

$$t_c(s) = \frac{1}{T} \sum_{k=1}^{k=10} \hat{t}(k\omega_c) e^{ik\omega_c s} \quad \theta_c(s) = \frac{1}{T} \sum_{k=1}^{k=10} \hat{\theta}(k\omega_c) e^{ik\omega_c s}$$

where the period $T = N_{Sec}/60$ is the sequence length (in minutes) and defines the domain of integration.

Since, even in healthy cases, the heart rate varies along the pullback, the peaks in the Fourier series are spread around the theoretic harmonic frequencies. The more irregularities in periodicity are, the more spread around the theoretic harmonic the Fourier development is. The harmonics less corrupted by noise are obtained by optical filtering (Klug & D.J.DeRosier, 1966). Optical filtering is a technique widely used in electron crystallography in order to discard harmonics corrupted with noise. Optical filtering selects only those harmonics presenting a prominent peak. The peakedness of an harmonic is given by the normalized difference between the amplitude achieved at the harmonic and an average of amplitudes in a neighborhood $I_{k\omega_c}$ centered at the harmonic:

$$OF(k\omega_c) = \frac{|F(k\omega_c)|}{S} - \frac{1}{N \times S} \sum_{x \in I_{k\omega_c} \setminus k\omega_c} |F(x)| \tag{3}$$

where F stands for either t or θ, $S = \sum_{x \in I_{k\omega_c}} |F(x)|$ and N is the number of harmonics in $I_{k\omega_c}$. Harmonics selected by optical filtering are the only contributions to the sums in (3).

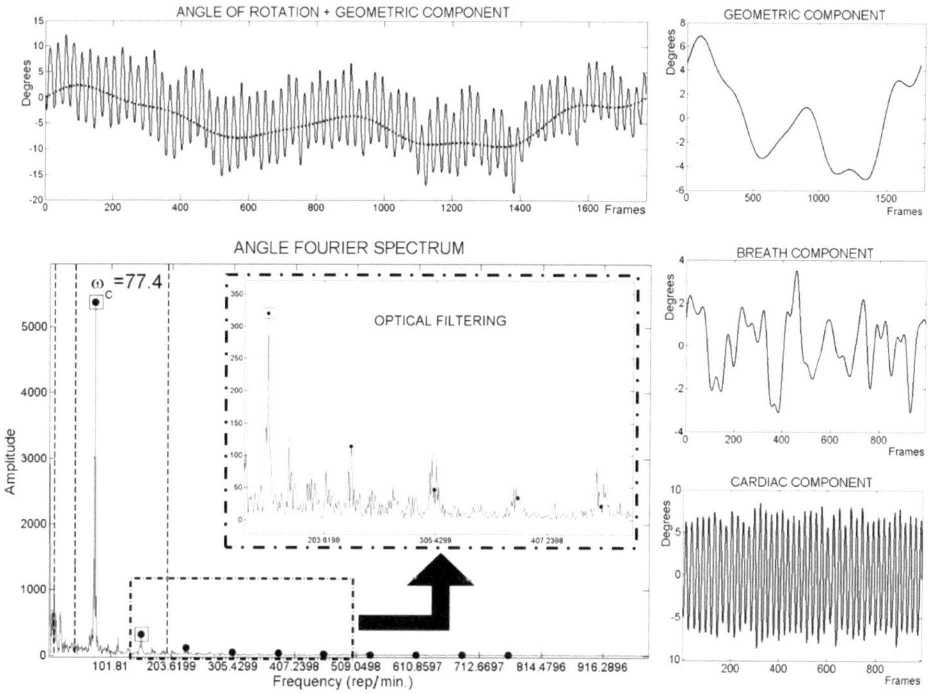

Fig. 8. Motion Decomposition. Rotation angle and its Fourier decomposition on the left; geometric, breathing and cardiac terms on the right.

Figure 8 shows the Fourier terms decoupling for the rotation angle in the top left plot. Vertical lines in the Fourier spectrum of the signal (bottom left plot) indicate the ranges defined for the 3 phenomena. Dots mark the 10 cardiac harmonics and squares the ones selected after optical filtering. The 3 components of the angle are shown in right plots.

Finally, the linear application mapping the artery at a given time to the artery at time zero is given by:

$$\begin{pmatrix} \tilde{x} \\ \tilde{y} \end{pmatrix} = \begin{pmatrix} \cos(\theta_c) & -\sin(\theta_c) \\ \sin(\theta_c) & \cos(\theta_c) \end{pmatrix} \begin{pmatrix} x - VCM_c^x \\ y - VCM_c^y \end{pmatrix} \tag{4}$$

for $VCM_c = (VCM_c^x, VCM_c^y)$ the cardiac component of the position of the vessel center of mass and θ_c the cardiac component of the angle of rotation in degrees.

3.2 Cardiac phase retrieval

The first step for modeling longitudinal motion in IVUS sequences is retrieving information about the cardiac phase. Following the general scheme shown in figure 9, our image-based algorithm to approach ECG sampling (Hernàndez-Sabaté et al., 2011) splits in the following three steps.

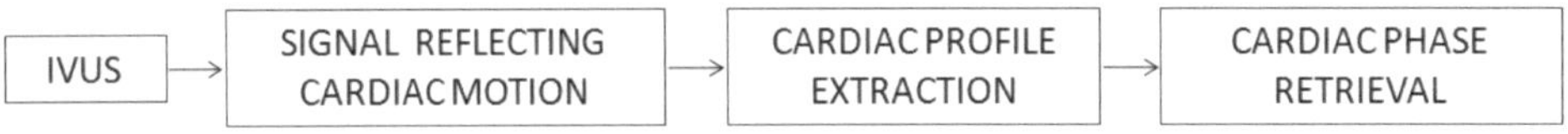

Fig. 9. Pipeline for Image-based Cardiac Phase Retrieval

1. **Extraction of Signal Reflecting Cardiac Motion:**
   By the physical coupling (Nadkarni et al., 2003), luminal area evolution is synchronized to other vessel cardiac phenomena, such as tissue motion or rigid motion. It follows that, since rigid in-plane motion comes from artery motion due to heart pumping, the angle of rotation is also synchronized to cardiac phase. In particular the periodic component, θ_c, given in Section 2 is a signal reflecting (pure) cardiac motion.
2. **Signal Filtering for Cardiac Profile Extraction:** Even in healthy subjects, cardiac frequency does not remain constant along the sequence. This artifact introduces (among other phenomena) irregularities in the Fourier transform of the cardiac motion profile. The irregularities distort the cardiac signal and corrupt the location of local extrema in the signal reflecting cardiac motion. Following the literature, we filter the cardiac profile with two families of band-pass filters centered at the cardiac frequency ω_c: Butterworth (B) (Zhu et al., 2003) and Gaussian-based (g) (Matsumoto et al., 2008).
   The Butterworth filter is defined as:
   $$B(\omega) = \frac{1}{\sqrt{1 + \left(\frac{|\omega| - \omega_c}{0.6\Delta\omega_c}\right)^{2n}}}$$
   where n is related to the filter decay and $\Delta\omega = \delta\omega_c$ to its support. Meanwhile, the Gaussian filter is defined as:
   $$g(\omega, \sigma) = \frac{1}{\sigma\sqrt{2\pi}} e^{-(|\omega| - \omega_c)^2/(2\sigma^2)}$$
   In this case, the decay cannot be handled (it is always exponential) and only its support might be tuned by its deviation σ.
   Figure 10 shows a signal reflecting cardiac motion filtered by a Butterworth filter with parameters $n = 2, \delta = 0.1$. In the top left image, we present the original filter. The Fourier transform is computed and shown in the bottom left image. The result of the product between its Fourier transform and the filter is shown in the bottom right image. The final result is shown in the top right image.
   The real part of the inverse Fourier transform of the filtered cardiac profile is a smooth signal suitable for cardiac phase retrieval. Regardless of the filter used we will denote it by $Filt$.

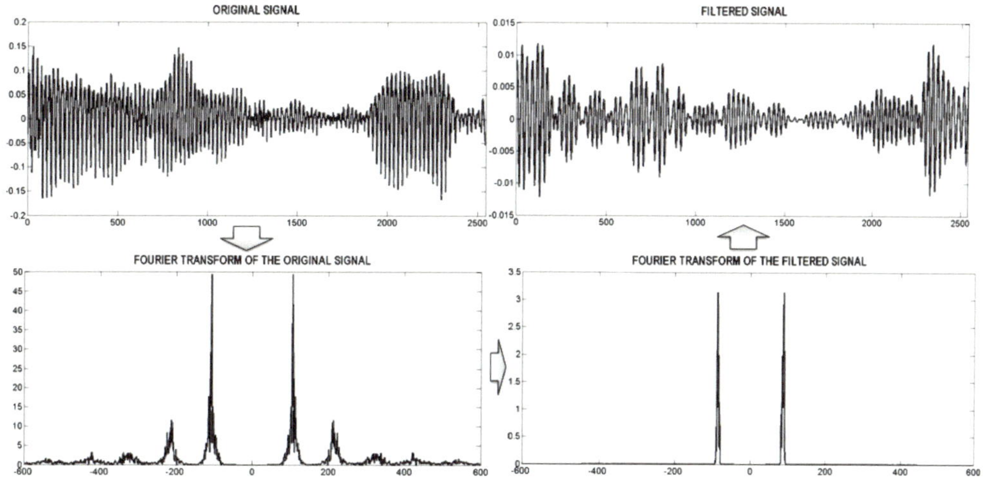

Fig. 10. Signal filtering with a Butterworth filter with parameters $n = 2; \delta = 0.1$

Figure 11 plots the rotation motion profile on a longitudinal cut (on the left) and the profile filtered on the same cut (on the right). Note that the most prominent minimums and maximums of the cardiac profile, on the left, correspond to the minimums and maximums of the filtered signal on the right, though it is necessary to filter the signal in order to extract the cardiac phase.

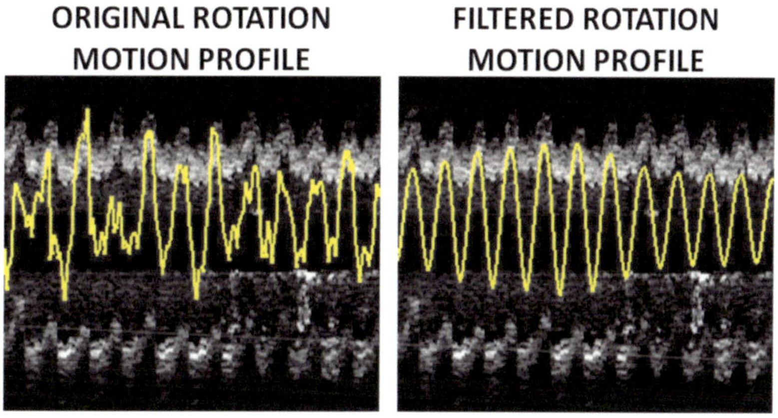

Fig. 11. Original rotation motion profile and the corresponding filtered one.

3. **Cardiac Phase Retrieval:** Maximums and minimums of the filtered signal give a sampling at end-systole and end-diastole and, thus, retrieve cardiac phase for each selected pixel. Extrema positions are computed in the Fourier domain using the equation:

$$\widehat{f'} = 2\pi i \omega \hat{f}$$

for speeding up the process, since $\hat{f}$ has already been computed.

3.3 Vessel structures detection

The strategy for media-adventitia (simply adventitia from now on) segmentation we suggest follows the general scheme presented in (Gil et al., 2006) summarized in figure 12. First, a pre-processing step simplifies the appearance of adventitia, as well as, enhances significant structures while removing noise and textured tissue. Second, the feature extraction task computes two different masks and, by combining them, we obtain those points that most probably correspond to the adventitia layer. Finally, a closing stage delineates the adventitia layer.

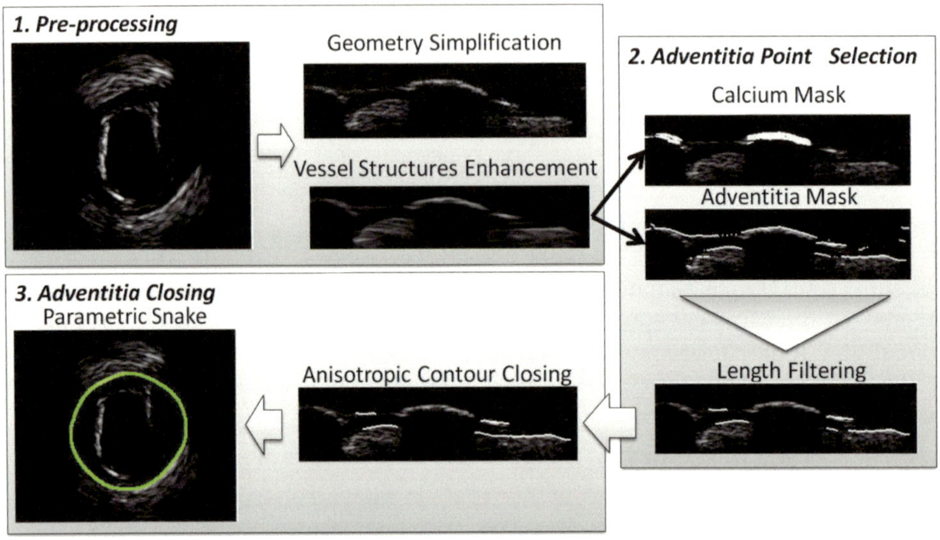

Fig. 12. Adventitia Detection Flow (Gil et al., 2006)

In the pre-processing step, in order to enhance significant structures while removing noise and textured tissue, some kind of filtering is necessary. The most extended way of preserving adventitia thin structure (Gil et al., 2006; Takagi et al., 2000) is by using anisotropic filtering, like the Structure Preserving Diffusion (SPD) introduced in (Gil et al., 2010). Given that such diffusions are computed by means of iterative schemes, the filtering step is, generally, the most time consuming task of the algorithm. For instance, the SPD filtering used in (Gil et al., 2006) takes about the half of the total time and it can consume up to 1.54 seconds per frame. We observe that, after rigid motion compensation, image pixel intensity, which is related to tissue density of mass, remains more uniform along frames. It follows that the mean of stabilized sequence blocks enhances vessel structures, while blurring texture and speckle. We propose replacing the SPD by the mean of stabilized sequences, namely MSS. The remaining steps of the process are the same reported in (Gil et al., 2006). Figure 13 shows the same image given in the general scheme of fig. 12 filtered using SPD diffusion and MSS. For a better comparison across filters, we show images in cartesian (top) and polar (bottom) domains.

4. Validation protocol

4.1 Sequence stabilization

The quality of sequence stabilization exclusively relies on the accuracy of the estimated parameters of rigid in-plane motion. Given that their accuracy has been assessed

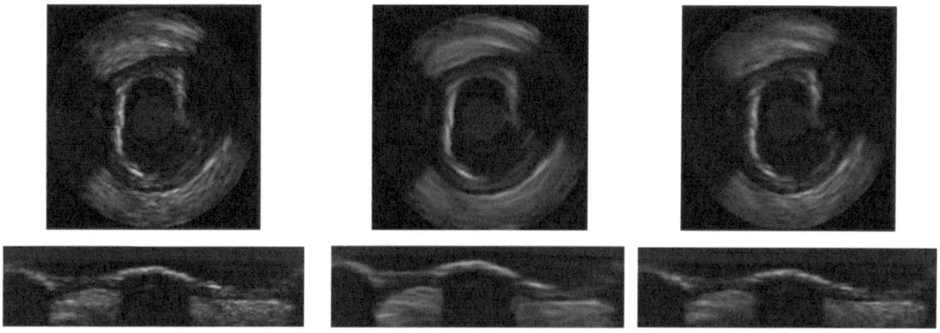

Fig. 13. Enhancement of vessel structures by using a diffusion filter (center images) and the mean of stabilized sequences (left images).

in (Hernàndez-Sabaté et al., 2009), we prefer only to visually illustrate the quality of stabilizations. Cardiac motion introduces a misalignment in IVUS images, as well as, irregular profiles in longitudinal cuts. Therefore, the quality of stabilizations will be visually checked by longitudinal cuts obtained from original sequences and after sequence stabilization.

4.2 Cardiac phase retrieval

For the assessment of cardiac phase retrieval, we have compared the automatic phase retrieval to a manual sampling of the sequence. Automatic samplings were compared to the frames achieving extrema lumen areas. These extrema were manually detected by exploring longitudinal cuts by selecting minimums and maximums of intima/lumen and media-adventitia transition profiles. The distances between each manual detected frame and the automatic one most close to it were computed. That is, if s^k and $\tilde{s}^k$ are frame positions in the sequence for a manual and automatic sampling respectively, we define their distance as the absolute differences between their positions:

$$E^k = |s^k - \tilde{s}^k|$$

The distances of all frames provide a distance map for each patient. As for in-plane dynamics, we retrieve a single quantity for each sequence (seq) by averaging E^k over all sampled frames (N):

$$E^1_{seq} = \frac{1}{N} \sum_{k=1}^{N} E^k$$

Statistical ranges (given by the mean $\pm$ the variance, $\mu \pm \sigma$) of errors for all patients indicate the accuracy of each of the method.

In order to detect if there are any significant differences among smoothing filters (that is, a best/worst performer), we have used the multiple comparison methodology (Nemenyi test) proposed in (Demsar, 2006). For each sequence (trial) the M filters (there are 12 in our case and might be considered as classifiers) are ranked according to their errors. The ranking assigns 1 to the best performer and M for the worst one. The average ranks are statistically compared to find out if there are any significant differences. The significance level for computing and comparing ranks in the Nemenyi test is 0.1.

Finally, we have checked the benefits of using dynamic quantities by comparing results to the ones obtained using gray-intensity cardiac signals (Hernàndez-Sabaté et al., 2011).

Therefore for the sake of a faithful comparison, the experimental set is the same used in (Hernàndez-Sabaté et al., 2011): 22 vessel segments 420-690 frames long (7-11.5 mm approximately) recorded with a Galaxy-BostonSci device at 40 MHz, with a rotating single transducer and constant pullback speed of 0.5 mm./s. The digitalization rate was 30 fps.

4.3 Vessel structures detection

The goal of this experiment is checking wether the rotation angle can produce accurate enough adventitia segmentations, while significantly reducing computational time. Therefore, we have compared segmentations obtained using MSS filtering to SPD diffusion (Gil et al., 2006) in terms of quality of the segmentations and computational cost.

In this case, ground truth is given by manual identification of the adventitia in IVUS images. Since discrepancies among experts provide a non-unique ground truth, we follow the same protocol described in (Gil et al., 2006), based on comparisons of inter-observer variability to manual segmentations. The accuracy has been assessed by means of absolute (in millimeters) and relative (in percent) distances. If $p = (x_p, y_p)$ denotes the points corresponding to an automatic contour, its absolute distance to the manual contour is defined as:

$$D(p) = min_{q \in \gamma} \sqrt{(x_p - x_q)^2 + (y_p - y_q)^2} \tag{5}$$

and relative distances correspond to the ratio:

$$RelD(p) = 100 \cdot \frac{D(p)}{d(q, O)}$$

for the origin O the center of mass of the manual contour and q the point achieving the minimum in (5). Absolute distances are given in mm and relative ones in percentages.

For each distance error, we compute its maximum and mean values on the automated contour to measure accuracy in positions.

- Maximum distance errors:

$$\begin{aligned} MaxD &= max_p(D(p) \cdot PixSze)) \\ RelMaxD &= max_p(RelD(p)) \end{aligned}$$

- Mean distance errors:

$$\begin{aligned} MeanD &= mean_p(D(p) \cdot PixSze)) \\ RelMeanD &= mean_p(RelD(p)) \end{aligned}$$

for PixSze denoting the image spatial resolution and p is any point on the automatically traced adventitia. The interval given by the mean $\pm$ standard deviation computed over the 4 experts contours indicate the statistical range of values for each of the automated errors (MaxD, RelMaxD, MeanD, RelMeanD). Inter-observer variability is obtained by computing the error measures for the models made every two independent observers and it, thus, quantifies discrepancy among experts.

Concerning computational time, we have considered maximums and ranges for the following tasks: Rigid In-plane Motion Estimation (RME), adventitia segmentation by means of Mean of Stabilized Sequences (MSS), adventitia segmentation by means of Structures Preserving Diffusion (SPD). For a better quantification of time improvement, we have also considered

the ratio between both segmentation techniques (SPD/MSS) and the ratio taking into account the time computation for Rigid In-plane Motion Estimation (SPD/(MSS+RME)).
Since we want to compare MSS filtering to the anisotropic filtering used in (Gil et al., 2006), the experimental setting is the same reported in (Gil et al., 2006). A total number of 5400 images extracted from 22 vessel segments of a length ranging from 4 to 6 mm (200-300 frames). Sequences were recorded with a Boston Scientific Clear View Ultra scanner at 40 MHz with constant pull-back at 0.5 mm/s and a digitalization rate of 25 frames/s.

5. Results

5.1 Sequence stabilization

Figure 14 shows two longitudinal cuts taken at the white lines on the IVUS left image and the same cut after sequence alignment. Each IVUS image cuts present the two main artifacts induced by vessel dynamics in *in vivo* pullbacks. The upper longitudinal cuts show the saw-tooth-shape pattern of the vessel intima wall (dark line) introduced by relative vessel-catheter translation. The profile of bottom cuts presents a structure misalignment due to the relative vessel-catheter rotation for an echo-shadowing calcified plaque. After sequence stabilization, the vessel wall profiles of upper cuts are straight and continuous, whereas calcium shows a uniform appearance.

5.2 Cardiac phase retrieval

As in (Hernàndez-Sabaté et al., 2011), the set of filters scanned, G_i for gaussian filters and B_i for Butterworth ones is the following.

$$G_1 : \{\sigma = 0.001\};\ G_2 : \{\sigma = 1.5\};\ G_3 : \{\sigma = 10\}$$

$$\begin{aligned} &B_1 : \{n = 1, \delta = 0.5\};\ B_2 : \{n = 1, \delta = 0.05\};\ B_3 : \{n = 1, \delta = 0.005\}; \\ &B_4 : \{n = 2, \delta = 0.5\};\ B_5 : \{n = 2, \delta = 0.05\};\ B_6 : \{n = 2, \delta = 0.005\}; \\ &B_7 : \{n = 4, \delta = 0.5\};\ B_8 : \{n = 4, \delta = 0.05\};\ B_9 : \{n = 4, \delta = 0.005\} \end{aligned}$$

As well, we have added the results of the angle output without filtering. Two Nemenyi tests have been performed, one (labeled TN_1) to detect differences across filters and another one (labeled TN_2) to compare the impact of the filtering with the angle itself. The first one only includes errors for B_i and G_i, while the second one incorporates the errors obtained by the angle θ_c. Tables 1 and 2, report the average ranks (the smaller, the better) reflecting each filter performance (table 1) and its comparison to the sampling obtained without filtering (table 2).

Filter Param.	G_1	G_2	G_3	B_1	B_2	B_3	B_4	B_5	B_6	B_7	B_8	B_9
Rank	8.12	5.53	6.15	5.71	5.24	7.47	6.06	5.44	7.94	5.56	6.68	8.12

Table 1. TN_1: Average rank of the filters set performance

Filter Param.	G_1	G_2	G_3	B_1	B_2	B_3	B_4	B_5	B_6	B_7	B_8	B_9	θ
Rank	8.29	5.65	6.27	5.82	5.35	7.59	6.18	5.56	8.06	5.68	6.79	8.29	11.47

Table 2. TN_2: Comparison of performance between the filters set and the sampling without filtering

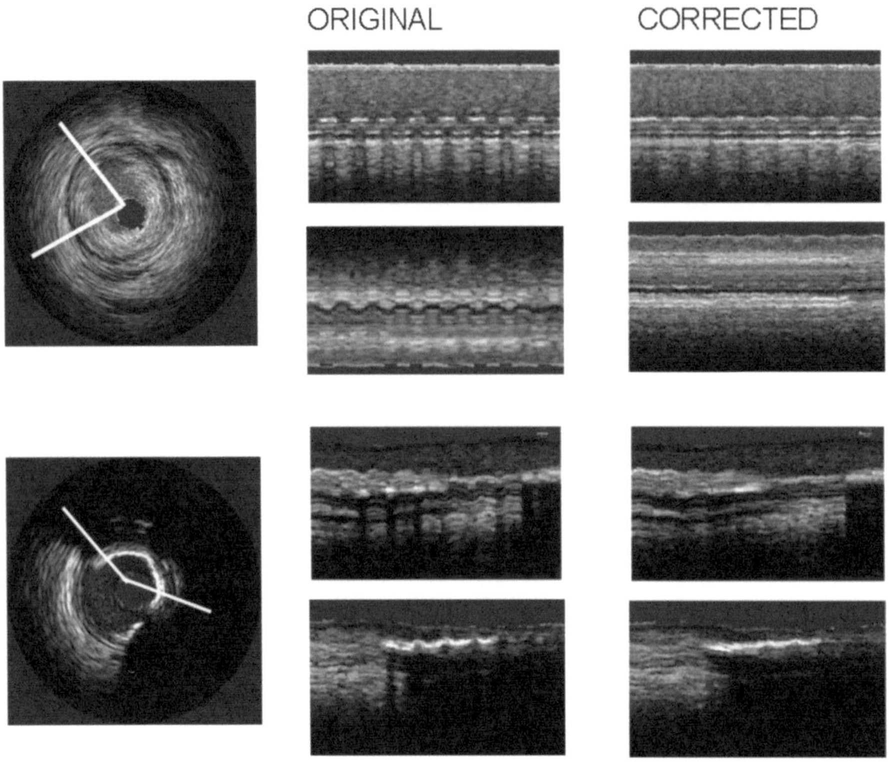

Fig. 14. Longitudinal cuts for sequences of two patients. The first column corresponds to a representative original frame, for each patient, with the angle of the longitudinal cuts. In the second column, the original longitudinal cut and the corrected one in the third column.

The Nemenyi critical difference (CD) for TN_1 is 3.75, while for TN_2 is 4.11. The test detects that the sampling without filtering is significatively worst than the filtered ones. However, the Nemenyi test also reports that there is not enough evidence of a significantly different performance among the filtered methods.

Figures 15 and 16 show the rank of samplings from left to right (the best is on the left) together with the critical difference in order to visually compare them. In figure 15 we can note that there is no significative difference among the filters. However, in figure 16, we can appreciate that the sampling without filtering is clearly separated from the rest.

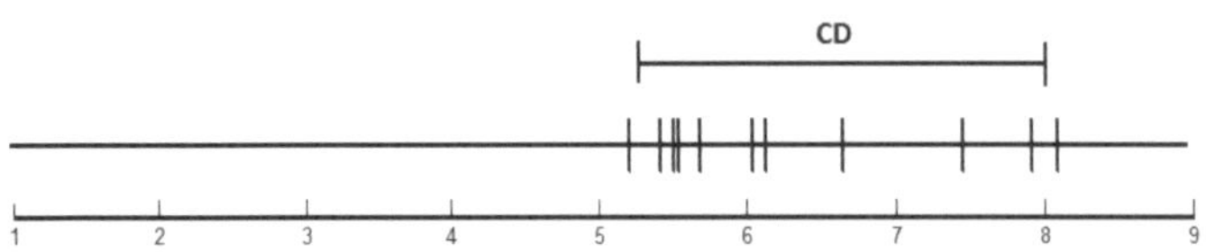

Fig. 15. Visually comparison of different filters using NT_1.

Table 3 reports the ranges, by the mean $\pm$ the variance ($\mu \pm \sigma$) of the 8 filters of the set with better ranks. Values in the first column are in frames, the ones of the second column are in seconds and the last column correspond to the values in millimeters. As figure 15 shows,

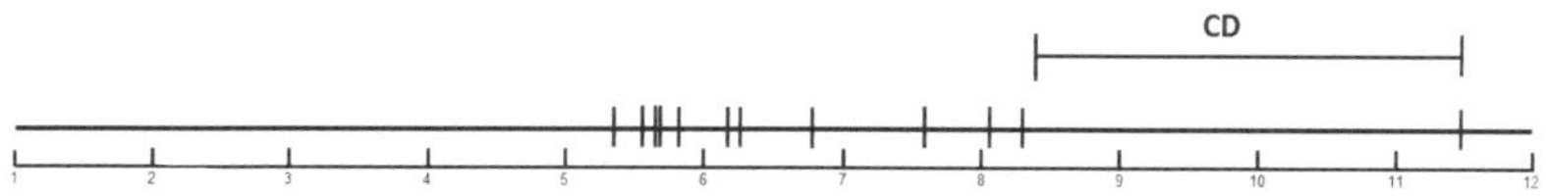

Fig. 16. Visually comparison of different filters to the sampling without filtering using NT_2.

there is no significative difference between them. The Butterworth filter with $n = 1$ and $\delta = 0.05$ achieves the best results with an error within 3.55 ± 1.80 frames, which corresponds to 0.06 ± 0.03 mm.

Method	Frames	Seconds	Millimeters
G_2	3.5601 ± 1.9804	0.1187 ± 0.0660	0.0593 ± 0.0330
G_3	3.6974 ± 1.8520	0.1232 ± 0.0617	0.0616 ± 0.0309
B_1	3.6416 ± 1.8747	0.1214 ± 0.0625	0.0607 ± 0.0312
B_2	3.5498 ± 1.7998	0.1183 ± 0.0600	0.0592 ± 0.0300
B_4	3.6824 ± 1.8478	0.1227 ± 0.0616	0.0614 ± 0.0308
B_5	3.7468 ± 1.5738	0.1249 ± 0.0525	0.0624 ± 0.0262
B_7	3.6660 ± 1.8423	0.1222 ± 0.0614	0.0611 ± 0.0307
B_8	4.0192 ± 1.6035	0.1340 ± 0.0534	0.0670 ± 0.0267

Table 3. Average Errors of the best set of filters

In order to compare the ranges of the approach proposed in this chapter to the ones presented in (Hernàndez-Sabaté et al., 2011) table 4 reports the ranges of the filters presented in table 3 in frames (1st column), seconds (2nd column) and millimeters (3rd column). We can observe that there is no significative difference as a Nemenyi test proves.

Method	Frames	Seconds	Millimeters
G_1	3.8644 ± 1.7497	0.1288 ± 0.0583	0.0644 ± 0.0292
G_2	3.8929 ± 1.6648	0.1298 ± 0.0555	0.0649 ± 0.0277
B_1	4.0240 ± 1.6105	0.1341 ± 0.0537	0.0671 ± 0.0268
B_2	$\mathbf{3.8972 \pm 1.8001}$	0.1299 ± 0.0600	0.0650 ± 0.0300
B_3	4.4488 ± 1.9458	0.1483 ± 0.0649	0.0741 ± 0.0324
B_4	3.8570 ± 1.7338	0.1286 ± 0.0578	0.0643 ± 0.0289
B_5	4.1506 ± 1.8597	0.1384 ± 0.0620	0.0692 ± 0.0310
B_7	3.8680 ± 1.7279	0.1289 ± 0.0576	0.0645 ± 0.0288
B_8	4.2071 ± 1.8385	0.1402 ± 0.0613	0.0701 ± 0.0306

Table 4. Average Errors of the best set of filters for the image-grey level evolution approach

Figure 17 shows the performance of our method for the Butterworth filtering in 4 large longitudinal cuts. The original cuts are in the left, while the cuts sampled at end diastole rate are in the right. For the first segment, we can notice the continuous profile for the lumen contour, while in the second and third segments, we can follow up the calcium plaques present in the vessel. In the four segment we can appreciate the continuous profile of two bifurcations at the upper side of the cut.

5.3 Vessel structures detection

Table 5 reports the inter-observer variability (INT-OBS) to ranges of automatic errors for SPD and MSS computed for all segments. The results for the MSS algorithm are slightly worse

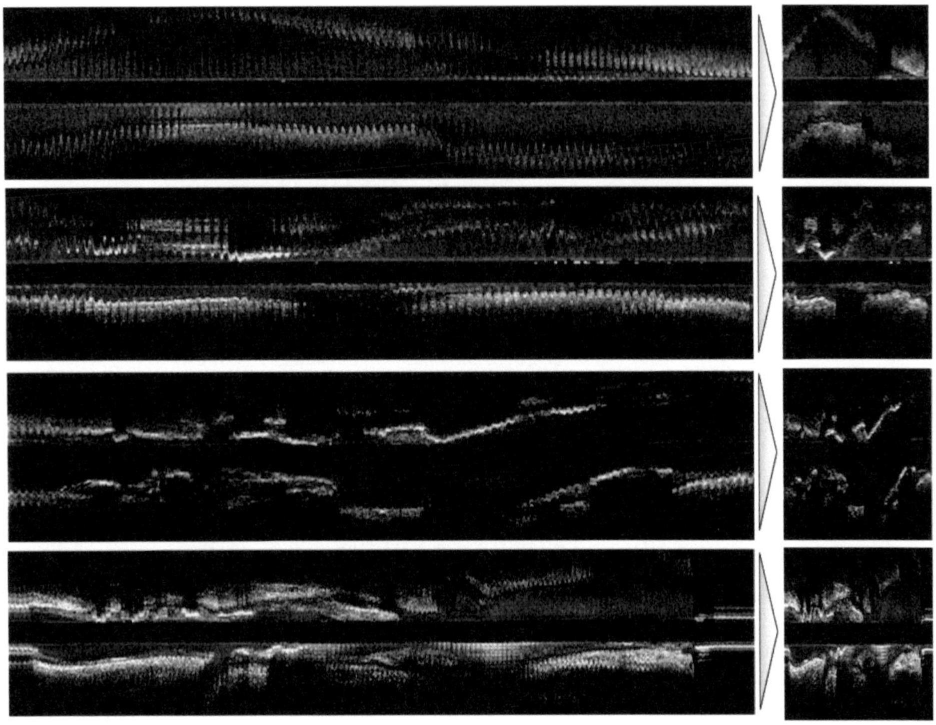

Fig. 17. Results of Image-based ECG sampling for two different longitudinal cuts.

than the ones from the SPD approach. However, note that they are still in the range of inter-observer variability.

	INT-OBS	SPD	MSS
MaxD (mm)	0.5386 ± 0.3075	0.5715 ± 0.2296	0.5988 ± 0.2047
RelMaxD (%)	0.4697 ± 0.2664	0.5122 ± 0.2344	0.5369 ± 0.1953
MeanD (mm)	0.2206 ± 0.1126	0.2265 ± 0.0688	0.2604 ± 0.0879
RelMeanD (%)	0.1888 ± 0.0945	0.1972 ± 0.0662	0.2387 ± 0.0808

Table 5. Performance Evaluation of the Adventitia Segmentation Strategies

Table 6 reports the computational times required for each task: Rigid In-plane Motion Estimation (RME), adventitia segmentation by means of Mean of Stabilized Sequences (MSS), adventitia segmentation by means of Structures Preserving Diffusion (SPD), the ratio between both segmentation techniques (SPD/MSS) and the ratio taking into account the time computation for Rigid In-plane Motion Estimation (SPD/(MSS+RME)). We can observe that the new approach proposed is almost 27 times faster (in average) than the vessel appearance

	RME	MSS	SPD	SPD/MSS	SPD/(MSS+RME)
Max	0.5412	0.0909	2.4379	32.2131	5.5228
Mean	0.3575 ± 0.0673	0.0797 ± 0.0057	2.1282 ± 0.1279	26.8792 ± 2.9042	4.9484 ±0.6193

Table 6. Times comparison of Adventitia Segmentation Strategies for each frame (in sec.)

diffusion approach. Although rigid in-plane motion estimation is useful for the whole integrative framework, we could take into account the time needed for computing it. Still, the new approach is 5 times faster (in average).

6. Discussions and conclusions

In this chapter we proposed an integrative framework for exploring vessel dynamics and structures, so that to obtain stable models of arteries. We showed the potential of vessel in-plane rigid dynamics to analyze and correct vessel in-plane rigid dynamics, retrieve cardiac phase and aid the automatic segmentation of adventitia layer.

In (Hernàndez-Sabaté et al., 2009) we already proved that rigid in-plane dynamics estimation contributes in a proper image misalignment correction. In this chapter we also showed the usefulness of this estimation for retrieving cardiac phase and we compared the method proposed to other vessel appearance-based models. There are two main advantages in using a dynamic quantity instead of the usual signals computed from image grey-level evolution (Barajas et al., 2007; Hernàndez-Sabaté et al., 2011; Matsumoto et al., 2008; Nadkarni et al., 2005). Firstly, since θ_c does not include non-cardiac phenomena (such as breathing) it requires less specific tuning of the band-pass filtering. Secondly, it is computationally faster. Although errors ranges seem to be worse for the new approach, a Nemenyi test reports that there is no significative differences. Concerning the usefulness of rigid dynamics for the contribution to the adventitia segmentation, the main improvement is the computational time. Nevertheless, the accuracy errors still keep within the range of inter-observer variability.

For that reasons, we can conclude that rigid in-plane dynamics estimation has a high potential for developing useful techniques for clinical practice, and reducing drastically the time computation, since they can be parallelizable.

7. References

Alliney, S. (1993). Spatial registration of multiespectral and multitemporal digital imagery using fast-fourier transform techniques, *IEEE PAMI* 15(5): 499–504.

Barajas, J., Caballero, K., Rodriguez, O. & Radeva, P. (2007). Cardiac phase extraction in IVUS sequences using 1-D gabor filters, *29th Annual International Conference of the IEEE EMBS*.

Bouma, C. J., Niessen, W. J., Zuiderveld, K. J., Gussenhoven, E. J. & Viergever, M. A. (1997). Automated lumen definition from 30 MHz intravascular ultrasound images, *Med. Image Anal* 1: 363–377.

Brathwaite, P., Chandran, K., McPherson, D. & Dove, E. (1996). Lumen detection in human IVUS images using region-growing, *Computers in Cardiology*, pp. 37–40.

Brathwaite, P. & McPherson, K. C. D. (1998). 3D IVUS border detection in highly diseased arteries with dissecting flaps, *Comp. in Card.*, pp. 157–160.

Brusseau, E., de Korte, C., Mastik, F., Schaar, J. & van der Steen, A. F. W. (2004). Fully automatic luminal contour segmentation in intracoronary ultrasound imaging: A statistical approach, *IEEE Trans. Med. Imag* 23(5).

Caballero, K., Barajas, J., Pujol, O., Salvatella, N. & Radeva, P. (2006). In-vivo IVUS tissue classification: A comparison between RF signal analysis and reconstructed images, *Progress in Pattern Recognition, Image Analysis and Applications*, Vol. 4225, pp. 137–146.

Céspedes, E., Korte, C. & van der Steen, A. (2000). Intraluminal ultrasonic palpation: assessment of local cross-sectional tissue stiffness, *Ultrasound Med. Biol.* 26: 385–396.

de Korte, C. L., Pasterkamp, G., van der Steen, A. F. W., Woutman, H. A. & Bom, N. (2000). Characterization of plaque components with intravascular ultrasound elastography in human femoral and coronary arteries in vitro, *Circulation* 102: 617–623.

Demsar, J. (2006). Statistical comparisons of classifiers over multiple data sets, *Journal of Machine Learning Research* 7: 1–30.

Dijkstra, J., Koning, G. & Reiber, J. (1999). Quantitative measurements in IVUS images, *Inter. Journal of Cardiovas. Imag.* 15(6): 513–522.

Dijkstra, J., Koning, G., Tuinenburg, J., Oemrawsingh, P. & Reiber, J. (2001). Automatic border detection in intravascular ultrasound images for quantitative measurements of the vessel, lumen and stent parameters, *Computer Assisted Radiology and Surgery - CARS 2001*, pp. 916–922.

Escalera, S., Pujol, O., Mauri, J. & Radeva, P. (2008). IVUS tissue characterization with sub-class error-correcting output codes, *Computer Vision and Pattern Recognition Workshops, 2008*, pp. 1–8.

Fuster, V. (1994). Mechanisms leading to myocardial infarction: Insights from studies of vascular biology, *Circulation* 90(4): 2126–2146.

Gil, D., Hernàndez, A., Rodriguez, O., Mauri, J. & Radeva, P. (2006). Statistical strategy for anisotropic adventitia modelling in IVUS, *IEEE Transactions on Medical Imaging* 25(6): 768–778.

Gil, D., Radeva, P. & Saludes, J. (2000). Segmentation of artery wall in coronary IVUS images: a probabilistic approach, *Intern. Conf. Pat. Recog.*, pp. 352–355.

Gil, D., Rodriguez-Leor, O., Radeva, P. & Mauri, J. (2008). Myocardial perfusion characterization from contrast angiography spectral distribution, *IEEE Trans. on Med. Imag.* 27(5): 641–649.

Gil, D., Hernàndez-Sabaté, A., Brunat, M., Jansen, S. & Martínez-Vilalta, J. (2010). Structure-preserving Smoothing of Biomedical Images, *Pattern Recognition* 44(9): 1842-1851.

Goldstein, H., Poole, C. & Safko, J. (2002). *Classical Mechanics*, 3rd edn, Addison Wesley.

Granada, J. F., Wallace-Bradley, D., Win, H. K., Alviar, C. L., Builes, A., Lev, E. I., Barrios, R., Schulz, D. G., Raizner, A. E. & Kaluza, G. L. (2007). In vivo plaque characterization using intravascular ultrasound virtual histology in a porcine model of complex coronary lesions, *Arteriosclerosis, Thrombosis, and Vascular Biology* 27: 387–393.

Haas, C., Ermert, H., Holt, S., Grewe, P., Machraoui, A. & Barmeyer, J. (2000). Segmentation of 3D intravascular ultrasonic images based on a random field model, *Ultrasound Med. Biol.* 26(2): 297–306.

Hansen, M., Møller, J. & Tøgersen, F. (2002). Bayesian contour detection in a time series of ultrasound images through dynamic deformable template models, *Biostatistics* 3(2): 213–228.

Hernàndez-Sabaté, A. (2009). *Exploring Arterial Dynamics and Structures in IntraVascular UltraSound Sequences*, PhD thesis, Universitat Autònoma de Barcelona.

Hernàndez-Sabaté, A., Gil, D., Fernandez-Nofrerias, E., Radeva, P. & Martí, E. (2009). Approaching rigid artery dynamics in IVUS, *IEEE Trans. Med. Imag.* 28(11): 1670–1680.

Hernàndez-Sabaté, A., Gil, D., Garcia-Barnés, J. & Martí, E. (2011). Image-based cardiac phase retrieval in intravascular ultrasound sequences, *IEEE Transaction on Ultrasonics, Ferroelectrics, and Frequency Control* 58(1): 60–72.

Holzapfel, G., Gasser, T. & Stadler, M. (2002). A structural model for the viscoelastic behavior of arterial walls: continuum formulation and finite element analysis, *Eur. J. Mech. A-Solids* 23: 1–162.

Kakadiaris, I., O'Malley, S., Vavuranakis, M., Carlier, S., Metcalfe, R., Hartley, C., Falk, E. & Naghavi, M. (2006). Signal-processing approaches to risk assessment in coronary artery disease, *IEEE Signal Processing Magazine* 23(6): 59–62.

Klingensmith, J., Shekhar, R. & Vince, D. (2000). Evaluation of three-dimensional segmentation algorithms for the identification of luminal and medial-adventitial borders in intravascular ultrasound, *IEEE Med. Imag.* 19(10): 996–1011.

Klug, A. & D.J.DeRosier (1966). Optical filtering of electron micrographs: reconstruction of one-sided images, *Nature* 212: 29–32.

Kuglin, C. & Hines, D. (1975). The phase correlation image alignment method, *Int. Conf. on Cybernetics and Society*, pp. 163–165.

Luo, Z., Wang, Y. & Wang, W. (2003). Estimating coronary artery lumen area with optimization-based contour detection, *IEEE Transactions on Medical Imaging* 22(4): 564–566.

Matsumoto, M. M. S., Lemos, P. A., Yoneyama, T. & Furuie, S. S. (2008). Cardiac phase detection in intravascular ultrasound images, *Medical Imaging 2008: Ultrasonic Imaging and Signal Processing*.

Mazumdar, J. (1992). *Biofluids Mechanics*, World Scientific Publishing.

Mendizabal-Ruiz, G., Rivera, M. & Kakadiaris, I. (2008). A probabilistic segmentation method for the identification of luminal borders in intravascular ultrasound images, *IEEE Conference on Computer Vision and Pattern Recognition. CVPR 2008.*, pp. 1–8.

Mintz, G. & Nissen, S. (2001). Clinical expert consensus document on standards for acquisition, measurement and reporting of intravascular ultrasound studies (IVUS), *JACC* 37(5): 1478–92.

Nadkarni, S. ., Boughner, D. . & Fenster, A. . (2005). Image-based cardiac gating for three-dimensional intravascular ultrasound imaging, *Ultrasound in Medicine and Biology* 31(1): 53–63.

Nadkarni, S., Austin, H. & et al (2003). A pulsating coronary vessel phantom for two and three-dimensional intravascular ultrasound studies., *Ultrasound Med. Biol.* 29(4): 621–628.

Nair, A., Kuban, B. D., Tuzcu, E. M., Schoenhagen, P., Nissen, S. E. & Vince, D. G. (2002). Coronary plaque classification with intravascular ultrasound radiofrequency data analysis, *Circulation* 106: 2200–2206.

Okubo, M., Kawasaki, M., Ishihara, Y., Takeyama, U. et al. (2008). Tissue characterization of coronary plaques: comparison of integrated backscatter intravascular ultrasound with virtual histology intravascular ultrasound, *Circulation* 72(10): 1631–9.

Olszewski, M. E., Wahle, A., Mitchell, S. C. & Sonka, M. (2004). Segmentation of intravascular ultrasound images: a machine learning approach mimicking human vision, *CARS*, pp. 1045–1049.

Oppenheim, A. & Willsky, A. (1997). *Signals and Systems*, 2n edn, Prentice-Hall.

Plissiti, M., Fotiadis, D., Michalis, L. & Bozios, G. (2004). An automated method for lumen and media-adventitia border detection in a sequence of IVUS frames, *IEEE Infor. Tech. Biomed.* 8(2): 131–141.

Pujol, O. & Radeva, P. (2005). *Handbook of Medical Image Analysis: Advanced Segmentation and Registration Models*, Kluwer Academic/ Plenum Publishers, chapter Supervised Texture Classification for Intravascular Tissue Characterization, pp. 57–110.

Ramírez, M. D. R. (2005). *A Physics-Based Image Modelling of IVUS as a Geometric and Kinematics System*, PhD thesis, Universitat Autònoma de Barcelona.

Rosales, M., Radeva, P., Mauri, J. & Pujol, O. (2004). Simulation model of intravascular ultrasound images, *MICCAI*, Vol. 3217, pp. 200–7.

Rotger, D., Radeva, P. & Rodriguez, O. (2006). Vessel tortuosity extraction from IVUS images, *Comp. in Card.*, pp. 689–692.

Sean M. O'Malley, Morteza Naghavi, I. A. K. (2006). Image-based frame gating for contrast-enhanced IVUS sequences, *International Workshop on Computer Vision for Intravascular and Intracardiac Imaging, International Workshop on CVIII, MICCAI.*

Sonka, M., Zhang, X., DeJong, S. C., Collins, S. M. & McKay, C. R. (1996). Automated detection of coronary wall and plaque borders in ECG-gated intravascular ultrasound pullback sequences (abstract), *Circulation* 94 (Suppl.).

Sonka, M., Zhang, X. & Siebes, M. (1995). Segmentation of intravascular ultrasound images: A knowledge based approach, *IEEE Med. Imag.* 14: 719–732.

Takagi, A., Hibi, K., Zhang, X., Teo, T. J., Bonneau, H. N., Yock, P. G. & Fitzgerald, P. J. (2000). Automated contour detection for high-frequency IVUS imaging: a technique with blood noise reduction for edge enhancement, *Ultrasound Med. Biol.* 26(6): 1033–1041.

Unal, G., Bucher, S., Carlier, S., Slabaugh, G., Fang, T. & Tanaka, K. (2006). Shape-driven segmentation of intravascular ultrasound images, *Proc. of the International Workshop on Computer Vision for Intravascular Imaging (CVII), MICCAI*, pp. 50–57.

von Birgelen, C., Mario, C., Li, W., Schuurbiers, J., Slager, C., de Feyter, P., Roelandt, J. & Serruys, P. (1996). Morphometric analysis in three-dimensional intracoronary ultrasound: An in vitro and in vivo study performed with a novel system for the contour detection of lumen and plaque, *Am. Heart Journal* 132: 516–527.

von Birgelen, C., Mintz, G. S., Nicosia, A., Foley, D. P., van der Giessen, W. J., Bruining, N., Airiian, S. G., Roelandt, J. R. T. C., de Feyter, P. J. & Serruys, P. W. (1997). Electrocardiogram-gated intravascular ultrasound image acquisition after coronary stent deployment facilitates on-line three-dimensional reconstruction and automated lumen quantification, *J. Amer. Coll. Cardiol.* 30: 436–443.

Waks, E., Prince, J. & Andrew, S. (1996). Cardiac motion simulator for tagged MRI, *Proceeding of MMBIA. IEEE.*

Wentzel, J., Krams, R., Schuurbiers, J. H., Oomen, J., Kloet, J., van der Giessen, W., Serruys, P. & Slager, C. (2001). Relationship between neointimal thickness and shear stress after wallstent implantation in human coronary arteries, *Circulation* 103(13): 1740–5.

Zhu, H., Oakeson, K. D. & Friedman, M. H. (2003). Retrieval of cardiac phase from IVUS sequences, *Medical Imaging 2003: Ultrasonic Imaging and Signal Processing*, Vol. 5035, pp. 135–146.